Biology of Sleep

Guest Editor

TEOFILO LEE-CHIONG Jr, MD

SLEEP MEDICINE CLINICS

www.sleep.theclinics.com

September 2012 • Volume 7 • Number 3

SAUNDERS an imprint of ELSEVIER, Inc.

W.B. SAUNDERS COMPANY
A Division of Elsevier Inc.

1600 John F. Kennedy Boulevard • Suite 1800 • Philadelphia, PA 19103-2899

http://www.sleep.theclinics.com

SLEEP MEDICINE CLINICS Volume 7, Number 3
September 2012, ISSN 1556-407X, ISBN-13: 978-1-4557-4911-9

Editor: Katie Hartner
Developmental Editor: Donald E. Mumford

Photocopying

Single photocopies of single articles may be made for personal use as allowed by national copyright laws. Permission of the Publisher and payment of a fee is required for all other photocopying, including multiple or systematic copying, copying for advertising or promotional purposes, resale, and all forms of document delivery. Special rates are available for educational institutions that wish to make photocopies for non-profit educational classroom use. For information on how to seek permission visit www.elsevier.com/permissions or call: (+44) 1865 843830 (UK)/(+1) 215 239 3804 (USA).

Derivative Works

Subscribers may reproduce tables of contents or prepare lists of articles including abstracts for internal circulation within their institutions. Permission of the Publisher is required for resale or distribution outside the institution. Permission of the Publisher is required for all other derivative works, including compilations and translations (please consult www.elsevier.com/permissions).

Electronic Storage or Usage

Permission of the Publisher is required to store or use electronically any material contained in this journal, including any article or part of an article (please consult www.elsevier.com/permissions). Except as outlined above, no part of this publication may be reproduced, stored in a retrieval system or transmitted in any form or by any means, electronic, mechanical, photocopying, recording or otherwise, without prior written permission of the Publisher.

Notice

No responsibility is assumed by the Publisher for any injury and/or damage to persons or property as a matter of products liability, negligence or otherwise, or from any use or operation of any methods, products, instructions or ideas contained in the material herein. Because of rapid advances in the medical sciences, in particular, independent verification of diagnoses and drug dosages should be made. Although all advertising material is expected to conform to ethical (medical) standards, inclusion in this publication does not constitute a guarantee or endorsement of the quality or value of such product or of the claims made of it by its manufacturer.

Sleep Medicine Clinics (ISSN 1556-407X) is published quarterly by Elsevier Inc., 360 Park Avenue South, New York, NY 10010-1710. Months of issue are March, June, September and December. Business and Editorial Offices: 1600 John F. Kennedy Blvd., Ste. 1800, Philadelphia, PA 19103-2899. Customer Service Office: 3251 Riverport Lane, Maryland Heights, MO 63043. Periodicals postage paid at New York, NY and additional mailing offices. Subscription prices are $174.00 per year (US individuals), $86.00 (US residents), $368.00 (US institutions), $214.00 (foreign individuals), $120.00 (foreign residents), and $406.00 (foreign institutions). Foreign air speed delivery is included in all *Clinics* subscription prices. All prices are subject to change without notice. **POSTMASTER:** Send change of address to *Sleep Medicine Clinics*, Elsevier Health Sciences Division, Subscription Customer Service, 3251 Riverport Lane, Maryland Heights, MO 63043. Customer Service: **Tel: 1-800-654-2452 (U.S. and Canada); 314-447-8871 (outside U.S. and Canada). Fax: 314-447-8029. E-mail: journalscustomerservice-usa@elsevier.com (for print support); journalsonlinesupport-usa@elsevier.com (for online support).**

Reprints. For copies of 100 or more of articles in this publication, please contact the Commercial Reprints Department, Elsevier Inc., 360 Park Avenue South, New York, NY 10010-1710. Tel.: 212-633-3812; Fax: 212-462-1935; E-mail: reprints@elsevier.com.

Printed and bound by CPI Group (UK) Ltd, Croydon, CR0 4YY

Transferred to Digital Print 2012

GOAL STATEMENT

The goal of *Sleep Clinics of North America* is to keep practicing physicians up to date with current clinical practice by providing timely articles reviewing the state of the art in patient care.

ACCREDITATION

The *Sleep Clinics of North America* is planned and implemented in accordance with the Essential Areas and Policies of the Accreditation Council for Continuing Medical Education (ACCME) through the joint sponsorship of the University of Virginia School of Medicine and Elsevier. The University of Virginia School of Medicine is accredited by the ACCME to provide continuing medical education for physicians.

The University of Virginia School of Medicine designates this enduring material activity for a maximum of 15 *AMA PRA Category 1 Credit*(s)™ for each issue, 60 credits per year. Physicians should only claim credit commensurate with the extent of their participation in the activity.

The American Medical Association has determined that physicians not licensed in the US who participate in this CME enduring material activity are eligible for a maximum of 15 *AMA PRA Category 1* Credit(s)™ for each issue, 60 credits per year.

Credit can be earned by reading the text material, taking the CME examination online at http://www.theclinics.com/home/cme, and completing the evaluation. After taking the test, you will be required to review any and all incorrect answers. Following completion of the test and evaluation, your credit will be awarded and you may print your certificate.

FACULTY DISCLOSURE/CONFLICT OF INTEREST

The University of Virginia School of Medicine, as an ACCME accredited provider, endorses and strives to comply with the Accreditation Council for Continuing Medical Education (ACCME) Standards of Commercial Support, Commonwealth of Virginia statutes, University of Virginia policies and procedures, and associated federal and private regulations and guidelines on the need for disclosure and monitoring of proprietary and financial interests that may affect the scientific integrity and balance of content delivered in continuing medical education activities under our auspices.

The University of Virginia School of Medicine requires that all CME activities accredited through this institution be developed independently and be scientifically rigorous, balanced and objective in the presentation/discussion of its content, theories and practices.

All authors/editors participating in an accredited CME activity are expected to disclose to the readers relevant financial relationships with commercial entities occurring within the past 12 months (such as grants or research support, employee, consultant, stock holder, member of speakers bureau, etc.). The University of Virginia School of Medicine will employ appropriate mechanisms to resolve potential conflicts of interest to maintain the standards of fair and balanced education to the reader. Questions about specific strategies can be directed to the Office of Continuing Medical Education, University of Virginia School of Medicine, Charlottesville, Virginia.

The faculty and staff of the University of Virginia Office of Continuing Medical Education have no financial affiliations to disclose.

The authors/editors listed below have identified no professional or financial affiliations for themselves or their spouse/partner:

Sabra M. Abbott, MD, PhD; Jennifer M. Arnold; Helen A. Baghdoyan, PhD; Cynthia Brown, MD (Test Author); Mary A. Carskadon, PhD; Christopher J. Davis, PhD; Jim Findley, PhD; Phil Gehrman, PhD; Martha U. Gillette, PhD; Namni Goel, PhD; Christian Guilleminault, MD, DBiol; Katie Hartner (Acquisitions Editor); Oskar G. Jenni, MD; James M. Krueger, PhD; Ralph Lydic, PhD; Vipin Malik, MD; Michael Perlis, PhD; Arman A. Savani, MD; Michael H. Silber, MBChB; Carlyle Smith, PhD; Daniel Smith, MD; John Arthur Trinder, PhD; Michael V. Vitiello, PhD; and Christopher J. Watson, PhD.

The authors/editors listed below identified the following professional or financial affiliations for themselves or their spouse/partner:

Karl Doghramji, MD is on the Advisory Board for UCB and Teva, and owns stock in Merck.

Sean Drummond, PhD receives reseach support from Actelion.

Marina Goldman, MD is a consultant for UCB.

Teofilo Lee-Chiong, Jr, MD (Guest and Consulting Editor) is employed by Respironics, and is an industry funded research/investigator for Respironics and Embla/Natus.

Dimitri Markov, MD is a consultant for UCB.

Wil Pigeon, PhD receives royalites from Ivy Press for self-help book on sleep.

Todd J. Swick, MD receives research support, is a consultant, and is on the Speakers' Bureau and Advisory Committee for Jazz Pharmaceuticals.

Disclosure of Discussion of Non-FDA Approved Uses for Pharmaceutical Products and/or Medical Devices.

The University of Virginia School of Medicine, as an ACCME provider, requires that all faculty presenters identify and disclose any off-label uses for pharmaceutical and medical device products. The University of Virginia School of Medicine recommends that each physician fully review all the available data on new products or procedures prior to clinical use.

TO ENROLL

To enroll in the Sleep Clinics of North America Continuing Medical Education program, call customer service at 1-800-654-2452 or visit us online at www.theclinics.com/home/cme. The CME program is available to subscribers for an additional fee of $114.00.

SLEEP MEDICINE CLINICS

Contributors

CONSULTING EDITOR

TEOFILO LEE-CHIONG Jr, MD
Professor of Medicine and Chief, Division
of Sleep Medicine, National Jewish Health;
Associate Professor of Medicine, University
of Colorado Denver School of Medicine,
Denver, Colorado

GUEST EDITOR

TEOFILO LEE-CHIONG Jr, MD
Professor of Medicine and Chief, Division
of Sleep Medicine, National Jewish Health;
Associate Professor of Medicine, University
of Colorado Denver School of Medicine,
Denver, Colorado

AUTHORS

SABRA M. ABBOTT, MD, PhD
Department of Molecular and Integrative
Physiology; College of Medicine, University of
Illinois at Urbana-Champaign, Urbana, Illinois;
Clinical Fellow in Medicine, Harvard Medical
School; Department of Internal Medicine,
Medical Resident, Massachusetts General
Hospital, Boston, Massachusetts

JENNIFER M. ARNOLD
Department of Molecular and Integrative
Physiology; College of Medicine, University
of Illinois at Urbana-Champaign, Urbana,
Illinois

HELEN A. BAGHDOYAN, PhD
Department of Anesthesiology, University
of Michigan, Ann Arbor, Michigan

MARY A. CARSKADON, PhD
Professor of Psychiatry and Human Behavior,
Director, E. P. Bradley Hospital Chronobiology
and Sleep Research Laboratory, Department
of Psychiatry and Human Behavior, Warren
Alpert Medical School of Brown University,
Providence, Rhode Island

AGOSTINHO DA ROSA, PhD
Stanford Outpatient Medical Center,
Redwood City, California

CHRISTOPHER J. DAVIS, PhD
Research Assistant Professor, Sleep and
Performance Research Center, WWAMI
Medical Education and Program in
Neuroscience, Washington State University,
Spokane, Washington

KARL DOGHRAMJI, MD
Professor of Psychiatry, Neurology, and
Medicine, Jefferson Medical College;
Director, Thomas Jefferson University
Sleep Disorders Center, Philadelphia,
Pennsylvania

SEAN DRUMMOND, PhD
Laboratory of Sleep & Behavioral
Neuroscience, UCSD and VA San Diego
Healthcare System, San Diego, California

JIM FINDLEY, PhD
Behavioral Sleep Medicine Program,
Department of Psychiatry, University of
Pennsylvania, Philadelphia, Pennsylvania

PHIL GEHRMAN, PhD
Behavioral Sleep Medicine Program,
Department of Psychiatry, University of
Pennsylvania, Philadelphia, Pennsylvania

MARTHA U. GILLETTE, PhD
Alumni Professor, Department of Cell and
Developmental Biology; Department of
Molecular and Integrative Physiology;
College of Medicine; Neuroscience Program,
University of Illinois at Urbana-Champaign,
Urbana, Illinois

NAMNI GOEL, PhD
Associate Professor, Division of Sleep and
Chronobiology, Department of Psychiatry,
Perelman School of Medicine, University of
Pennsylvania, Philadelphia, Pennsylvania

MARINA GOLDMAN, MD
Instructor, Department of Psychiatry,
University of Pennsylvania, Philadelphia,
Pennsylvania

**CHRISTIAN GUILLEMINAULT, MD, DM,
DBiol**
Professor, Stanford Outpatient Medical
Center, Redwood City, California

CHAD C. HAGEN, MD
Sleep Medicine Program, Stanford University,
Redwood City, California

OSKAR G. JENNI, MD
Director, Child Development Center, University
Children's Hospital Zurich, Steinwiesstrasse,
Zurich, Switzerland

JAMES M. KRUEGER, PhD
Regent's Professor, Sleep and Performance
Research Center, WWAMI Medical Education
and Program in Neuroscience, Washington
State University, Spokane, Washington

TEOFILO LEE-CHIONG Jr, MD
Section of Sleep Medicine, National Jewish
Medical and Research Center, Denver, Colorado

RALPH LYDIC, PhD
Department of Anesthesiology, University
of Michigan, Ann Arbor, Michigan

VIPIN MALIK, MD
Section of Sleep Medicine, Division of Critical
Care and Hospital Medicine, National Jewish
Medical and Research Center, Denver, Colorado

DIMITRI MARKOV, MD
Assistant Professor, Department of Psychiatry
and Human Behavior; Assistant Professor,
Department of Medicine, Jefferson Medical
College, Philadelphia, Pennsylvania

MICHAEL PERLIS, PhD
Behavioral Sleep Medicine Program,
Department of Psychiatry, University of
Pennsylvania, Philadelphia, Pennsylvania

WIL PIGEON, PhD
Sleep and Neurophysiology Research
Laboratory, Department of Psychiatry,
University of Rochester, Rochester, New York

OLGA PRILIPKO, MD, PhD
Sleep Medicine Program, Stanford Outpatient
Medical Center, Redwood City, California

AMAN A. SAVANI, MD
Fellow, Neurology center, Chevy Chase, Maryland

MICHAEL H. SILBER, MBChB
Professor of Neurology, Mayo Clinic College
of Medicine; Center for Sleep Medicine and
Department of Neurology, Mayo Clinic,
Rochester, Minnesota

CARLYLE SMITH, PhD
Professor Emeritus of Psychology, Department
of Psychology, Trent University, Peterborough,
Ontario, Canada

DANIEL SMITH, MD
Section of Sleep Medicine, National Jewish
Medical and Research Center, Denver, Colorado

TODD J. SWICK, MD, FAAN, FAASM
University of Texas School of Medicine-
Houston; Apnix Sleep Diagnostics-Memorial
Sleep Center, Houston, Texas; North Cypress
Medical Center Sleep Disorders Center,
Cypress, Texas

JOHN TRINDER, PhD
Professor of Psychology, Melbourne School
of Psychological Sciences, University of
Melbourne, Melbourne, Victoria, Australia

MICHAEL V. VITIELLO, PhD
Professor, Department of Psychiatry and
Behavioral Sciences, University of Washington,
Seattle, Washington

CHRISTOPHER J. WATSON, PhD
Department of Anesthesiology, University
of Michigan, Ann Arbor, Michigan

Contents

Wakefulness, rapid eye movement (REM) sleep, and non-REM (NREM) sleep are characterized by specific changes in electroencephalography, eye movements, and muscle activity. The discharge of brainstem and cortical neuronal groups have state specific firing rates resulting in the cycling of wakefulness, non-REM and REM sleep. Cholinergic, monoaminergic and hypocretin neurons have their highest discharge rates during wakefulness. GABAergic, galaninergic, glutamatergic and melanin concentrating hormone containing neurons are most active during non-REM and REM sleep. Cholinergic neurons resume firing during REM sleep. The neurons within the suprachiasmatic nucleus generate the circadian rhythm. The understanding of the orchestration of these state specific neuronal groups with the timing of sleep onset/offset and REM on/REM off is the key to unlocking the mystery of the function of sleep.

The cyclic repetition of sleep and wakefulness states is essential to the basic functioning of all higher animals including human beings. As our understanding of the neurobiology of sleep increases, we no longer view it as a passive state, that is, sleep as merely the absence of wakefulness. In fact, sleep is an active neurobehavioral state, which is maintained through a highly organized interaction of neurons and neural circuits in the central nervous system. This article reviews the circadian rhythms and the neurobiological mechanisms underlying sleep and wakefulness.

This review explains the neurobiology of circadian timekeeping, describing what is known about the master pacemaker for circadian rhythmicity, how biologic systems provide input to the endogenous biologic timing, and how the pacemaker influences physiology and behavior. We discuss how the circadian system can adapt to a changing environment by resetting the circadian clock in the face of a variety of inputs. The genetics of circadian timekeeping are discussed, highlighting what is known about heritable disorders in circadian timing and how circadian genetics have been used to study timekeeping. The role of the clock in peripheral tissues is discussed.

The circadian biological clock interacts with sleep homeostatic drive. This article reviews the genetic underpinnings of sleep timing, duration, and homeostasis in healthy adult sleepers. Individual differences in circadian and sleep measures as well as in neurobehavioral performance have motivated recent studies using candidate gene approaches to predict baseline responses as well as responses to sleep loss. Results from this growing database point to several important circadian and noncircadian genetic biomarkers involved in differential vulnerability to sleep loss. Actively searching for other potential genetic biomarkers will allow effective prediction of response and use of countermeasures in response to sleep loss.

Sleep States, Memory Processing, and Dreams   455

Carlyle Smith

There are 2 basic types of memory, declarative and nondeclarative, subserved by different neural systems. Within these 2 memory types, there are several distinct subtypes. Efficient memory consolidation is differentially benefited by different stages of posttraining sleep, depending on the type or subtype of learning task involved. As sleep is accompanied by dreams (sleep mentation), dreams may also be involved with the memory consolidation of recently learned material. An examination of this hypothesis suggests that dreams may reflect the ongoing process of memory consolidation, but results do not support the idea that dreaming enhances this process.

Neuropharmacology of Sleep and Wakefulness: 2012 Update   469

Christopher J. Watson, Helen A. Baghdoyan, and Ralph Lydic

The development of sedative/hypnotic molecules has been empiric rather than rational. The empiric approach has produced clinically useful drugs, but for no drug is the mechanism of action completely understood. All available sedative/hypnotic medications have unwanted side effects, and none of these medications creates a sleep architecture that is identical to the architecture of naturally occurring sleep. This article reviews recent advances in research aiming to elucidate the neurochemical mechanisms regulating sleep and wakefulness. One promise of rational drug design is that understanding the mechanisms of sedative/hypnotic action will significantly enhance drug safety and efficacy.

Staging Sleep   487

Michael H. Silber

Various schemas have been suggested to describe the different electrophysiologic patterns of human sleep. The Rechtschaffen and Kales method was used from 1968 until the publication of the American Academy of Sleep Medicine (AASM) *Manual for the Scoring of Sleep and Associated Events* in 2007. This article reviews the development of sleep staging. The development of the new AASM manual and the scientific background underlying the choice of staging criteria are reviewed. The rules for the different stages of wakefulness are described, as well as variations recommended for scoring sleep in children. Recent studies evaluating the AASM method are reviewed.

Respiratory Physiology During Sleep   497

Vipin Malik, Daniel Smith, and Teofilo Lee-Chiong Jr

The respiratory system provides continuous homeostasis of partial pressures of arterial oxygen, carbon dioxide, and pH levels during constantly changing physiologic conditions. This system responds promptly to subtle variations in metabolism.

Modifications occur in the regulation and control of respiration with the onset of sleep, which differ with specific sleep stages. These alterations can lead to sleep-related breathing disorders and limit the usual respiratory compensatory changes to specific disease states. This article reviews the normal physiology of respiration in both awake and sleep states, and discusses the effects of common disease processes and medications on the respiratory physiology of sleep.

Non–rapid eye movement sleep is associated with reduced sympathovagal tone. The effect is characterized by reduced sympathetic vasomotor tone, downward resetting of the baroreflex, marginally increased baroreceptor reflex sensitivity, and increased parasympathetic activity. However, a central cardiac effect of the sympathetic nervous system remains unproven. The direction of influence between sleep mechanisms and the autonomic nervous system also remains uncertain. Sleep deprivation seems to have only minor effects on sympathovagal balance. However, the effects of obstructive sleep apnea are substantial and are likely to mediate many of the pathophysiologic processes associated with the disorder.

Our knowledge of cytokine sleep mechanisms has led to a view of brain organization of sleep positing that sleep is a local property of neural networks. Cortical columns oscillate between functional states; the sleeplike state of cortical columns is promoted by multiple cytokines. Cytokine-mediated sleep mechanisms support the hypothesis that sleep serves a synaptic-connectivity function and is tightly coupled to cerebral metabolism. Cytokine release from glia is enhanced by neuronal activity via adenosine triphosphate signaling and, in turn, these cytokines activate nuclear factor κ B, adenosine, and other downstream mechanisms thereby linking activity to local changes in state.

Knowledge of what constitutes normal sleep behavior during development is a prerequisite for understanding sleep disorders in children and adolescents. This article (1) describes normal sleep patterns in children and adolescents, (2) depicts sleep stages and sleep electrophysiology in children, and (3) identifies changes in sleep-wake (homeostatic) and circadian regulatory processes across early human development. Three basic principles should guide our consideration of sleep during childhood and adolescence: first, sleep patterns exhibit large variability among children; second, sleep behavior must be viewed within a biopsychosocial framework; and third, sleep may provide undisturbed insights into the developing brain.

Many high-functioning older adults are satisfied with their sleep, even though it is of objectively poorer quality than that of younger adults. When the various factors that can disrupt sleep are screened out, aging adults can expect to undergo little change in their sleep relative to those in the early to middle adult life span. Nevertheless, even successfully aging older adults can expect on average to be earlier to bed and to rise, and to be less tolerant of circadian phase shifts, such as those induced by jet lag, than younger similarly health adults.

Foreword
Biology of Sleep

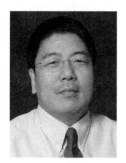

Teofilo Lee-Chiong Jr, MD
Consulting Editor

Kindly reflect on this for a moment: should sleeping and waking be considered yin and yang forces—ie, 2 opposite principles believed to exist in all things, such as black and white or hot and cold—or are they more like an ebb and flow, a waning and waxing, or a contraction and expansion of the daily rhythm of biological life?

Waking, rapid eye movement (REM) sleep and non-REM (NREM) sleep are each generated and maintained by precise sets of neurotransmitters located in definite neural networks within the brain, and each is associated with state-determined changes in physiologic processes. However, are they the *only* specific types of human existence, or are they, instead, interrelated expressions of a unitary human consciousness?

Do we distinguish among the different states of waking, REM sleep, and NREM sleep simply because they are noticeably distinct using currently available measuring devices? Perhaps waking, REM sleep, and NREM sleep are merely electroencephalographic representations of existence.

Are there other states of existence that will remain undefined until we possess more advanced techniques for identifying them? Recall that it was not until the 1950s that REM sleep was discovered and recognized to be different from NREM sleep and waking; prior to this, humans were thought to simply to be "awake" or "not awake." Would new imaging modalities or nano-neurotechnology reveal other domains embedded within REM sleep, other realms scattered among NREM sleep, or other extensions of the waking terrain?

If we were to begin this search for the ">3" versions of human existence, where do we start? Maybe the interstices between waking, REM sleep, and NREM sleep might offer clues. Often neglected, these state transitions may explain how, and more importantly why, one state gains relative dominance over others, and in so doing, comes to exist. Another avenue of inquiry may be the altered states of consciousness—eg, psychosis, drug-induced hallucinations, daydreaming, déjà vu, fugue, eureka moments, mystical (religious) experiences, or prolonged sleep deprivation. Should these different manifestations of consciousness be thought of as "abnormal" states or as truly unique expressions of being?

Finally, must the contemporary concept of *states* be abandoned, and should human existence be conceived as a continuum with no artificial divisions within its whole but only having different "appearances" because of different functions throughout the 24-hour day? This idea has some parallels in clinical sleep medicine: insomnia is characterized by both nighttime sleep disturbance and daytime hyperarousal; narcolepsy results from impairments in both sleep and alertness, and parasomnias break the boundaries between waking, REM sleep, and NREM sleep.

Sleep Med Clin 7 (2012) xi–xii
http://dx.doi.org/10.1016/j.jsmc.2012.07.001
1556-407X/12/$ – see front matter

I do not know if these questions are answerable. What I do believe, however, is that answering these questions is essential if we are to understand better the functions of waking-sleep and the full implications of our existence. Are future sleep-wake researchers to remain mere navigators using established maps, consensus statements, and practice guidelines, or are we to become intrepid explorers of the uncharted vastness of possibilities?

Teofilo Lee-Chiong Jr, MD
Division of Sleep Medicine
National Jewish Health
University of Colorado Denver School of Medicine
1400 Jackson Street, Room J221
Denver, CO 60206, USA

E-mail address:
Lee-ChiongT@NJC.ORG

The Neurology of Sleep: 2012

Todd J. Swick, MD[a,b,c],*

KEYWORDS

- Sleep • Wakefulness • REM/non-REM • Sleep/Wake Control

KEY POINTS

- The 3 behavioral states of wakefulness, rapid eye movement (REM) sleep, and non-REM (NREM) sleep are characterized by specific changes in electroencephalography, eye movements, and muscle activity (age dependent).
- The transitions to and from sleep are not discrete phenomena but rather a continuum.
- The discharge of brainstem and cortical neuronal groups have state specific firing rates resulting in the cycling of wakefulness, non-REM and REM sleep. Cholinergic, monoaminergic and hypocretin neurons have their highest discharge rates during wakefulness. GABAergic, galaninergic, glutamatergic and melanin concentrating hormone containing neurons are most active during non-REM and REM sleep. Cholinergic neurons resume firing during REM sleep.
- The neurons within the suprachiasmatic nucleus generate the circadian rhythm by means of oscillatory protein synthesis via several clock genes.
- The understanding of the orchestration of these state specific neuronal groups with the timing of sleep onset/offset and REM on/REM off is the key to unlocking the mystery of the function of sleep.

By virtue of its study of the brain, neurology is the primary medical science for the elucidation of the anatomy, physiology, and pathology, and ultimately the function, of sleep.

HISTORICAL CONTEXT

The Greco-Roman concepts of sleep were based on their belief that there were gods and goddesses who controlled both the minor and major events of people's lives. They identified the goddess of night (Nyx) who had 2 sons: Hypnos (the god of sleep) and his brother, Thanantos (the god of death). Hypnos sprinkled drops of poppy milk into people's eyes so that the opium would make them fall asleep, and then fanned the sleeping person with his wings to enable them to sleep in comfort. As late as the beginning of the Common Era, Ovid wrote that Hypnos lived with his thousand children, the dreams, in a cave in the Caucasus. The River of Lethe (the river of forgetfulness) was thought to run through this cave.[1]

In ancient Greece, if a citizen was unable to sleep because of his "problems", he would visit one of the many sanitariums dedicated to Asclepios (the Greek god of medicine), where he would spend 3 weeks in rest, thought, and meditation, soothed by gentle music and then, having his balance restored, he would be able to sleep again (predating the concept of "managed care").[2]

From the Middle Ages to the Renaissance, small but discrete changes in the conceptualization of sleep came about. Lucretius, the Epicurean poet and philosopher described, "sleep as the absence of wakefulness."[3] This was the prevailing view through the centuries. As medical science advanced with the discovery of the circulatory system and as the young field of neurology was being explored, there was renewed interest in the science of sleep and wakefulness.

A version of this article originally appeared in *Neurologic Clinics of North America Volume 23, Issue 4*.
[a] University of Texas School of Medicine-Houston, Houston, TX, USA; [b] Apnix Sleep Diagnostics-Memorial Sleep Center, Houston, TX, USA; [c] North Cypress Medical Center Sleep Disorders Center, Cypress, TX, USA
* Neurology and Sleep Medicine Consultants, 7500 San Felipe, Suite 525, Houston, TX 77063.
E-mail address: tswick@houstonsleepcenter.com

In 1866, the Surgeon General of the United States, William A. Hammond,[4] wrote a treatise *On Wakefulness: With an Introductory Chapter on the Physiology of Sleep* and argued against the prevailing opinion of his day that sleep began as a consequence of congestion of the cerebral vessels. He pointed out several discrepancies in observations pertaining to the physiology/pathophysiology of sleep that were quoted in contemporary textbooks of medicine:

1. Stupor never occurs in the healthy individual, whereas sleep is a necessity of life.
2. It is easy to awaken a person from sleep, whereas it is often impossible to arouse a person from stupor.
3. In sleep, the mind is active and, in stupor, it is as if it were dead.
4. Congestion of cerebral vessels causes stupor, not sleep.

Hammond[4] also disputes another nineteenth century physician (Dr Arthur Durham) who wrote: "During sleep, the brain is in a comparatively bloodless condition and the blood in the encephalic vessels is not only diminished in quantity but moves with diminished rapidity. Whatever increases the activity of the cerebral circulation tends to preserve wakefulness and whatever decreases the activity of the cerebral circulation and, at the same time, is not inconsistent with the general health of the body tends to induce and favor sleep."

Although still surrounded by myth and imperfect science, the concept of the neural control of sleep was established. From 1916 to 1928, the world was ravaged by an epidemic of influenza, with tens of thousands of deaths involving numerous neurologic signs and symptoms. During the acute phase of the illness, some patients exhibited severe insomnia and many more had severe hypersomnia, whereas numerous survivors developed signs and symptoms of parkinsonism.

In 1917 Constantin von Economo[5] published his first paper on encephalitis lethargica and, on December 3, 1929, he gave a presentation before the College of Physicians and Surgeons of Columbia University in New York City entitled *Sleep as a Problem of Localization*. He stated that patients with insomnia had lesions in the anterior portion of their hypothalamus and that patients with hypersomnia had lesions in the posterior aspect of the hypothalamus. He designated this area of the interbrain as the center for regulation of sleep.[5,6] These observations contradicted the prevailing concept espoused by such luminaries as Lhermitte and Dejerine that sleep cannot be localized.

In 1928, Hans Berger[7] showed that the brain produced clearly identifiable electrical activity that could be recorded using surface electrodes, and that there existed a different pattern of electrical activity of the brain during consciousness compared with sleep.

In 1935, Frederic Bremer[8] reported on the effects of transection of the brainstem of cats at the pontine-midbrain level (cerveau isolé) versus transection at the medullary–spinal cord level (encéphale isolé). He found that the cerveau isolé animals maintained a continuous sleeplike state with synchronous slow wave activity, whereas the encéphale isolé cats looked awake and their electroencephalograms (EEGs) contained both synchronous and desynchronized activity resembling sleep/wake cycling. Bremer[8] went on to hypothesize that sleep was a passive process and that wakefulness required a high level of continuous sensory input from the periphery to maintain activity within the cerebral hemispheres.[8]

The work of Bremer[8] rekindled research concerning the observations of Santiago Ramón y Cajal[9] and James Papez.[10] In 1909, Ramón y Cajal described an extensive network of neurons that both ascended and descended through the brain stem. This finding was further refined by Papez[10] who, in 1926, published a more complete description of the reticular formation and its caudal projections into the spinal cord in cats.[9,10]

In 1942, Morison and Dempsey[11] published a series of papers that described a diffuse nonspecific thalamocortical recruiting system. They differentiated this nonspecific system from the primary sensory input (ie, specific system; described by Lorente de No[12] in 1938) acting through direct thalamic relays.[11,12]

In 1949, Moruzzi and Magoun[13] identified the ascending reticular activating system "whose direct stimulation activates or desynchronizes the EEG, replacing high-voltage slow waves with low-voltage fast activity." They went on to state that "the effect is exerted generally on the cortex and is mediated, in part, at least, by the diffuse thalamic projection system."

Thus, by the middle of the twentieth century, it was established that sleep and wakefulness are different states that are controlled by the brain, and that sleep is not a passive period devoid of activity. Jouvet and colleagues[14–16] showed that the brainstem contains the site of rapid eye movement (REM) sleep neural activity by way of placing mechanical lesions at discrete levels of the brainstem in cats. Transections at a level just above the midbrain-pons junction preserved the appearance of REM sleep activity, whereas transections in the pons abolished the appearance of REM sleep.

With the discovery of REM and non-REM (NREM) sleep by Aserinsky and Kleitman[17,18] in 1955 and REM/NREM cycling by Dement and Kleitman[19] in 1957, researchers could devote their medical and scientific careers to the study of normal and pathologic sleep and wakefulness.[17–19]

SLEEP AND WAKE STATES

Humans exist in 1 of 3 behavioral states during normal functioning:

1. Wakefulness
2. NREM sleep
3. REM sleep

These states are characterized by specific changes in EEG, eye movements, and muscle activity (age dependent). Wakefulness is characterized by well-recognized patterns on surface EEG recording. α activity (8–12 Hz waves of <50 μV amplitude) occurs when individuals are resting with their eyes closed. The rhythms are most evident in the parieto-occipital areas of the head. α activity is attenuated or blocked by attention, especially visual (eye opening) and mental effort. Eye movements are purposeful and conjugate. Muscle tone is variable but is never absent (**Fig. 1**).

The transition to and from sleep is not a discrete phenomenon but a continuum. However, criteria have been set that allow for the clinical and research separation of individual sleep states in a reproducible fashion.[20] Drowsiness (current designation is stage N1 as per the newest American Academy of Sleep Medicine [AASM] *Manual for the Scoring of Sleep and Associated Events*[21]) can also be produced by boredom and/or fatigue and is characterized by EEG changes of gradual or rapid α dropout (<50% of the epoch contains α frequencies) with δ-range rhythms (from 4.5–7.5 Hz) appearing and can be mixed with very low-voltage faster (15-Hz to 25-Hz) activity as well. Deepening of drowsiness is characterized by increasing slow activity with transients of 2 to 4 Hz and 4.5 to 7 Hz. The hallmark of deep drowsiness is the appearance of vertex sharp waves, which can appear as an isolated event or can occur in trains of events. Accompanying the slowing of the background rhythm is the appearance of slow-rolling eye movements and moderately increased muscle tone.

It has been said that then first true stage of sleep is stage N2 sleep. This stage is characterized by the presence of sleep spindles, which have a frequency of 12 to 14 Hz with progressively increasing, and then progressively decreasing, amplitude lasting 0.5 to 2 seconds. Sleep spindles are thought to arise from generators located in the reticular nucleus of the thalamus[22,23] and develop

as brainstem nuclei, particularly the cholinergic neurons, diminish their firing rates. It is thought that sleep spindles represent the electrical signature of cerebral deafferentation, which occurs when primary sensory pathways are gated.

The second hallmark of stage N2 sleep is the appearance of K complexes. K complexes are evoked cortical responses to arousing stimuli and are characterized by a sharp negative wave followed by a slower positive wave with a minimum duration of 0.5 seconds (there is no voltage criterion). Slow eye movements generally persist for only a brief time after the appearance of sleep spindles and K complexes, and electromyograms (EMGs) show persistence of moderate muscle tone.[24]

The third component of NREM sleep is deep sleep, also known as slow wave sleep (SWS) or stage N3. Here, the background rhythm is at its slowest frequency of the sleep period. Eye movements are absent and the EMG tone remains increased but less than in stage N1 and N2. Stage N3 is defined as δ activity comprising more than 20% of a recording epoch (30 seconds). The overall pattern of the EEG is one of high-voltage, synchronous slow wave activity over the entire brain, with a frequency of 0.5 Hz to 2 Hz and peak-to-peak amplitude of greater than 75 μV, measured over the frontal regions. Cortical cells that are governed by cells in the dorsal thalamus and transmitted via the array of the thalamocortical projections generate these waves. As the dorsal and reticulothalamic nuclei become more hyperpolarized, sleep spindles diminish and slower δ waves increase. The appearance of the very-low-frequency slow waves marks the virtual cessation of firing of the cholinergic neurons in the brainstem.

REM sleep or paradoxic sleep (PS), designated as stage R, represents the time of cortical activation as shown by a rapid transition to a higher frequency rhythm of the EEG (rapid, low-voltage, irregular activity). REMs occur in phasic bursts and there is the occurrence of large burst potentials that originate in the pons and pass rapidly to the lateral geniculate body and then to the occipital lobe (PGO-waves).[25] There is a marked reduction in skeletal muscle tone (REM sleep atonia) except for the diaphragm and the extraocular eye muscles by way of activation of the medial medulla, which inhibits motor neurons by the release of glycine onto spinal and brainstem neurons, producing hyperpolarization and inhibition.

The timing of sleep onset and offset and the timing of non-REM and REM sleep cycling changes over our lifetime but certain generalizations can be observed. Typically there is rapid descent into N3 sleep at the beginning of the night

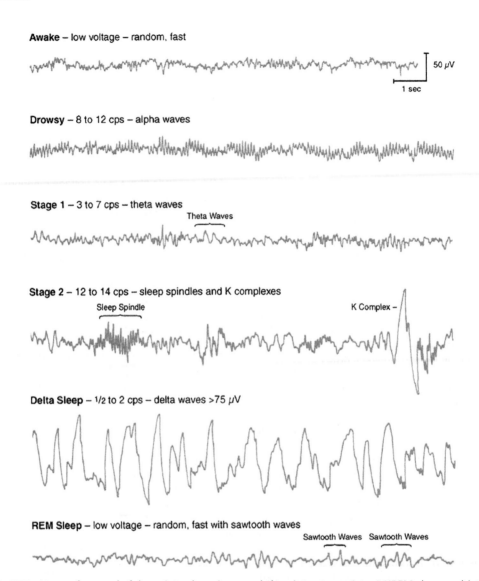

Fig. 1. EEG patterns from wakefulness into drowsiness and then into stages 1 to 4 NREM sleep and into REM sleep. Sleep spindles and K complexes are noted in stage 2 sleep and sawtooth waves are seen in REM sleep. cps, cycles per sec = Hz. (*Adapted from* Hauri P. The sleep disorders. Curr Concepts 1982;7; with permission.)

and the first REM period typically starts 90 minutes after sleep onset. Thereafter REM sleeps recurs approximately every 90 minutes through the night with each subsequent REM episode lasting longer than the preceding one. Slow wave sleep (N3) on the other hand is concentrated at the beginning of the major sleep period and decreases as the night progresses (**Fig. 2**).

ASCENDING RETICULAR SYSTEM

As noted previously, Moruzzi and Magoun[13] identified the reticular activating system as having a significant role in the maintenance of wakefulness and its EEG correlates.[13] The neurons of

the reticular activating system receive input from a wide range of neural networks including visceral, somatic, and special sensory systems. The inputs travel through 2 pathways: a dorsal pathway to the thalamic nuclei and a ventral pathway to the hypothalamus. The mediating neurotransmitters include acetylcholine, serotonin (5-HT), noradrenalin, dopamine (DA), histamine, and hypocretin (orexin [ORX]).

Acetylcholine

Steriade and colleagues[26] first identified groups of cells in the pons-midbrain junction projecting to the thalamus that increased their firing rate

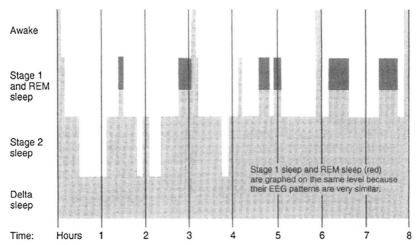

Fig. 2. Sleep hypnogram showing the course of sleep stages over the nocturnal sleep period for this young adult (aged 20–30 years). Note the rapid descent into SWS (δ sleep) at the beginning of the nights and the 90-minute cycling if REM sleep. Note that most of SWS, or δ sleep, takes place in the first half of the night and REM sleep increases in period length as the night progresses, with the longest REM episode occurring just before sleep offset. (*Adapted from* Hauri P. The sleep disorders. Curr Concepts 1982;8; with permission.)

approximately a minute before the first change to a desynchronized state was seen on the EEG. These cells were identified as cholinergic neurons in the laterodorsal tegmental nuclei (LDT) and pedunculopontine tegmental nuclei (PPT). They send fibers via the dorsal pathway to the thalamus where they project specifically to the intralaminar nuclei, the thalamic relay nuclei, and the reticular nucleus. It is thought that this cholinergic input to the reticular nucleus of the thalamus is of particular importance in the activation of thalamocortical transmission. When active, the cholinergic projections allow flow of information through the thalamus, to and from the cerebral cortex, and promote cortical desynchronization (thalamocortical activation). It has been shown that the activity of the LDT-PPT neurons changes with the appearance of each of the states of sleep and wakefulness. During wakefulness, the neurons fire rapidly. With the onset of stage N1 and N2, the LDT-PPT neurons slow their firing rate and, in N3, the neurons become quiet. During REM sleep,

Table 1
State-specific firing rates of brainstem and cortical neuronal groups

Site	Neurotransmitter	Wakefulness	Non-REM Sleep	REM Sleep
Basal forebrain	Acetylcholine	++++	+	++++
LDT/PPT	Acetylcholine	++++	+++ → 0	++++
Dorsal and median raphe	5-HT	++++	++	0
Locus coeruleus	Norepinephrine	++++	++	0
TMN	Histamine	++++	++	0
Lateral hypothalamus	Hypocretin/orexin	++++	+	0
Ventrolateral preoptic area/median preoptic area	GABA/galanin	0	++++	++++
Ventrolateral periaqueductal gray/lateral pontine tegmentum	Dopamine	++++	++	0
Sublaterodorsal nucleus	GABA/glutamate	0	0	++++
Lateral hypothalamus	Melanin-concentrating hormone	0	0	++++

Abbreviation: GABA, γ-aminobutyric acid.

their activity suddenly becomes active again, when they are released from monoamine-mediated inhibition (**Table 1**).[27–31]

There is a mixed population of noncholinergic (γ-aminobutyric acid [GABA]ergic) and cholinergic neurons in the basal forebrain (magnocellular preoptic nucleus in the substantia innominata, medial septal nucleus, and the nucleus of the diagonal band of Broca). These neurons send projections throughout the cortex, hippocampus, and amygdala and, to a lesser extent, the thalamus. Firing rates are highest during wakefulness and REM sleep and are lowest during NREM sleep.[32]

Monoaminergic Systems

The second branch of the reticular activating system is the branch that innervates the hypothalamus via the ventral route. The neurons that make up these fibers are monoaminergic and include the noradrenergic locus coeruleus (LC), the serotoninergic dorsal raphe (DR) and median raphe (MR) nuclei, dopaminergic neurons of the ventrolateral periaqueductal gray matter (vlPAG), and the histaminergic neurons originating in the tuberomammillary nucleus (TMN).[33–36] These neurons then send fibers back to the basal forebrain, the ventral preoptic area (VPOA), and subsequently the cerebral cortex.

Like the cholinergic PPT-LDT neurons, the monoaminergic neurons, noradrenergic LC, 5-HT raphe, dopaminergic neurons (vlPAG), and His (TMN) also have a state-specific firing rate. These collectively fire fastest during wakefulness, slow down during NREM sleep, and nearly stop firing during REM sleep (see **Table 1**).[30,31] The specific monoamines are all associated with the maintenance of wakefulness.

Norepinephrine and Histamine

Norepinephrine (NE) is released during wakefulness[37] and pharmacologic manipulation with NE or NE-agonist drugs uniformly produces an increase in waking behavior and activity of inhibitory mechanisms on sleep production. Likewise, histamine, a major wakefulness-promoting neurotransmitter, has its highest activity during wakefulness, with decreasing activity during NREM sleep, and its lowest levels during REM sleep. Histamine blockers promote sleep onset and increase N2 sleep.[38] New studies investigating H_3 receptor agonists suggest that these moieties stimulate autoinhibitory receptors on histamine and other aminergic neurons and produce augmentation of sleep onset.[39]

5-HT

Studies on the physiologic effects of 5-HT on sleep and wake behavior have been controversial, with conflicting reports that 5-HT both promotes sleep and induces wakefulness. Most recent evidence shows that 5-HT promotes wakefulness with an increase in sleep-onset latency and a decrease in REM sleep. The separate 5-HT agonist moieties, 1A, 1B, 2, and 3 5-HT all exhibit the same wakefulness-promoting responses. Clinical observations suggest that downregulation of 5-HT signaling may be the cause of the hypersomnia seen when selective serotonin reuptake inhibitor are first initiated in depressed patients.[40,41]

DA

DA and its role in sleep/wake regulation remain unclear. From a pharmacologic standpoint, the release of DA and its reuptake inhibition by powerful stimulants such as amphetamines shows its wakefulness-promoting properties.[42–44] DA blockers have long been known for their sleep-inducing effects (eg, chlorpromazine and haloperidol). Recent reports concerning the sleep of patients with Parkinson disease, in which there is a deficiency in DA in the substantia nigra and the ventral tegmental area, show similarities to patients with narcolepsy (ie, fragmented nocturnal sleep, early onset REM periods, and multiple sleep latent testing [MSLT]), showing pathologic daytime sleepiness. However, a confound has been noted that some patients (both with Parkinson disease and those who are being treated with DA receptor agonists for restless legs syndrome) have on occasion experienced unintentional sudden sleep attacks. One possible explanation for this incongruity is that low doses of DA receptor agonists bind to autoinhibitory receptors on DA neurons, further decreasing DA signaling and thus decreasing the wakefulness drive.[45]

REM sleep behavior disorder, a disorder characterized by lack of REM sleep atonia with resultant nocturnal dream enactment behavior, has been described as a possible biologic marker for the subsequent development of the α-synucleinopathies (Parkinson disease, Lewy body dementia, and multiple system atrophy), with some cases having a 50-year latency between the onset of the sleep disorder and the appearance of the neurologic disorder.[46,47]

Hypocretin (Orexin)

The recent discovery of excitatory sleep/wake neuropeptides Hypocretin R1 (HcrtR1) and Hypocretin R2 (HcrtR2) also known as ORX-1 and ORX-2, has added significant insight into the regulation of the sleep/wake state as well as offering causal explanations for the cause of narcolepsy.[48–51] HcrtR1 and HcrtR2 are produced from the same precursor, preprohypocretin (ppHcrt), by a small cluster of neurons in the lateral hypothalamus.[52] These neurons have diffuse projections to many brain regions including adjacent cell groups of the hypothalamus, the limbic system, the periaqueductal gray, DR nucleus, and lateral parabrachial nucleus. These areas of the hypothalamus receive dense input from GABAergic, glutamatergic, and cholinergic neurons.

The lateral hypothalamus contains 2 distinct populations of neurons. Hcrt-containing neurons are active during wakefulness, particularly during periods of increased psychomotor activity, and decrease in firing during NREM sleep. They cause an increase in firing rates of neurons in the TMN, LC, and raphe nuclei. During REM sleep, Hcrt neurons are quiet with occasional burst discharges linked to phasic muscle twitches (**Fig. 3**).[53]

More than 90% of narcoleptics with cataplexy have low or undetectable levels of HcrtR1 in their cerebrospinal fluid (CSF; ($\leq$110 pg/mL) and post-mortem analysis of brains of patient's with narco-lepsy had a marked reduction in the number of hypocretin neurons.[54,55] The hypocretin neurons are activated by glutamate, which in turn increases the amount of glutamate in the surrounding cells of the hypothalamus, and creates a positive feedback system to sustain the firing of the hypocretin neurons.

Recent studies have suggested that the hypocre-tin moieties, HcrtR1 and HcrtR2, perform distinct functions in terms of modulation of sleep and its constituent parts based on which of the Hcrt moiety–specific G-protein-coupled cell surface receptors (GPCRs) it is bound to. Although both moieties mediate excitatory responses, HcrtR1 is a selective neuropeptide for HcrtR1 receptors, whereas HcrtR2, having a high affinity for both HcrtR1 and HcrtR2 receptors, binds to both specific and nonspecific receptors, signifying that the 2 moieties perform separate functions.[49] It seems that HcrtR1 is responsible for maintenance of sleep and wake episodes and HcrtR2 is involved in the maintenance of skeletal muscle tone while awake.[56]

NREM AND REM SLEEP

With the idea that the governance of sleep and wake states can be localized, the search for specific sleep-promoting areas was intensified.

GABA and Galanin

Sleep-active neurons in the ventrolateral preoptic area (VLPO) and the median preoptic area (MnPO) have been shown to be instrumental in the onset and maintenance of sleep. The neurons in the VLPO and MnPO contain the inhibitory neurotransmitters GABA and galanin. They inner-vate all the wake-promoting centers (LDT/PPT, LC, DR, TMN, and lateral hypothalamus) and are thought to inhibit arousal during sleep.[57,58]

The sleep-active neurons in the VLPO fire fast-est during NREM sleep, slow significantly during REM sleep, and are silent during wakefulness.[59–61] The MnPO neurons begin to discharge just before NREM sleep starts, which has led to the hypoth-esis that MnPO neurons begin the onset of sleep, whereas VLPO neurons are necessary for the maintenance of sleep.[31]

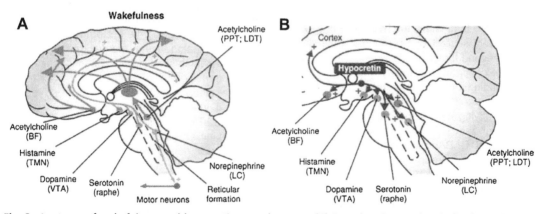

Fig. 3. Anatomy of wakefulness and hypocretin neural groups. (*A*) Dorsal and ventral reticular formations are shown with the dorsal cholinergic system (*blue*) sending fibers into the thalamus (*green*) and basal forebrain. The thalamus then projects out over the cortex by way of the thalamocortical projections. The ventral aminergic pathway is associated with wakefulness. (*B*) The hypocretin cell group in the lateral and posterior hypothalamus sends excitatory neurons to the cholinergic and monoaminergic groups of the reticular formation (all awake-promoting cell groups). BF, basal forebrain; VTA, ventral tegmental area. (*Adapted from* España RA, Scammell TE. Sleep neurobiology for the clinician. Sleep 2004;27:812; with permission.)

Melanin-Concentrating Hormone (MCH)

The hypothalamus contains another set of neurons that contain melanin-concentrating hormone (MCH). Recent research has shown that MCH facilitates both NREM and REM sleep states; however, there is more robust REM activity when MCH neurons are firing.[62] There is also evidence to suggest that these neurons actively inhibit the ascending monoaminergic systems to suppress wakefulness through feedback to the same monoaminergic cell groups that are stimulated by the Hcrt neurons.[62]

New observations have been made concerning the control of REM sleep. One area of interest has involved the sublaterodorsal nucleus (SLD), also called the subcoeruleus (LCα). These small clusters of cells are located ventral to the LC and produce either GABA or glutamate. These clusters contain a subset of cells that project to the ventromedial medulla and ventral horn of the spinal cord and is active during REM sleep. Experimental studies have shown that activation of the SLD region produces atonia and REM sleep–like EEG activity. There is also evidence that the SLD neurons may be strongly inhibited by REM sleep–suppressing neurons in the midpons. These GABAergic cells are located in an arc starting in the ventral part of the periaqueductal gray (vlPAG) in the mesopontine tegmentum and extending out into the lateral pontine tegmentum (LPT). The vlPAG/LPT inhibits the SLD, and the SLD may in turn inhibit the vlPAG/LPT, giving rise to the REM-on/REM-off flip-flop switch (discussed later).[31]

The understanding of the orchestration of the timing of sleep onset and then the initiation of the ultradian rhythm of REM and NREM sleep is the ultimate goal of sleep research. Von Economo[5] hypothesized that, within the hypothalamus, there are 2 distinct sites: 1 that promotes wakefulness and the second that promotes sleep. Recent findings have confirmed his theory and offer a better understanding of sleep onset and maintenance mechanisms.

By identifying modulators of the histaminergic neurons of the TMN, Sherin and colleagues[57] showed that GABAergic inputs that originate in the ventrolateral preoptic (VLPO) area and the extended VLPO (eVLPO) area of the hypothalamus inhibit the TMN. In addition to GABA, the eVLPO neurons also contain the inhibitory neuropeptide, galanin.[27] There are also inhibitory efferents to other monoaminergic nuclei such as the raphe nuclei and the LC. Thus, by inhibiting the wake-promoting action of these monoaminergic amines, the VLPO/eVLPO helps promote the onset of sleep. However, these same monoaminergic cell groups also supply

efferents back to the VLPO/eVLPO. There is also input from hypocretin-containing cells in the lateral hypothalamus. This reciprocal innervation facilitates control of the sleep/wake switch. In addition, known sleep-inducing substances (somnogens) such as adenosine and prostaglandin D2 increase activity in the VLPO/eVLPO, which in turn promotes sleep, allowing more modulatory input to the sleep/wake control.[63–66] This scenario has led to the hypothesis that there is a bistable sleep-wake switch through which the VLPO/eVLPO and arousal systems are reciprocally inhibited.[67]

The firing rates of VLPO/eVLPO neurons increase during sleep and get progressively faster as sleep deepens (SWS). This increased firing causes further inhibition of arousal centers, which allows less interrupted, and thereby deeper, sleep. In the opposite scenario, wakefulness causes inhibition of the VLPO/eVLPO, which ensures full wakefulness without letting drowsiness cause diminished cognitive abilities. Saper and colleagues described this as a sleep/wake flip-flop switch that has built-in stability with each half of the mechanism strongly inhibiting the other, thus avoiding intermediate states.[31,67–69] Full change of state requires overwhelming forces such as accumulated homeostatic sleep drive coupled with the appropriate circadian influence to drive the switch into its opposite configuration.

This model can explain how the behavioral states of wakefulness and sleep can transition from one to the other and maintain the state regardless of constantly changing homeostatic forces that accumulate and dissipate during the course of a day as well as allowing the circadian influences to ensure 24-hour rhythmicity. However, if 1 side of the switch is weakened, the affected side becomes less able to inhibit the other, thereby moving the system to a less stable midpoint (analogous to the fulcrum on a seesaw) with which smaller perturbations may trigger a state transition.

Once sleep onset occurs, a second set of neuronal interactions takes place that account for NREM/REM cycling. Firing of VLPO/eVLPO neurons increases as sleep gets deeper. A transition occurs during REM sleep when REM-on neurons located in and near the cholinergic neural group of the LDT/PPT start to release acetylcholine into the thalamus producing cortical desynchrony. The aminergic neurons of the TMN, DR, MR, and LC become silent (most likely mediated through afferents in the area of the eVLPO or MCH activity).

In 1975, Hobson and colleagues[70] proposed that the cycling of REM and NREM sleep came about because of reciprocal discharge by 2 brainstem neuronal groups. They theorized that, because cholinergic REM-on neurons were active during REM sleep at the same time that the noradrenergic LC and serotoninergic raphe were silent, there had to be a feedback mechanism that could account for this on/off effect. They termed this phenomenon reciprocal interaction, in which the cholinergic neurons activate reticular formation neurons in a positive feedback fashion to produce onset of REM sleep.[70] REM sleep is turned off by the inhibitory activity of REM-off aminergic neurons (raphe and LC cell groups) that become active at the conclusion of an REM cycle (REM-off neurons are thought to be recruited by REM-on activity). REM-off activity decreases in SWS and becomes minimal at the onset of REM sleep because of negative autofeedback as well as adenosine inhibition. At the same time, GABA stimulation from the hypothalamus is important for the maintenance of the REM period. Thus, decreasing REM-off activity disinhibits REM-on neurons and allows the onset of another REM sleep episode.[71]

This concept of a brainstem flip-flop switch for REM-on/REM-off physiology has recently been updated by Saper and colleagues,[67] proposing that the switch is set between 2 groups of GABAergic neurons located in the mesopontine tegmentum. It is their contention that the mutually inhibitory GABAergic populations more readily explain the sharp transitions into and out of REM sleep as well as explaining the increased frequency of transitions when either side is weakened (as in narcolepsy). They think that the cholinergic/monoaminergic interactions still have an important modulatory role in the process but are not parts of the switch itself.

The REM-on area in addition to GABA also contains 2 groups of glutamatergic neurons. One set of these neurons projects to the basal forebrain allowing desynchronization of the EEG, whereas the other projects to the medulla and spinal cord producing inhibition of the interspinal neurons via glycinergic and GABAergic mechanisms to produce REM-related muscle atonia (**Figs. 4** and **5**).[72]

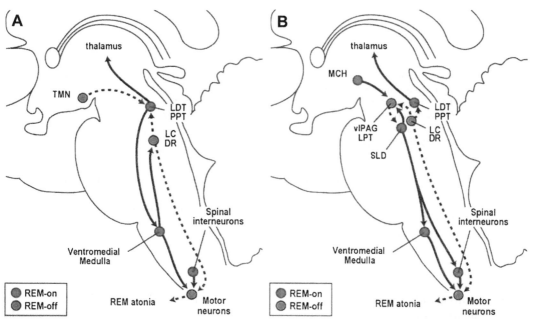

Fig. 4. Anatomic pathways that control REM-on and REM-off sleep. (*A*) The classic perspective on REM sleep control postulating a reciprocal interaction between the cholinergic and aminergic systems. REM sleep–active cholinergic neurons in the LDT/PPT activate thalamocortical signaling and drive atonia by exciting neurons in the ventromedial medulla that inhibit motor neurons. During REM sleep, monoaminergic neurons including the LC, DR, and TMN become silent, which disinhibits the LDT/PPT and lessens the excitation of motor neurons by NE and 5-HT. (*B*) Recent observations have expanded on the classic view of REM sleep control. In this model, mutual inhibition between REM sleep-on neurons of the SLD and REM sleep-off neurons of the ventrolateral periaqueductal gray (vlPAG) and LPT is thought to regulate transitions into and out of REM sleep. During REM sleep, SLD neurons activate GABA/glycine neurons in the ventromedial medulla and spinal cord that inhibit motor neurons. At most times, the vlPAG/LPT inhibits the SLD but, during REM sleep, the vlPAG/LPT may be inhibited by neurons containing MCH and other neurotransmitters. Solid lines depict pathways that are active during REM sleep and dashed lines are pathways that are inactive during REM sleep. (*Adapted from* España RA, Scammell TE. Sleep neurobiology from a clinical perspective. Sleep 2011;34:851; with permission.)

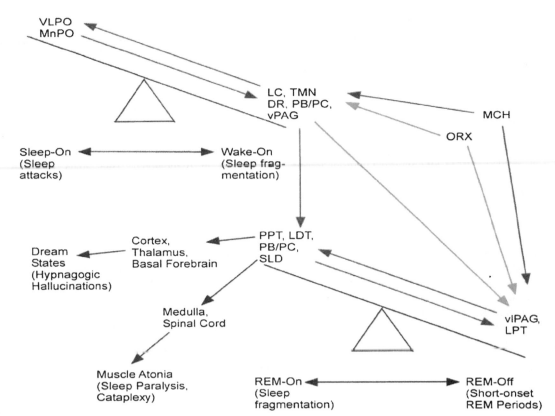

Fig. 5. Wake-sleep and REM-NREM flip-flop switches stabilized by the orexin system. The wake-promoting and sleep-promoting neurons are shown as components of a counterbalanced switch (flip-flop) at the upper left and the REM-on and REM-off populations at the lower right. *Red arrows*, inhibitory projections; *green arrows*, excitatory projections. The monoaminergic arousal neurons that inhibit the VLPO during wakefulness also inhibit the REM-on neurons at the same time as exciting the REM-off neurons in this switch, thus making it almost impossible for normal individuals to transition directly from wakefulness to an REM state. If there is loss of orexin signaling (eg, narcolepsy), both switches become destabilized and their normal balanced relationship is disrupted, so that the clinical presentation of REM intrusion into wakefulness becomes possible (cataplexy, sleep paralysis, hypnagogic hallucinations). The clinical phenomena of narcolepsy (when each population of wake-promoting, sleep-promoting, or REM-promoting neurons fires at the wrong time) are identified in parentheses. The neurons that contain MCH have the same targets as the orexin neurons but exert the opposite effect (mainly inhibitory) and have the opposite activity pattern (REM active). Hence, their net effect is to reinforce the influence of the orexin neurons. (*Adapted from* Saper CB, Fuller PM, Pedersen NP, et al. Sleep state switching. Neuron 2010;68:1035; with permission.)

CIRCADIAN RHYTHM
Suprachiasmatic Nucleus

Circadian rhythms are biologic activities that recur approximately every 24 hours. In the absence of external timing cues (zeitgebers), some of these processes remain rhythmical and run freely with an approximate 24-h period (*circa*, about; *deis*, day). In mammals, the suprachiasmatic nucleus (SCN) is the pacemaker for maintaining circadian sleep-wake cycles, body temperature changes, hormonal releases, and cyclic behavioral patterns. The SCN is located in the ventromedial hypothalamus immediately dorsal to the optic chiasm.

In mammals, the most important stimulus for the time-locked regulation of the circadian rhythm is light. The SCN has a direct afferent connection from the retina via the retinohypothalamic tract (RHT).[73] Activation is via a unique class of melanopsin-containing photopigment cells in the retinal ganglia, providing the main input for photic entrainment. The putative neurotransmitter in the RHT is the excitatory amino acid, glutamate.[74]

Nonphotic entrainment remains controversial. It is generally thought that nonphotic input to the SCN is mediated by thalamic input under the influence of serotoninergic neurons.[75] However, there are also afferents from the histaminergic TMN, cholinergic inputs from multiple forebrain and brain-stem regions, in particular, the pedunculopontine tegmentum.[76]

There are diffuse projections from the paraventricular nucleus of the thalamus and inputs from the hypothalamus itself, via the geniculohypothalamic tract (GHT). It is thought that input from the GHT is critical in nonphotic entrainment. The GHT originates from cells in the intergeniculate leaflet (IGL), which is located between the dorsal and ventral lateral geniculate nuclei in the thalamus.[77] The IGL has inputs from the retina, the noradrenergic LC, and the serotonergic raphe.[78] Efferents project to the contralateral IGL, the SCN and the peri-SCN area, the pineal, the accessory optic system the superior colliculus, the zona incerta, and the pretectum.

Besides glutamate, other neurotransmitters associated with the SCN include GABA, neuropeptide Y (NPY), Met-enkephalin, and orphanin-FQ.[79] NPY has been shown to phase shift circadian rhythms, and injecting antiserum to NPY into the SCN area can block its effect. 5-HT input from the median raphe nucleus goes directly into the SCN. However, serotonergic input from the DR comes via projections to the IGL, which then feed into the SCN via NPY.[80]

Efferents from the SCN project to 4 main areas. One group of fibers goes dorsally to the paraventricular area of the thalamus and the posterior hypothalamus. A second group of efferents go to nuclei located rostral to the SCN; in particular, the medial preoptic area (MPOA). The third group of fibers runs caudally from the SCN to the anterior, medial, and lateral hypothalamic areas. The fourth group of fibers runs dorsal to the optic tracts into the ventral lateral geniculate nucleus (vLGN). Thus there are extensive innervations from the SCN back into the hypothalamus and thalamus to control a complex series of interactions involving hormonal, behavioral, and temperature control.[81]

CLOCK GENES

The neurons within the SCN generate the circadian rhythm by means of oscillatory protein synthesis via several clock genes. The first gene, *Period* (*Per*), which encodes a clock component protein, PER, was discovered in 1971.[82] Since then, at least 8 genes have been identified that are involved with mammalian clock regulation. There are 3 *Per* genes (*mPer1, mPer2,* and *mPer3*), 2 *Cryptochrome* genes (*mCry1* and *mCry2*), *Clock* gene, *Bmal1* or *Mop3*, and *Ckle*.[82] Through a series of experiments that studied mutations of these clock genes and the resultant physiologic and behavioral changes

that they produced, Daan and colleagues[83] proposed a model that explains the negative feedback control that produces the 24-hour rhythms and also allows for adjustment to seasonal changes in the change in the length of daylight with a morning oscillator (M) that phase advances the circadian rhythm by sensing light at dawn, and an evening oscillator (E) that phase delays the rhythm keyed to decreasing light at dusk.

Within the nucleus of an SCN neuron, the CLOCK and BMAL1 proteins form a heterodimer that binds to the promoters of the *Per1* and *Per2* genes and activates their transcription. The PER1 and PER2 proteins, after phosphorylation in the cytoplasm, interact with clock gene products; CRY1 and CRY2 proteins. These *Cry* genes have opposite effects of the *Per1* and *Per2* genes. It has also been observed that *Per1* (M) and *Per2* (E) gene expression have different light responsiveness. Thus, the clock can be seen as an oscillator that is stabilized by 2 regulatory loops. The first is M, which is sensitive to dawn and the reappearance of sunlight, and the second is E, tracking the fading of light. Following the modulation by the CRY1 proteins, the PER1/CRY1 heterodimer would be transported back into the nucleus and would turn off the transcription of CLOCK/BMAL1, thereby inhibiting *Per1* and *Cry1* transcription. Likewise, the PER2/CRY2 heterodime would regulate *Per2* and *Cry2* transcription.[84]

HOMEOSTATIC AND CIRCADIAN SLEEP/WAKE INTERACTIONS

Before the SCN was identified as the master clock, the main theories of why humans sleep had to do with maintenance of physiologic equilibrium (ie, the concept of homeostasis).[85] Several examples of these theories are:

1. Sleep allowed brain energy to be restored after being depleted during the waking and thinking hours.
2. During the day, toxic products built up in the brain and sleep either facilitated their removal or detoxified these substances.
3. Sleep onset occurred when hypnotoxins caused brain system deactivation.
4. Habit and suggestion controlled sleep onset and offset.
5. Control of the biologic processes of sleep and wakefulness were extrinsic in origin.

In 1913, Legendre and Pieron[86] found that CSF of sleep-deprived dogs instilled into the ventricular system of non–sleep-deprived dogs induced sleep. This led to the hypothesis that there is a sleep factor that builds up within the central nervous system when there is sleep loss and/or accumulates after repeated bouts of insufficient sleep and then dissipates during the sleep state.

In 1982, Borbely and Tobler[85] proposed a 2-process model of sleep regulation with a homeostatic force that builds as wakefulness progresses and declines during sleep (process S) that is opposed by a circadian process (process C), which is independent of sleep and waking. Edgar and colleagues[87] further refined this theory in 1993 with the inclusion of the role of the SCN in the initiation and maintenance of wakefulness along with the active opposition of the homeostatic sleep force during waking hours (**Fig. 6**).

There is now evidence that adenosine may be one of, if not the, main sleep-inducing factors or somnogens responsible, at least in part, for the homeostatic sleep force (process S). Adenosine levels in the basal forebrain increase with sleep deprivation and then decrease rapidly during the subsequent sleep period, which may explain why caffeine, an adenosine A1 receptor blocker, is able to augment alertness. It seems that adenosine promotes sleep by direct inhibition of wake-promoting neural groups and by disinhibiting the sleep-promoting VLPO neurons.[63]

Adenosine may not be the only somnogen present. Infectious processes can induce sleep. Sleep is also induced by cytokines such as interferon-α, interlukin-1β, and tumor necrosis factor-α.[88] Cytokines also induce the production of prostaglandin D_2 (PGD_2), which promotes REM and NREM sleep.[89]

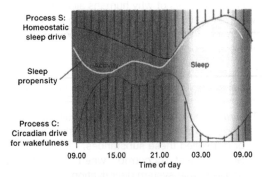

Fig. 6. Summary of sleep process C and sleep process S. The interaction of the circadian and homeostatic drives produces a sleep propensity curve that is biphasic. There is a higher sleep propensity in the midafternoon and a more robust period at night. The sleep onset occurs just after the sleep gate opens, and sleep offset occurs just after the nadir of body temperature. (*Data from* Edgar DM, Dement W, Fuller CA. Effect of SCN lesions on sleep in squirrel monkeys: evidence for opponent processes in sleep-wake regulation. J Neurosci 1993;13:1075.)

The postulates of defining biologic rhythms and their control can be summarized as follows:

1. The environment does not impose the processes, they are an intrinsic part of the biologic makeup of the organism.
2. They persist in the absence of all known extrinsic influences.
3. They retain a 24-hour periodicity when there is an acute change in the periodicity of the environment.
4. Following an acute and sustained temporal change, there is a slow phase recovery.
5. The rhythms do not revert immediately after having been synchronized to a new periodicity.
6. When external time cues are removed, there is a slow drift away from the 24-hour cycle.

To better understand the interaction of the 2 processes, several experimental paradigms were developed. One such set of experiments involved sleep deprivation studies in which sleep was eliminated for extended periods. Even though the overall sleep pressure increased, there was still a discernible 24-hour cycle with increased sleep propensity during what would ordinarily be the subject's nighttime and increased alertness during the subject's day.[90] Several studies showed that there are 2 times of increased sleep propensity; 1 less robust period during the early afternoon and a second, more powerful, period at night. All studies showed that the greatest increase in sleepiness occurred in the early morning, whereas the least sleepiness occurred in the early evening.[91]

A second set of experiments involved sleep displacement in which sleep-onset times were shifted. When sleep was shifted by 12 hours, there was a significant increase in wakefulness in beginning of the sleep period, which was accompanied by a shift of REM sleep to the first third to half of the night (REM sleep is normally maximal during the second half of the night). Thus, there was a decrease in the first REM latency and an increase in wakefulness after sleep onset (WASO).[92] This corresponds with the clinical problem of shift workers, who, after working at night, report fragmented and nonrestorative sleep when their rest cycle takes place during the day.

Some of the earliest work involved temporal isolation studies in which subjects were placed in environments where there were no discernible cues to the external environment (ie, all zeitgebers were removed). The sleep/wake cycle tended to increase to slightly less than 25 hours and the diurnal temperature curve behaved similarly; this was called a free-running rhythm.[93]

It had been known for some time that the sleep/wake cycle is synchronized with the ambient light/dark cycle, with the peak rectal temperature occurring in the late afternoon to early evening. The nadir occurs in the second half of the sleep period. However, after several days in a free-running environment, the temperature peak advanced to the first half of the activity period and the nadir changed to the first half of the sleep period. In these subjects, sleep onset occurred close to the temperature minimum, and sleep offset took place on the rising limb of the temperature cycle. The total amount of sleep was reduced even when the sleep pressure was increasing, as measured by the total amount of prior wakefulness.

Another significant observation of these temporal isolation subjects was that many of them had a spontaneous dissociation of their temperature cycles from their rest/activity cycles after several days. This response is called internal desynchronization.

Zulley and colleagues[94] found that, in internally desynchronized subjects, the circadian temperature curve not only influenced the duration of sleep but also the propensity for falling asleep. Czeisler and colleagues[95] showed that the timing of REM sleep depends on the circadian phase of the temperature cycle at sleep onset and not on the amount of prior wakefulness. Further studies showed that there were 2 zones of high probability to go to sleep and there were 2 zones of a low probability to fall asleep.[95]

These findings led to what seemed to be a paradoxic conclusion: that it is most difficult to fall asleep shortly before what, in most people, would be their regular bedtime. The 2 zones of highest sleep propensity were further analyzed using nap times in internally desynchronized subjects. Zulley and Campbell[96] found that naps clustered at 2 circadian phases, 1 at the temperature nadir and a second at a point halfway between 2 successive temperature nadirs. They explained this by the existence of not only a primary sleep period but also a secondary circadian sleep period that, under normally entrained conditions, corresponds with the early afternoon.[96]

FORCED DESYNCHRONY

Another experimental paradigm used a forced day length close to, but not exactly, that of a 24-hour time period (eg, 22.7 or 25.3 hours). The duration of wakefulness between successive sleep periods remained constant but sleep onset occurred at different circadian phases. The net effect was to allow the body temperature rhythm to run free and to separate the circadian-dependent processes from the homeostatic processes.

Using the forced desynchrony protocol, it was established that the human circadian clock is closer to the environmental diurnal day/night cycle (24 hours ± 10 minutes) and it is the same for all age groups. Thus, the concept that aging brings on circadian changes was successfully challenged.[97]

Sleep pressure, as measured by sleep-onset latency, is maximal near the nadir of core body temperature, which is close to the usual wake time in normally entrained conditions. The drive to maintain wakefulness is strongest during the evening hours near the temperature maximum, which, as described previously, is close to the usual sleep-onset time. Thus the paradox: the pressure to maintain wakefulness is highest just before sleep onset and the maximal drive for sleep is just before waking. The teleologic explanation is that wakefulness is maintained right up to the point of sleep onset and sleep is maintained through the night until sleep offset.

Lavie[98] described a forbidden zone for sleep. Strogatz[99] also described this as the wake-maintenance zone.[99,100] This zone corresponds with the period just before sleep onset when wakefulness is being countered by an increasing circadian drive for sleep. There then occurs an abrupt transition from low sleep propensity during the evening period to the high-propensity night period. This time frame has been called the nocturnal sleep gate and has been found to be phase locked to the dark-phase hormone, melatonin. The opening of the sleep gate occurs approximately 2 hours after the onset of the nocturnal secretion of melatonin.[101]

AGENTS OF ENTRAINMENT
Light

Light exposure in the early morning hours (just after the body temperature minimum) caused an advance in the sleep/wake cycle, whereas exposure to light in the early evening, before the temperature minimum, caused a delay in the sleep/wake cycle. This light exposure does not have to be at the brightness level of sunlight and even artificial incandescent light can cause phase shifts if exposure is present at critical times. It has also been showed that non–sleep/wake circadian rhythms are shifted by light exposure with changes in urine production, cortisol production, and melatonin secretion. All these rhythms showed a stable temporal relationship to temperature rhythms after light-induced phase shifts.[102,103]

Melatonin

Melatonin is synthesized from circulating tryptophan, transformed to 5-HT, and then converted into melatonin in the pineal gland. There is no pineal storage of melatonin; as it is secreted, it is distributed through the circulation. Maximum plasma concentrations occur between 3:00 and 4:00 AM and, during the day, levels are almost undetectable. Even in temporal isolation, melatonin continues to express its circadian rhythm. The rhythmicity of melatonin secretion is driven by the SCN through connections to the paraventricular nuclei and then to a multisynaptic pathway that courses through the upper part of the cervical spinal cord, synapsing on preganglionic cell bodies of the superior cervical ganglia (SCG) of the cervical sympathetic chains. The SCG then sends noradrenergic neuronal projections directly to the pineal gland.[104]

Melatonin synthesis is limited to the dark period and is inhibited by light. Exogenous melatonin exerts phase-shifting effects on the endogenous production of melatonin in humans. Melatonin administered in the morning (time of shutdown of natural melatonin production) caused phase-shift delay of the endogenous rhythm, and phase advances occurred when melatonin was administered before onset of the endogenous production.

It is hypothesized that the endogenous cycle of melatonin secretion is involved in the regulation of the sleep/wake cycle not by actively promoting sleep but by inhibiting the SCN wakefulness-producing mechanism.[105,106]

In this way, the evening onset of melatonin secretion, which coincides with the maximum point of the SCN-driven arousal cycle, inhibits the circadian drive for waking, thereby enabling the sleep-onset structures to be activated, unopposed by the drive for wakefulness.

REFERENCES

1. Leadbetter R. Nyx, . Encyclopedia mythica. Rome (Italy): Pantheon; 1999.
2. Poortvliet R, Huygun W. What is sleep? The book of the sandman and the alphabet of sleep. New York: Harry N Abrams; 1989.
3. Rouse W, Smith M. Lucretius: on the nature of things. Cambridge (MA): Harvard University Press; 1992. p. 34.
4. Hammond W. Physiology of sleep: on wakefulness. Philadelphia: JB Lippincott; 1866. p. 2–38.
5. von Economo C. Sleep as a problem of localization. J Nerv Ment Dis 1930;71:249–59.
6. Aldrich M. Neurology of sleep. Sleep medicine. New York: Oxford University Press; 1999. p. 27–38.
7. Berger H. Ueber das elektroenkephalogram des menschen. J Psychol Neurol 1930;40:160–79.
8. Bremer F. Cerveau "isole" et physiologie du sommeil. C R Soc Biol (Paris) 1935;118:1235–41.
9. Ramón y Cajal S. Histologie du systeme nerveux de l'homme et des vertebres maloine. Paris: Oxford University Press; 1911.
10. Papez J. Reticulo-spinal tracts in the cat, Narchi method. J Comp Neurol 1926;41:365–99.
11. Morison R, Dempsey E. Mechanism of thalamo-cortical augmentation and repetition. Am J Physiol 1942;38:297–308.
12. de No L. The cerebral cortex: architecture, intracortical connections and motor projections. In: Fulton J, editor. Physiology of the nervous system. London: Oxford University Press; 1938. p. 291–339.
13. Moruzzi G, Magoun H. Communications: brain stem reticular formation and activation of the EEG. Electroencephalogr Clin Neurophysiol 1949; 1:455–73.
14. Jouvet M, Michel F. Correlations electromyographiques du sommeil chez le chat decortique et mesencephalique chronique. C R Seances Soc Biol Fil 1959;153:422–5.
15. Jouvet M, Michel F, Courjon J. Sur un stade d'activity electrique cerebral rapide au cours du sommeil physiologique. C R Seances Soc Biol Fil 1959;153:1024–8.
16. Jouvet M, Mounier D. Effects des lesions de la formation reticulaire pontine sur le sommeil du chat. C R Seances Soc Biol Fil 1960;154:2301–5.
17. Aserinsky E, Kleitman N. Regularly occurring periods of eye movements and concomitant phenomena during sleep. Science 1953;118:273–4.
18. Aserinsky E, Kleitman N. Two types of ocular motility occurring in sleep. J Appl Physiol 1955;8: 11–8.
19. Dement W, Kleitman N. Cyclic variations in EEG during sleep and their relation to eye movements, body motility and dreaming. Electroencephalogr Clin Neurophysiol 1957;9:673–90.
20. Rechtschaffen A, Kales A. A manual of standardized terminology, techniques and scoring system for sleep stages of human subjects. Los Angeles (CA): Brain Information Service/Brain Research Institute; 1968.
21. Iber C, Ancoli-Israel S, Chesson A, et al. The AASM manual for the scoring of sleep and associated events. Westchester (IL): American Academy of Sleep Medicine; 2007.
22. Steriade M, Gloor P, Llinas R. Basic mechanisms of cerebral rhythmic activities. Electroencephalogr Clin Neurophysiol 1990;76:481–508.
23. Pare D, Steriade M, Deschenes M, et al. Physiological characteristics of anterior thalamic nuclei, a group devoid of inputs from reticular thalamic nucleus. J Neurophysiol 1987;57:1669–85.
24. Colrain I. The K-complex: a 7 decade history. Sleep 2005;28:255–73.
25. Buzsaki G, Traub R. Physiological basis of EEG activity. In: Engel J, Pedley TA, editors. Epilepsy:

a comprehensive textbook. New York: Raven Press; 1997. p. 819–32.

26. Steriade M, Datta S, Pare D, et al. Neuronal activities in brain-stem cholinergic nuclei related to tonic activation processes in thalamocortical systems. J Neurosci 1990;10:2541–59.

27. Pace-Schott E, Hobson J. The neurobiology of sleep: genetics, cellular physiology and subcortical networks. Nat Rev Neurosci 2002;3:591–605.

28. Steriade M. Arousal: revisting the reticular activating system. Science 1996;272:225–6.

29. Armstrong D, Saper C, Levey A, et al. Distribution of cholinergic neurons in rat brain: demonstrated by the immunocytochemical localization of choline acetyltransferase. J Comp Neurol 1983;216:53–68.

30. España R, Scammell T. Sleep neurobiology for the clinician. Sleep 2004;27:811–20.

31. España R, Scammell T. Sleep neurobiology from a clinical perspective. Sleep 2011;34:845–58.

32. Detari L, Rasmussin D, Semba K, et al. The role of the basal forebrain neurons in tonic and phasic activation of the cerebral cortex. Prog Neurobiol 1999;58:249.

33. Tork I. Anatomy of the serotonergic system. Ann N Y Acad Sci 1990;600:9–34.

34. Koella W. Serotonin and sleep. Exp Med Surg 1969;27:157–68.

35. Schonrock B, Busselberg D, Haas H. Properties of tuberomammillary histamine neurons and their response to galanin. Agents Action 1991;33:135–7.

36. Yang Q, Hatton G. Electrophysiology of excitatory and inhibitory afferents to rat histaminergic tuberomammillary nucleus neurons from hypothalamic and forebrain sites. Brain Res 1997;773:162–72.

37. Morrison J, Foote S. Noradrenergic and serotoninergic innervation of cortical, thalamic and tectal visual structures in old and new world monkeys. J Comp Neurol 1986;243:117–38.

38. Tasaka K, Chung Y, Sawada K. Excitatory effect of histamine on the arousal system and its inhibition by H1 blockers. Brain Res Bull 1989;22:271–5.

39. Mignot E, Taheri S, Nishino S. Sleeping with the hypothalamus: emerging therapeutic targets for sleep disorders. Nat Neurosci 2002;5(Suppl):1071–5.

40. Hillarp N, Fuxe K, Dahlstrom A. Demonstration and mapping of central neurons containing dopamine, noradrenaline, and 5-hydroxytryptamine and their reactions to psychopharmaca. Pharmacol Rev 1966;18:727–39.

41. Dzoljic M, Ukponmwan O, Saxena P. 5-HT1-like receptor agonists enhance wakefulness. Neuropharmacology 1992;31:623–33.

42. Nishino S, Mao J, Sampathkumaran R, et al. Increased dopaminergic transmission mediates the wake-promoting effects of CNS stimulants. Sleep Res Online 1998;1:49–61.

43. Wisor J, Nishino S, Sora I, et al. Dopaminergic role in stimulant-induced wakefulness. J Neurosci 2001;21:1787–94.

44. Isaac S, Berridge C. Wake-promoting actions of dopamine D1 and D2 receptor stimulation. J Pharmacol Exp Ther 2003;307:386–94.

45. Rye D. The two faces of eve: dopamine's modulation of wakefulness and sleep. Neurology 2004;63(8 Suppl 3):S2–7.

46. Claassen D, Josephs K, Ahlskog J, et al. REM sleep behavior disorder preceding other aspects of synucleinopathies by up to half a century. Neurology 2010;75:494–9.

47. Comella C. Sleep disorders in Parkinson's disease. Curr Treat Options Neurol 2008;10:215–21.

48. De Lecea L, Kilduff T, Peyron C, et al. The hypocretins: hypothalamus-specific peptides with neuroexcitatory activity. Proc Natl Acad Sci U S A 1998;95:322–7.

49. Sakurai T, Amemiya A, Ishii M, et al. Orexins and orexin receptors: a family of hypothalamic neuropeptides and G protein-coupled receptors that regulate feeding behavior. Cell 1998;92:573–85.

50. Methippara M, Alam N, Szymusiak R, et al. Effects of lateral preoptic area application of orexin-A on sleep-wakefulness. Neuroreport 2000;11:3423–6.

51. Espāna R, Baldo B, Kelley A, et al. Wake-promoting and sleep-suppressing actions of hypocretin (orexin): basal forebrain sites of action. Neuroscience 2001;106:699–715.

52. Kilduff T, Peyron C. The hyporetin/orexin ligand-receptor system: implications for sleep and sleep disorders. Trends Neurosci 2000;23:359–65.

53. Lee M, Hassani O, Jones B. Discharge of identified orexin/hypocretin neurons across the sleep-waking cycle. J Neurosci 2005;25:6716–20.

54. Siegel J, Moore R, Thannickal T, et al. A brief history of hypocretin/orexin and narcolepsy. Neuropsychopharmacology 2001;25(Suppl 5):S14–20.

55. Thannickal T, Moore R, Nienhuis R, et al. Reduced number of hypocretin neurons in human narcolepsy. Neuron 2000;27:469–74.

56. Kiyashchenko L, Mileykovskiy B, Lai Y, et al. Increased and decreased muscle tone with orexin (hypocretin) microinjections in the locus coeruleus and pontine inhibitory area. J Neurophysiol 2001;85:2008–16.

57. Sherin J, Shiromani P, McCarley R, et al. Activation of ventrolateral preoptic neurons during sleep. Science 1996;271:216–9.

58. Gong H, McGinty D, Guzman-Marin R, et al. Activation of c-fos in GABAergic neurones in the preoptic area during sleep and in response to sleep deprivation. J Physiol 2004;556:935–46.

59. Szymusiak R, Alam N, Steininger T, et al. Sleep-waking discharge patterns of ventrolateral preoptic/anterior hypothalamic neurons in rats. Brain Res 1998;803:178–88.

60. Takahashi K, Lin J, Saki K. Characterization and mapping of sleep-waking specific neurons in the basal forebrain and preoptic hypothalamus in mice. Neuroscience 2009;161:269–92.

61. Suntsova N, Szymusiak R, Alam N, et al. Sleep-waking discharge patterns of median preoptic nucleus neurons in rats. J Physiol 2002;543:665–77.

62. Torterolo P, Lagos P, Monti J. Melanin-concentrating hormone: a new sleep factor? Front Neurol 2011;2:1–12.

63. Porkka-Heiskanen T, Strooker R, Thakkar M, et al. Adenosine: a mediator of the sleep-inducing effects of prolonged wakefulness. Science 1997; 276:1265–8.

64. Tanase D, Martin W, Baghdoyan H, et al. G protein activation in rat ponto-mesencephalic nuclei is enhanced by a combined treatment with a mu opioid and an adenosine A1 receptor agonist. Sleep 2001;24:52–61.

65. Chamberlin N, Arrigoni E, Chou T, et al. Effects of adenosine on GABAergic synaptic inputs to identified ventrolateral preoptic neurons. Neuroscience 2003;119:913–8.

66. Ueno R, Ishikawa Y, Nakayama T, et al. Prostaglandin D2 induces sleep when microinjected into the preoptic area of conscious rats. Biochem Biophys Res Commun 1982;109:576–82.

67. Lu J, Sherman D, Devor M, et al. A putative flip-flop switch for control of REM sleep. Nature 2006;441: 589–94.

68. Saper C, Chou T, Scammell T. The sleep switch: hypothalamic control of sleep and wakefulness. Trends Neurosci 2001;24:726–31.

69. Saper C, Scammell T, Lu J. Hypothalamic regulation of sleep and circadian rhythms. Nature 2005; 437:1257–63.

70. Hobson J, McCarley R, Wyzinski P. Sleep cycle oscillation: reciprocal discharge by two brainstem neuronal groups. Science 1975;189:55–8.

71. McCarley R. Mechanisms and models of REM sleep control. Arch Ital Biol 2004;142:429–67.

72. Curtis D, Hosli L, Johnston G, et al. The hyperpolarization of spinal motor neurons by glycine and related amino acids. Exp Brain Res 1968;5:235–58.

73. Johnson R, Moore R, Morin L. Loss of entrainment and anatomical plasticity after lesions of the hamster retinohypothalamic tract. Brain Res 1988; 460:297–313.

74. Berson D, Dunn F, Tako M. Phototransduction by retinal ganglion cells that set the circadian clock. Science 2002;295:1070–3.

75. Morin L. Serotonin and the regulation of mammalian circadian rhythmicity. Ann Med 1999;31:12–33.

76. Bina K, Rusak B, Semba K. Localization of cholinergic neurons in the forebrain and brainstem that project to the suprachiasmatic nucleus of the hypothalamus in rat. J Comp Neurol 1993;335:295–307.

77. Moore R, Card J. Intergeniculate leaflet: an anatomically and functionally distinct subdivision of the lateral geniculate complex. J Comp Neurol 1994;344:403–30.

78. Morin L. The circadian visual system. Brain Res Rev 1994;67:102–27.

79. Harrington M, Mistlberger R. Anatomy and physiology of the mammalian circadian system. In: Kryger M, Roth T, Dement W, editors. Principles and practice of sleep medicine. 2nd edition. Philadelphia: WB Saunders; 2000. p. 334–45.

80. Biello S, Janik D, Mrosovsky N. Neuropeptide Y and behaviorally induced phase shifts. Neuroscience 1994;62:273–9.

81. Watts A, Swanson L. Efferent projections of the suprachiasmatic nucleus, II: studies using retrograde transport of fluorescent dyes and simultaneous peptide immunochemistry in the rat. J Comp Neurol 1987;258:230–52.

82. Konopka R, Benzer S. Clock mutants of *Drosophila melanogaster*. Proc Natl Acad Sci U S A 1971;68: 2112–6.

83. Daan S, Beersma D, Borbely A. Timing of human sleep recovery process gated by a circadian pacemaker. Am J Physiol 1984;246:161–83.

84. Albrecht U. Functional genomics of sleep and circadian rhythm. Invited review: regulation of mammalian circadian clock genes. J Appl Physiol 2002;92:1348–55.

85. Borbely A, Trobler I. Endogenous sleep-promoting substances and sleep regulation. Physiol Rev 1989;69:605–58.

86. Legendre R, Pieron H. Le probleme des facteurs du sommeil. Resultats d'injections vasculaires et intracerebrales de liquids insomniques. C R Soc Biol (Paris) 1910;68:1077–9.

87. Edgar D, Dement W, Fuller C. Effect of SCN lesions on sleep in squirrel monkeys: evidence for opponent processes in sleep-wake regulation. J Neurosci 1993;13:1065–79.

88. Spath-Schwalbe E, Lange T, Perras B, et al. Interferon-alpha acutely impairs sleep in healthy humans. Cytokine 2000;12:518–21.

89. Besedovsky L, Lange T, Born J. Sleep and immune function. Pflugers Arch 2012;463(1):121–37.

90. Blake M. Time of day effects on performance in a range of tasks. Psychon Sci 1967;9:349–50.

91. Webb W, Agnew H, Williams R. Effects on sleep of a sleep period time displacement. Aerosp Med 1971;42:152–5.

92. Aschoff J, Wever R. Spotanperiodik des menschen bei ausschluss aller zeitgeber. Naturwissenschaften 1962;49:337–42.

93. Zulley J. Distribution of REM sleep in entrained 24 hour and free-running sleep-wake cycles. Sleep 1980;2:377–89.

94. Zulley J, Wever R, Aschoff J. The dependence of onset and duration of sleep on the circadian rhythm of rectal temperature. Pflugers Arch 1981;391: 314–8.

95. Czeisler C, Zimmerman J, Ronda J, et al. Timing of REM sleep is coupled to the circadian rhythm of body temperature in man. Sleep 1980;2: 329–46.

96. Zulley J, Campbell S. Napping behavior during spontaneous internal desynchronization: sleep remains in synchrony with body temperature. Hum Neurobiol 1985;4:123–6.

97. Lavie P. Sleep-wake as a biological rhythm. Annu Rev Psychol 2001;52:277–303.

98. Lavie P. Ultrashort sleep-waking schedule: III. 'Gates' and 'forbidden zones' for sleep. Electroencephalogr Clin Neurophysiol 1986;63:414–25.

99. Strogatz S. The mathematical structure of the human sleep wake cycle. New York: Springer-Verlag; 1986.

100. Liu X, Uchiyama M, Shibui K, et al. Diurnal preference, sleep habits, circadian sleep propensity and melatonin rhythm in healthy human subjects. Neuroscience Let 2000;280:199–202.

101. Froberg J. Twenty-four-hour patterns in human performance, subjective and physiological variables and differences between morning and evening types. Biol Psychol 1977;5:119–34.

102. Czeisler C, Allan J, Strogatz S, et al. Bright light resets the human circadian pacemaker independent of the timing of the sleep-wake cycle. Science 1986;244:1328–33.

103. Czeisler C, Kronauer R, Allan J, et al. Bright light induction of strong (type 0) resetting of the human circadian pacemaker. Science 1989;244: 1328–33.

104. Arendt J. Melatonin and the mammalian pineal gland. London: Chapman-Hall; 1995.

105. Lewy A, Ahmed S, Jackson J, et al. Melatonin shifts human circadian rhythms according to a phase-response curve. Chronobiol Int 1992;9:380–92.

106. Lavie P. Melatonin: role in gating nocturnal rise in sleep propensity. J Biol Rhythms 1997;12:657–65.

Normal Sleep and Circadian Rhythms
Neurobiological Mechanisms Underlying Sleep and Wakefulness

Dimitri Markov, MD[a],*, Marina Goldman, MD[b],
Karl Doghramji, MD[a]

KEYWORDS

• Circadian rhythms • Sleep • Wakefulness • Neurobiological mechanisms

KEY POINTS

• Sleep is a neurobehavioral state, maintained through a highly organized interaction of neurons and neural circuits in the central nervous system.
• Sleep plays an important role in the regulation of central nervous system and body physiologic functions.
• Reduction or disruption of sleep can affect numerous functions varying from thermoregulation to learning and memory during the waking state.

INTRODUCTION

The cyclic repetition of sleep and wakefulness states is essential to the basic functioning of all higher animals including human beings. As our understanding of the neurobiology of sleep increases, we no longer view it as a passive state, that is, sleep as merely the absence of wakefulness. In fact, sleep is an active neurobehavioral state, which is maintained through a highly organized interaction of neurons and neural circuits in the central nervous system (CNS).

Defining Sleep

Sleep physicians define human sleep on the basis of a person's observed behavior and accompanying physiologic changes in the brain's electrical activity as it transitions between wakefulness and sleep. Behaviorally, human sleep is characterized by reclined position, closed eyes, decreased movement, and decreased responsivity to internal and external environment. The responsiveness to stimuli is not completely absent; a sleeper continues to process some sensory information during sleep; and meaningful stimuli are more likely to produce arousals than nonmeaningful ones. For example, a sound of one's own name is more likely to arouse a sleeper than some other sound, and the cry of her baby is more likely to arouse a sleeping mother than a cry of another infant.

Constituents of Sleep

Sleep consists of two strikingly different states, rapid eye movement (REM) and non–rapid eye movement (NREM) sleep. The NREM sleep can be further subdivided into 3 stages.

Polysomnography is the gold-standard technique that simultaneously records the 3 physiologic measures that define the main stages of sleep and wakefulness: muscle tone, recorded

A version of this article originally appeared in *Psychiatric Clinics of North America, Volume 29, Issue 4*.
[a] Thomas Jefferson University Sleep Disorders Center, 211 South Ninth Street, Suite 500, Philadelphia, PA 19107, USA; [b] University of Pennsylvania Treatment Research Center, 3900 Chestnut Street, Philadelphia, PA 19104, USA
* Corresponding author.
E-mail address: dimitri.markov@jefferson.edu

through an electromyogram (EMG); eye movements, recorded through an electro-oculogram (EOG); and brain activity, recorded through an electroencephalogram (EEG).[1,2] The clinical polysomnogram, whose purpose is to detect findings that are characteristic of certain sleep disorders, includes the following in addition to these 3 variables: monitors for air flow at the nose and mouth; respiratory-effort strain gauges placed around the chest and abdomen; and noninvasive oxygen saturation monitors that function by introducing a beam of light through the skin. Other parameters include the electrocardiogram and EMG of the anterior tibialis muscles, which are intended to detect periodic leg movements. Finally, a patient's gross body movements are continuously monitored by audiovisual means.

The EEG pattern of drowsy wakefulness consists of low-voltage rhythmic alpha activity (8–13 cycles per second [Hz]). In stage 1 of NREM sleep (N1), the low-voltage mixed frequency theta waves (4–8 Hz) replace the alpha rhythm of wakefulness. Slow asynchronous eye movements are seen on the EOG in the beginning of stage 1 sleep and disappear in a few minutes. The muscle activity is highest during wakefulness and diminishes as sleep approaches. Individuals with behavioral characteristics of sleep and polysomnographic characteristics of stage 1 sleep may or may not perceive themselves as sleeping. Stage N1 is viewed as a shallow sleep, during which an individual can be easily aroused. With transition to stage N2, EEG patterns termed sleep spindles and K complexes appear on the EEG. Sleep spindles are 12- to 14-Hz synchronized EEG waveforms with duration of up to 1.5 seconds. Sleep-spindle waves arise as a result of synchronization of groups of thalamic neurons by a γ-aminobutyrate (GABA)-ergic thalamic spindle pacemaker. The origin of K complexes is not known. With the onset of stage N2 the arousal threshold increases, and more intense stimulus is needed to arouse a sleeper. Stages 3 and 4 of NREM sleep are defined by a synchronized high-amplitude (more than 75 μV) and slow (0.5–2 Hz) delta-wave EEG pattern. Stage N3 is referred to as deep sleep, delta sleep, or slow-wave sleep (SWS). By definition, delta waves account for more than 20% of EEG activity during the stage 3 and greater than 50% of EEG activity during stage N3 sleep. SWS is associated with higher arousal threshold than are lighter stages of NREM sleep. No eye movements are detected on the EOG during stages 2, 3, and 4 of NREM sleep. The EMG tracks continued decline in muscle tone as NREM sleep deepens from stages 1 to 4.

The cortical EEG pattern of REM sleep is characterized by low voltage and fast frequencies (alpha or 8–13 Hz). This EEG pattern is referred to as activated or desynchronized, and is also seen in the state of relaxed wakefulness (with eyes closed). Activated refers to an active mind (dreams) and the EEG pattern characteristic of wakefulness. Paradoxically, individuals in REM, while activated, are behaviorally less responsive than during the wake state.[3,4] Desynchronized refers to the random-appearing wave pattern seen on the REM sleep EEG, in contrast to the synchronized uniform wave pattern seen on the NREM sleep EEG.[3,4] To be scored as REM sleep, a polysomnographic tracing must contain an activated EEG pattern as well as muscle atonia (EMG) and the presence of rapid eye movements (EOG). REM sleep can be further subdivided into 2 stages: tonic and phasic. The tonic stage is continuous, and shows muscle atonia and desynchronized EEG as the 2 main features. Superimposed on the tonic stage of REM are intermittent phasic events, which include bursts of rapid eye movements, and irregularities of respiration and heart rate.[5]

Sleep Architecture

Sleep typically begins with a shallow stage 1 of NREM (N1) and deepens to NREM stages 2, and 3, which are followed by the first brief episode of REM in approximately 90 minutes. After the first sleep cycle, NREM and REM sleep continue to alternate in a predictable fashion, each NREM-REM cycle lasting approximately 90 to 120 minutes.[1] In the course of the night, sleep cycles recur 3 to 7 times. Stage 1 of NREM, which lasts only a few minutes, serves as a transition from wakefulness to sleep, and later during sleep serves as a transition between REM-NREM sleep cycles. Typically stage N1 constitutes 2% to 5% of total sleep time. An increase in the amount or percentage of stage N1 sleep may be a sign of sleep disruption. The brief first period of stage 1 NREM sleep is followed by the "deeper" stage N2, which lasts for approximately 10 to 20 minutes. Stage N2 sleep normally constitutes 45% to 55% of the total sleep time. Stage N2 sleep progresses to stage N3, also known as "deep sleep" or slow wave sleep. Stage N3 constitutes about 15% of the total sleep time. Stages 3 of NREM sleep predominate during the first third of the night. The first REM period is brief and occurs approximately 90 minutes after sleep onset; subsequent REM cycles occur approximately 90 to 120 minutes apart. REM sleep episodes become longer as the night progresses, and the longest REM periods are found in the last third of the night.[6,7] NREM sleep accounts for 75% to 80%, and REM sleep accounts for 20% to 25%

of the total sleep time.[1,6,8–10] These proportions commonly vary with age (see the section Effects of Age).

PHYSIOLOGIC FUNCTIONS IN SLEEP
Autonomic Nervous System during Sleep

The parasympathetic drive is higher during all stages of sleep than in relaxed wakefulness. The sympathetic drive increases significantly during phasic REM, decreases slightly during tonic REM, and remains relatively unchanged during relaxed wakefulness and NREM sleep. The net effect is the dominance of the parasympathetic tone during NREM and tonic REM sleep and the sympathetic dominance during phasic REM.[11–13]

Regulation of Body Temperature

The energy expenditure is lower during NREM sleep than during wakefulness. The body temperature is maintained at a lower set point in NREM than in wakefulness. During REM sleep, thermoregulatory responses of shivering and sweating are absent, and thermal regulation appears to cease (as in poikilothermic organisms).[11–13]

Control of Respiration and Cardiovascular Function During Sleep

The predominance of the parasympathetic tone and decreased energy expenditure during NREM sleep are responsible for decreased ventilation during this stage. The respiration rate in NREM sleep is regular, and cardiovascular changes are consistent with decreased energy expenditure. By contrast, breathing patterns and heart rate during REM sleep are irregular.[11–13] The irregularities in cardiovascular parameters increase the risk of myocardial infarctions during REM sleep in vulnerable individuals. The changes in ventilation, respiration, and upper airway tone make REM sleep a vulnerable period for individuals with obstructive sleep apnea (**Table 1**).

EFFECTS OF AGE

Age is likely the strongest factor that affects sleep continuity and the distribution of sleep stages through the night. The sleep pattern of newborn infants dramatically differs from that of adults. During the first year of life, infants sleep twice as much as adults and, unlike adults, enter sleep through REM. During the first year of life, REM sleep constitutes as much as 50% of the total sleep time; the percentage occupied by REM sleep decreases to adult levels of 20% to 25% by age 3 years, and remains at that level until old age. NREM-REM cycles, controlled by the ultradian process, are present at birth, but the 50- to 60-minute cycle periods in newborns are shorter than the approximately 90-minute periods in adults. SWS is not present at birth, but develops by the age of 2 to 6 months. The amount of SWS

Table 1
Physiologic changes with stages of sleep

Parameter	NREM	REM
Heart	Decreases	Irregular with increases and decreases
Blood pressure	Unchanged and stable	Irregular with increases and decreases
Respiration	Decreased rate	Irregular rate in phasic stage
Ventilation	Decreased tidal volume Decreased hypoxic response	Decreased tidal volume in phasic stage Decreased hypoxic response
Upper airway muscle tone	Decreased	Further decreased
Temperature	Preserved thermoregulation	Increased temperature and poikilothermia
Pupils	Constricted	Constricted in tonic stage Dilated in phasic stage
Gastrointestinal	Failure of inhibition of acid secretion; prolonged acid clearance	Failure of inhibition of acid secretion
Nocturnal penile tumescence/ clitoral enlargement	Infrequent	Frequent

Data from Chokroverty S. Physiologic changes in sleep. In: Chokroverty S, editor. Sleep disorders medicine: basic science, technical considerations, and clinical aspects. Boston: Butterworth Heinemann; 1999. p. 95–126; and Catesby JW, Hirshkowitz, M. Assessment of sleep-related erections. In: Kryger MH, Roth T, Dement WC, editors. Principles and practice of sleep medicine. Philadelphia: Elsevier Saunders; 2005. p. 1394–402.

steadily declines from maximal levels in the young to almost nonexistent amounts in the elderly.[6,12,14] In addition to loss of SWS, sleep changes in the elderly include sleep fragmentation, increased percentage of stage 1 sleep, and decreased ability to maintain continuous sleep at night and wakefulness during the day. Contrary to commonly held beliefs, the need to sleep does not decrease with advancing age; what changes in the elderly is the ability to maintain sleep (**Fig. 1**).[12,14,15]

HOW MUCH SLEEP DOES ONE NEED?

One needs a sufficient amount of sleep to feel alert, refreshed, and avoid falling asleep unintendedly during the waking hours. Most young adults average between 7 and 8 hours of sleep nightly, but there is a significant individual and night-to-night variability in these figures. Genetics play a role in determining sleep length, and voluntary sleep reduction plays a significant role in determining how much sleep a person actually gets. Sleep restriction results in daytime sleepiness, and daytime sleepiness suggests that an individual's sleep needs have not been met.[6]

REGULATION OF SLEEP AND WAKEFULNESS
The Drives

Experimental studies in humans and animals led to the development of the two-process model, which accounts for regulation of sleep and wake time.

According to the model, sleep is regulated by 2 basic processes: a homeostatic process, which depends on the amount of prior sleep and wakefulness, and a circadian process, which is driven by an endogenous circadian pacemaker, generating near 24-hour cycles of behavior. An ultradian process within sleep is believed to control the alternation between REM and NREM sleep every 90 to 120 minutes. It is hypothesized that the interaction of homeostatic and circadian processes is responsible for helping humans to maintain wakefulness during the day and consolidated sleep at night (**Fig. 2**).

Homeostatic Regulation of Sleep

Virtually all organisms have an absolute need to sleep. Human beings cannot remain awake voluntarily for longer than 2 to 3 days, and rodents cannot survive without sleep for longer than a few weeks.[12,16] The homeostatic factor represents an increase in the need for sleep (sleep pressure) with increasing duration of prior wakefulness. The presence of homeostatic factor is best demonstrated through sleep-deprivation studies. When a normal amount of sleep is reduced the homeostatic drive is increased, leading to increased sleep pressure and sleepiness during the day as well as increased deep sleep at night. When normal sleep is preserved, the homeostatic factor represents a basic increase in sleep propensity during waking hours. The pull of this drive builds up during

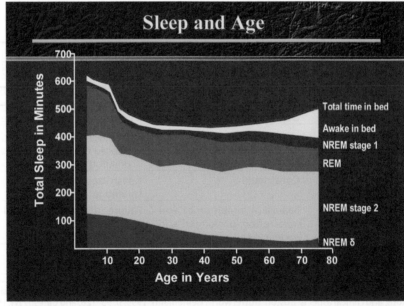

Fig. 1. Sleep and age. (*From* Williams RL, Karacan I, Hurrsch CJ. EEG of human sleep: clinical applications. New York: Wiley and Sons; 1974; with permission.)

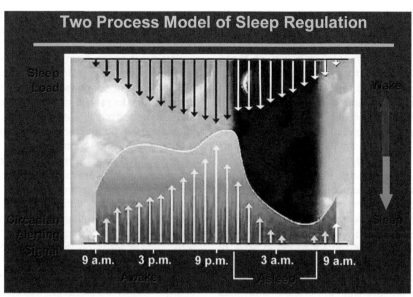

Fig. 2. Two-process model of sleep regulation. (*Data from* Edgar DM, Dement W, Fuller CA. Effect of SCN lesions on sleep in squirrel monkeys: evidence for opponent processes in sleep-wake regulation. J Neurosci 1993;13: 1065–79.)

wakefulness and reaches its peak at sleep time. Its strength declines during sleep, with the lowest point (nadir) on awakening in the morning.

It is also useful to differentiate sleepiness from tiredness or fatigue. A tired or fatigued individual does not necessarily have a propensity to fall asleep given an opportunity to do so. A sleepy individual is not only anergic but will fall asleep given the opportunity to do so.

Circadian Rhythms

Human beings have an endogenous circadian pacemaker with an intrinsic period of slightly longer than 24 hours.[17] Virtually all living organisms exhibit metabolic, physiologic, and behavioral circadian (ie, about 24-hour) rhythms. The most obvious circadian rhythm is the human sleep-wake cycle. Examples of other circadian rhythms include the release of cortisol, thyroid-stimulating hormone, and melatonin. Most mammalian tissues and organs contain mechanisms capable of expressing their function in accordance with the circadian rhythm. The "master biological clock," which regulates sleep-wake and all other circadian rhythms, resides in the suprachiasmatic nuclei (SCN) of the hypothalamus. SCN are bilaterally paired nuclei located slightly above the optic chiasm in the anterior hypothalamus.

Circadian clocks are normally synchronized to environmental cues (zeitgebers) by a process called entrainment. The process of entrainment

of SCN cells is mediated through glutamate stimulating the *N*-methyl-D-aspartate (NMDA) receptor.[18] Light hitting the retina activates the release of glutamate through the retinohypothalamic tract projecting to the SCN.[19] In most mammals and human beings, the light-dark cycle is the most potent entraining stimulus. The modulation of the SCN by both environmental cues and neurotransmitters/hormones is phase dependent. For example, when a patient is exposed to light at night it shifts the circadian clock back, whereas light exposure in the early morning shifts the clock forward. Melatonin is effective in shifting the circadian clock only when given at dawn or at dusk but not during the daytime hours. Cholinergic activation of the muscarinic receptors affects the circadian clock only at night.[20,21]

Circadian information from the SCN is transmitted to the rest of the body after input from the hypothalamus. Thus body-organ responses (eg, sleep-wake cycle, core body temperature, the release of cortisol, thyroid-stimulating hormone, and melatonin) to the circadian rhythm is controlled by the SCN and modulated by the hypothalamus. The release of melatonin from the pineal gland, signaled by the circadian rhythm, peaks at dawn and dusk. The SCN contains melatonin receptors, and the circadian clock can be reset by melatonin through a feedback mechanism.[17,20,22] In the absence of environmental cues (eg, under conditions of sensory deprivation), the endogenous rhythmicity of a circadian pacemaker persists independently of the light-dark cycle.[20,23] The genes of the SCN cells, through transcription/translation, are responsible for maintaining the 24-hour clock. Experimental mutation of these genes in animals produces prolonged or shortened circadian periods, whereas in humans such mutations result in abnormal circadian rhythms.[20] For example, polymorphisms in the PERIOD3 (PER3) gene have been linked to specific variations in the circadian rhythm. "Morning types" were more frequently homozygous for the PER35/5 (a genetic variant found in 10% of the population where the nucleotide coding sequence is repeated 5 times), and they were more susceptible to decline in executive function following sleep deprivation. Individuals homozygous for the PER34/4 (a genetic variant found in 50% of the population where the nucleotide coding sequence is repeated 4 times) were more likely to express an evening preference and less impacted by sleep deprivation.[24]

NEUROTRANSMITTERS INVOLVED IN SLEEP AND WAKEFULNESS

Adenosine, which has been identified as a possible mediator of the homeostatic sleep process, is an endogenous sleep-producing substance.[12,20,25–27] A breakdown product of adenosine triphosphate (ATP), adenosine is believed to be a homeostatic sleep factor that mediates the transition from prolonged wakefulness to NREM sleep. Adenosine mediates this transition by inhibiting arousal-promoting neurons of the basal forebrain. Caffeine is believed to promote wakefulness by blocking adenosine receptors. ATP is an important energy reserve in neurons. Adenosine accumulates in certain areas of the brain when neurons consume energy in the form of ATP during prolonged wakefulness. In animal studies, adenosine levels in the brain increased during sleep deprivation and returned to baseline during sleep.[16,28,29] Other substances hypothesized to be involved in promoting sleep and contributing to the homeostatic factor include proinflammatory cytokines (interleukin-1),[20,21] prostaglandin D_2, and growth hormone–releasing hormone.[30]

Cholinergic neurons have a dual role; some promote sleep and others promote wakefulness. The serotonergic, noradrenergic, and histaminergic wakefulness-promoting neurons have a discharge pattern nearly opposite to that of the cholinergic sleep-promoting neurons. The discharge rate of serotonergic, noradrenergic, and histaminergic neurons is fastest during wakefulness, decreases during NREM sleep, and virtually stops firing during REM sleep. In addition, newly discovered peptides called hypocretins (also known as orexins) are thought to regulate wakefulness by interacting with histaminergic, aminergic, and cholinergic systems (**Fig. 3**).

Acetylcholine

Cholinergic neurons that originate in the laterodorsal and pedunculopontine tegmental nuclei (LDT/PPT) of the midbrain reticular formation reach the cortex by ascending through the thalamus

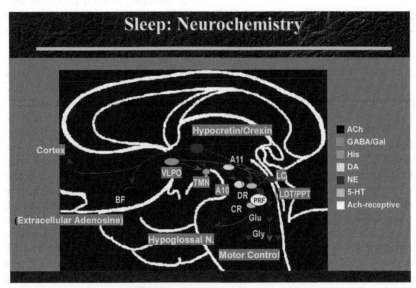

Fig. 3. Neurochemistry of sleep. BF, basal forebrain cholinergic nuclei; CR, caudal raphé; LDT/PPT, laterodorsal tegmental nuclei/pedunculopontine tegmental nuclei; PRF, pontine reticular formation; TMN, tuberomammillary nucleus; VLPO, ventrolateral preoptic nucleus. (*Courtesy of* E. Mignot, Stanford University.)

and hypothalamus. These midbrain LDT and PPT areas contain 2 interspersed subsets of cholinergic neurons. One subset is responsible for the fast-frequency and low-voltage EEG pattern of cortical activation that appears in both REM sleep and restful wakefulness. These neurons are called wake/REM-on neurons.[31] The second subset is responsible for generations of REM sleep. These latter cholinergic neurons are called REM-on cells. The 3 physiologic components of REM sleep (muscle atonia, rapid eye movements, EEG activation/desynchronization) are controlled by different nuclei located in the pontine reticular formation (PRF). The REM-on cholinergic neurons promote REM sleep by sending excitatory input to the PRF. This process causes the rapid firing of the PRF, which in turn produces the 3 cardinal physiologic components of REM sleep. The PRF is shut off during NREM sleep.

Cholinergic neurons that project from the basal forebrain to the cerebral cortex and limbic areas are part of the vigilance-waking system. The side effects produced by anticholinergic medications likely result from a disruption of both the vigilance-wake–producing cholinergic neurons and the wake/REM-on cholinergic neurons.

Serotonin and Norepinephrine

Serotonergic neurons originate in the dorsal raphé nucleus (DRN) and noradrenergic neurons originate in the locus coeruleus (LC). Both sets of neurons act as suppressants of REM sleep (REM-off cells) by inhibiting REM-promoting cholinergic neurons and by sending inhibitory input to the PRF. Serotonin and norepinephrine neurons promote cortical activation during wakefulness by rapid firing.[32] Recently, the noradrenergic wake-promoting system was also found to have an important role in the cognitive function of learning during the waking state. Activity of the noradrenergic system triggers an increase in the expression of genes associated with memory formation and learning.[20] The serotonergic system was not found to have this close link to cognitive function.

During the NREM sleep period, at the beginning of the first sleep cycle, the serotonergic and noradrenergic neurons significantly reduce their firing rate. This process removes the inhibition from the REM-on cholinergic neurons; leading to the first REM sleep period approximately 90 minutes later.

Hypocretin

Hypocretins (also called orexins) are 2 neuropeptides (hypocretin 1 and hypocretin 2) with key roles in regulation of arousal and metabolism. These compounds bind to their corresponding receptors

(Hcrtr1 and Hcrtr2) throughout the brain and spinal cord. Hypocretins are produced by hypothalamic neurons that surround the fornix bilaterally and exist in the dorsolateral hypothalamus. These hypothalamic regions are implicated in the control of nutritional balance, blood pressure, and temperature regulation, as well as endocrine secretion and arousal. Hypocretins likely play a role in all these functions.[33]

The hypocretin-producing neurons in the hypothalamus receive direct input from the SCN (the circadian rhythm clock) and project to the posterior hypothalamus (TMN-histamine), basal forebrain (cholinergic vigilance-wake area), thalamus, LC, DRN (noradrenergic and serotonergic REM-off cells), LDT, and PRF (cholinergic REM-on cells and muscle atonia).[33,34] In accordance with circadian rhythmic control of hypocretin levels (through SCN input), their concentration is highest during the waking period. Hypocretin levels also increase during a period of forced sleep deprivation. It remains unclear whether this increase during sleep deprivation represents hypocretin actually opposing and attempting to override the sleep drive or producing a stress response to sleep deprivation. Hypocretin input to the brainstem REM-on cells controls the switch into REM by reducing the firing rate of the REM-on cells during the wake period.[33]

Histamine

Antihistaminergic drugs that cross the blood-brain barrier are known to produce sedation. The neurotransmitter histamine plays a key role in the maintenance of wakefulness. Histaminergic neurons originate from the tuberomammillary nucleus (TMN) of the posterior hypothalamus, and project diffusely throughout the brain. In the cortex, histamine facilitates cortical arousal. Histaminergic neurons fire most rapidly during cortical activation in the wake state and turn off during REM sleep.[32,35]

Hypothalamus

The role of the hypothalamus as a key area of the brain involved in the regulation of sleep and wakefulness was recognized after the pandemic of encephalitis lethargica swept the world in the early 1900s. Thought to be a viral infection of the brain, encephalitis lethargica induced severe sleep abnormalities in affected individuals. Most patients exhibited profound and prolonged sleepiness while some suffered from a severe insomnia. Those afflicted by sleepiness were discovered to have lesions in the posterior hypothalamus; those afflicted by insomnia were found to have lesions in the anterior hypothalamus.[26,36]

Since this clinical observation more than 70 years ago, several human and animal studies have further elucidated the role of the hypothalamus in the regulation of sleep. In accordance with these original observations, the ventrolateral preoptic nucleus (VLPO) in the anterior hypothalamus has been established as the key sleep-inducing region, with the TMN of the posterior hypothalamus being one of the important wakefulness-promoting regions of the brain.

The anterior hypothalamus contains GABAergic cells. Activity of GABAergic cells in the VLPO region is implicated in production of NREM sleep while the GABAergic cells in the area adjacent to the VLPO is thought to promote REM sleep by inhibiting the noradrenergic (LC) and serotonergic (DRN) REM-off nuclei of the brainstem.[26] The rapid firing of the anterior hypothalamus region during sleep leads to inhibition of the LC and DRN in the brainstem, in effect taking the "noradrenergic and serotonergic brakes" off the hypothalamic sleep generator, thus reinforcing the sleep state.[36]

The posterior hypothalamus/TMN receives histaminergic input and has hypocretin receptors (hctr2). Both histamine and hypocretin produce activation of the TMN cells, which leads to sustained wakefulness.[26] At the same time, hypocretin activates the noradrenergic and serotonergic cells in the brainstem, which send inhibitory signals to the anterior hypothalamus. This process in effect takes the "GABAergic brakes" off the hypothalamic wakefulness generator, thus reinforcing the wake state.

From the viewpoint of evolutionary advantage, it may be important for most animals to be either in the fully awake or the fully asleep state and to spend little time in the transition state between sleep and wakefulness. The anterior and posterior regions of the hypothalamus work through a system of mutual inhibition in what has been referred to as a flip-flop switch (like a light switch).[36] The hypothalamic sleep switch is quickly turned on and off, with both positions being equally stable. It is hypothesized that the circadian, homeostatic, and ultradian drives are responsible for flipping the hypothalamic switch into the sleep and wake positions. The hypocretin tone, which is also influenced by the circadian and homeostatic drives, helps to stabilize the hypothalamic switch in the wake position and prevent intrusion of REM sleep into the waking state.[26,36] When the hypocretin tone is reduced, as in narcolepsy, this stability of the wake state is impaired, resulting in abnormal shifts from wake to REM states (eg, cataplexy, sleep paralysis).

PHARMACEUTICALS AND RECREATIONAL DRUGS

All drugs that cross the blood-brain barrier may affect sleep. Selective serotonin reuptake inhibitors, tricyclic antidepressants, serotonin norepinephrine reuptake inhibitors, and monoamine oxidase inhibitors suppress REM sleep; acute withdrawal from these antidepressants is likely to produce a rebound increase in REM sleep. Barbiturates increase SWS and suppress REM. Benzodiazepines suppress SWS and do not affect REM. Psychostimulants, such as amphetamine and cocaine, increase sleep latency, fragment sleep, and suppress REM sleep.[6,12,14]

SLEEPING AND DREAMING

Several theories attempt to explain the biological function of sleep, none of which is preeminent. One such theory posits that sleep serves a restorative function for the brain and body. Normal sleep is subjectively associated with feeling refreshed on awakening. REM sleep is associated with increased CNS synthesis of proteins and is critical for the CNS development of infants/young humans/animals. Growth-hormone secretion is increased while cortisol secretion is decreased during sleep. All of these facts can be used to support the restorative theory of sleep.[37] Another theory of sleep function proposes that sleep has a central role in reinforcement and consolidation of memory. Sleep-deprivation experiments have highlighted the important role of REM sleep in memory function.[37] Yet another theory suggests that sleep is important for thermoregulatory function. Experiments have demonstrated that total sleep deprivation results in thermoregulatory abnormalities, NREM sleep maintains thermoregulatory function, and REM sleep is associated with impaired thermoregulatory responses (shivering, sweating, and so forth).[37]

Since the mid-1950s, when REM sleep was identified, sleep research has focused on understanding the physiology of dreams. Most dreams (about 80%) occur during REM sleep; the remainder occurs during NREM sleep. REM sleep dreams are more complex, have more emotional valence, can be bizarre, and are easier to recall. NREM sleep dreams are more logical and realistic, but more difficult to recall possibly because awakening from NREM sleep leaves a person feeling more confused and disoriented than awakening from REM sleep. During REM sleep, neuronal signals originating from the brainstem are transmitted to the cerebral hemispheres, and stimulate the cortical association areas to produce images that comprise our dreams.

SUMMARY

Sleep is a vital, highly organized process regulated by complex systems of neuronal networks and neurotransmitters. Sleep plays an important role in the regulation of CNS and body physiologic functions. Sleep architecture changes with age and is easily susceptible to external and internal disruption. Reduction or disruption of sleep can affect numerous functions varying from thermoregulation to learning and memory during the waking state.

REFERENCES

1. Sinton CM, McCarley RW. Neurophysiological mechanisms of sleep and wakefulness: a question of balance. Semin Neurol 2004;24(3):211–23.
2. Iber C, Anvoli-Israel S, Chesson AL. The AASM manual for the scoring of sleep and associated events: The American Academy of Sleep Medicine. Weschester: IL; 2007.
3. Doghramji K. The evaluation and management of sleep disorders. In: Stoudemire A, editor. Clinical psychiatry for medical students. Philadelphia: J.B. Lippincott Company; 1998. p. 783–818.
4. Siegel JM. REM sleep. In: Kryger MH, Roth T, Dement WC, editors. Principles and practice of sleep medicine. Philadelphia: Elsevier Saunders; 2005. p. 120–35.
5. Catesby JW, Hirshkowitz M. Assessment of sleep-related erections. In: Kryger MH, Roth T, Dement WC, editors. Principles and practice of sleep medicine. Philadelphia: Saunders; 2005. p. 1394–402.
6. Carskadon MA, Dement WC. Normal human sleep: an overview. In: Kryger MH, Roth T, Dement WC, editors. Principles and practice of sleep medicine. Philadelphia: Elsevier Saunders; 2005. p. 13–23.
7. Markov D, Jaffe F, Doghramji K. Update on parasomnias: a review for psychiatric practice. Psychiatry 2006;3(7):69–76.
8. Carskadon MA, Rechtschaffen A. Monitoring and staging human sleep. In: Kryger MH, Roth T, Dement WC, editors. Principles and practice of sleep medicine. Philadelphia: Elsevier Saunders; 2005. p. 1359–77.
9. Chokroverty S. An overview of sleep. In: Chokroverty S, editor. Sleep disorders medicine: basic science, technical considerations, and clinical aspects. Boston: Butterworth Heinemann; 1999. p. 7–20.
10. Walczak T, Chokroverty S. Electroencephalography, electromyography, and electro-oculography: general principles and basic technology. In: Chokroverty S, editor. Sleep disorders medicine: basic science, technical considerations, and clinical aspects. Boston: Butterworth Heinemann; 1999. p. 175–203.
11. Chokroverty S. Physiologic changes in sleep. In: Chokroverty S, editor. Sleep disorders medicine: basic science, technical considerations, and clinical aspects. Boston: Butterworth Heinemann; 1999. p. 95–126.
12. Roth T, Roehrs T. Sleep organization and regulation. Neurology 2000;54(5 Suppl 1):S2–7.
13. Parmeggiani PL. Physiology in sleep. In: Kryger MH, Roth T, Dement WC, editors. Principles and practice of sleep medicine. Philadelphia: Elsevier Saunders; 2005. p. 185–91.
14. Roth T. Characteristics and determinants of normal sleep. J Clin Psychiatry 2004;65(Suppl 16):8–11.
15. Bliwise DL. Normal aging. In: Kryger MH, Roth T, Dement WC, editors. Principles and practice of sleep medicine. Philadelphia: Elsevier Saunders; 2005. p. 24–38.
16. Porkka-Heiskanen T, Strecker RE, Thakkar M, et al. Adenosine: a mediator of the sleep-inducing effects of prolonged wakefulness. Science 1997;276(5316): 1265–8.
17. Czeisler CA, Duffy JF, Shanahan TL, et al. Stability, precision, and near-24-hour period of the human circadian pacemaker. Science 1999;284(5423): 2177–81.
18. Hattar S, Liao HW, Takao M, et al. Melanopsin-containing retinal ganglion cells: architecture, projections, and intrinsic photosensitivity. Science 2002; 295(5557):1065–70.
19. Berson DM, Dunn FA, Takao M. Phototransduction by retinal ganglion cells that set the circadian clock. Science 2002;295(5557):1070–3.
20. Pace-Schott EF, Hobson JA. The neurobiology of sleep: genetics, cellular physiology and subcortical networks. Nat Rev Neurosci 2002;3(8):591–605.
21. Brzezinski A. Melatonin in humans. N Engl J Med 1997;336(3):186–95.
22. Reiter RJ. Melatonin: clinical relevance. Best Pract Res Clin Endocrinol Metab 2003;17(2):273–85.
23. Reppert SM, Weaver DR. Molecular analysis of mammalian circadian rhythms. Annu Rev Physiol 2001;63:647–76.
24. Dijk D-J, Archer SN. PERIOD3, circadian phenotypes, and sleep homeostasis. Sleep Medicine Reviews 2010;14:151–60.
25. Borbely AA, Achermann P. Sleep homeostasis and models of sleep regulation. J Biol Rhythms 1999; 14(6):557–68.
26. Mignot E, Taheri S, Nishino S. Sleeping with the hypothalamus: emerging therapeutic targets for sleep disorders. Nat Neurosci 2002;5(Suppl):1071–5.
27. Borbely AA, Achermann P. Sleep homeostasis and models of sleep regulation. In: Kryger MH, Roth T,

Dement WC, editors. Principles and practice of sleep medicine. Philadelphia: Elsevier Saunders; 2005. p. 405–17.

28. Boutrel B, Koob GF. What keeps us awake: the neuropharmacology of stimulants and wakefulness-promoting medications. Sleep 2004;27(6):1181–94.

29. Porkka-Heiskanen T, Alanko L, Kalinchuk A, et al. Adenosine and sleep. Sleep Med Rev 2002;6(4): 321–32.

30. McGinty D, Szymusiak R. Sleep-promoting mechanisms in mammals. In: Kryger MH, Roth T, Dement WC, editors. Principles and practice of sleep medicine. Philadelphia: Elsevier Saunders; 2005. p. 169–84.

31. McCarley RW. Sleep neurophysiology: basic mechanisms underlying control of wakefulness and sleep. In: Chokroverty S, editor. Sleep disorders medicine: basic science, technical considerations, and clinical aspects. Boston: Butterworth Heinemann; 1999. p. 21–50.

32. Jones BE. Basic mechanisms of sleep-wake states. In: Kryger MH, Roth T, Dement WC, editors. Principles and practice of sleep medicine. Philadelphia: Elsevier Saunders; 2005. p. 136–53.

33. Sutcliffe JG, de Lecea L. The hypocretins: setting the arousal threshold. Nat Rev Neurosci 2002;3(5): 339–49.

34. Peyron C, Tighe DK, van den Pol AN, et al. Neurons containing hypocretin (orexin) project to multiple neuronal systems. J Neurosci 1998;18(23): 9996–10015.

35. Siegel JM. The neurotransmitters of sleep. J Clin Psychiatry 2004;65(Suppl 16):4–7.

36. Saper CB, Chou TC, Scammell TE. The sleep switch: hypothalamic control of sleep and wakefulness. Trends Neurosci 2001;24(12):726–31.

37. Chokroverty S. An overview of normal sleep. In: Chokroverty S, Wayne AH, Walters AS, editors. Sleep and movement disorders. Philadelphia: Butterworth Heinemann; 2003. p. 23–43.

Biological Timekeeping

Martha U. Gillette, PhD[a,b,*], Sabra M. Abbott, MD, PhD[b,c,d],
Jennifer M. Arnold[b]

KEYWORDS

- Biological rhythms • Sleep • Circadian • Suprachiasmatic nucleus

KEY POINTS

- Circadian rhythms are regulated by the suprachiasmatic nucleus in the hypothalamus, which receives input about environmental light, sleep-wake state, and activity status. These stimuli also provide output signals to regulate the timing of rest/activity and behavioral cycles.
- Clock gene proteins are now being used as molecular tools to further study clocks in all tissues, and how the suprachiasmatic nucleus synchronizes and aligns these various body clocks to environmental cycles and imposed work schedules.
- Circadian rhythm sleep disorders as well as sleep phenotypes are correlated with abnormalities in the genes regulating circadian rhythms.

The daily transitions between light and darkness have significantly shaped the evolution of most living species, from unicellular organisms to mammals. Superimposed on the daily light-dark cycle is a seasonal influence that changes the relative durations of day and night over the course of a year. Be they day-active or night-active, all organisms organize their behaviors in the 24-hour world, adapting to the availability of food and changing temperature, rearing their young, and avoiding predators. To optimize survival, they must be able to anticipate environmental transitions and to adjust to changes in night length or transition times that may occur.

Adaptation to these needs occurred through the emergence of a circadian system capable of aligning behavioral, physiologic, and metabolic processes with this light-dark cycle. The circadian system organizes body systems so that they occur in 24-hour rhythms. Rather than simply reflecting the external day-night cycle, these rhythms in behaviors persist in the absence of exogenous timing cues, such as light, food availability, or social cues. Every organism expresses an endogenous rhythm that varies slightly from 24 hours, making it circadian, or "about a day." Uninterrupted, this circadian rhythm persists.

These circadian rhythms can be observed in outputs, such as the patterning of the sleep-wake cycle. In humans, core body temperature is often used as a marker of circadian phase. In addition, numerous endogenous hormones oscillate with a predictable phase relationship to day and night (reviewed by Van Cauter[1]). Hormonal rhythms show complex waveforms as a result of combined effects of the circadian pacemaker, organismic

A version of this article originally appeared in *Sleep Medicine Clinics Volume 4, Issue 2*.
This work was supported by the following past and present grants from the National Institutes of Health: HL67007, HL086870, HL092571Z ARRA, NS22155, and NS35859 (MUG), F30 NS047802 and GM07143 (SMA), and GM007283 (JMA).
[a] Department of Cell & Developmental Biology and the Neuroscience Program, University of Illinois at Urbana-Champaign, 601 South Goodwin Avenue, Urbana, IL 61801, USA; [b] Department of Molecular and Integrative Physiology and the College of Medicine, 407 S. Goodwin Avenue, University of Illinois at Urbana-Champaign, Urbana, IL 61801, USA; [c] Harvard Medical School, 25 Shattuck Street, Boston, MA 02115, USA; [d] Massachusetts General Hospital, 55 Fruit Street, Boston, MA 02114, USA
* Corresponding author. Department of Cell & Developmental Biology and the Neuroscience Program, University of Illinois at Urbana-Champaign, 601 South Goodwin Avenue, Urbana, IL 61801.
E-mail address: mgillett@life.illinois.edu

state, such as activity level, sleep, and feeding, and the pulsatile nature of secretion. Nevertheless, clear diurnal patterns of secretion have been reported.[2] Plasma melatonin,[3,4] growth hormone,[5] prolactin,[6] thyrotropin-releasing hormone,[7] luteinizing hormone,[8] and leptin[9–11] are all increased during the night, in antiphase to adrenocorticotropic hormone and cortisol.[12,13] These oscillations in hormone secretion continue in a constant environment, and, therefore, are clock-regulated. Circadian rhythmicity seems to be present at virtually every level of function studied. Maintenance of a constant *milieu intérieur* may be a consequence of a balance among rhythmic, mutually opposed control mechanisms.[2]

This review explains the neurobiology of circadian timekeeping, describing what is known about the master pacemaker for circadian rhythmicity, how various biologic systems can provide input to the endogenous biologic timing, and how the pacemaker can, in turn, influence the physiology and behavior of the individual. We discuss how the circadian system can adapt to a changing environment by resetting the circadian clock in the face of a variety of inputs, including changes in light, activity and the sleep-wake cycle. We then discuss the genetics of circadian timekeeping, highlighting what is currently known about heritable disorders in circadian timing and how circadian genetics have been used to study timekeeping. The role of the clock in peripheral tissues is also discussed.

THE CIRCADIAN CLOCK

In mammals, circadian rhythms are regulated by a paired set of nuclei located at the base of the hypothalamus, directly above the optic chiasm, hence their name: the suprachiasmatic nuclei (SCN) (**Fig. 1**). Multiple experiments have shown the role of the SCN as a central pacemaker for circadian rhythms. Lesioning studies found that damage to the SCN disrupts rhythmicity in corticosterone levels, drinking, and wheel-running behavior.[14,15] This finding provided the initial evidence that the central pacemaker for the mammalian clock lay within the SCN.

In later work, it was found that transplanting fetal SCN tissue into the third ventricle of animals in which the SCN had been lesioned could restore rhythmicity.[16] Furthermore, if fetal SCN tissue from a wild-type hamster was implanted into the third ventricle of a hamster with a genetic alteration that shortened free-running period, the new free-running period resembled that of the SCN donor rather than the host animal. This evidence suggested that not only was the SCN

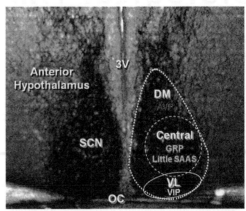

Fig. 1. Anatomy of the mammalian SCN. This medial, transverse section of the rat anterior hypothalamus shows the bilateral SCN stained darkly with an antibody to an endogenous peptide. The paired SCN are at the base of the brain, flanking the third ventricle (3V) and positioned directly above the optic chiasm (OC). The major subdivisions of the SCN are delineated. The dorsomedial SCN (DM) is marked by neurons expressing arginine vasopressin (AVP), whereas neurons of the ventrolateral SCN (VL) express vasoactive intestinal peptide (VIP). A central region contains neurons that express gastrin-releasing peptide (GRP) and little SAAS.

necessary for generating rhythms but also the period of this rhythmicity was an intrinsic property of the SCN cells, and the presence of SCN was sufficient to drive the rhythms for the entire animal.[17]

In the mouse, each SCN measures approximately 300 μm medial to lateral, 350 μm dorsal to ventral, and spans approximately 600 μm from rostral to caudal end. One SCN contains a total of approximately 10,500 cells.[18] The rodent SCN has several peptidergic subregions (see **Fig. 1**). The central region of the SCN contains small neurons that show positive staining for gastrin-releasing peptide (GRP) colocalized with γ-amino butyric acid (GABA), and the newly discovered peptide, little SAAS.[18–21] The ventrolateral region of the SCN contains neurons that stain predominately for vasoactive intestinal peptide (VIP), but a population of calretinin cells is also seen here. The dorsomedial region of the SCN contains larger neurons that contain arginine vasopressin (AVP), met-enkephalin, and angiotensin II.[18,20,21] There are topographic connections between all regions of the nucleus, as well as communication between the 2 nuclei of the animal.[22]

The human SCN is not as compact as the rodent, but has a similar peptidergic organization. The dorsal and medial regions contain neurophysin/vasopressin neurons. The central region contains calbindin, synaptophysin, and VIP neurons, whereas the ventral and rostral regions contain synaptophysin, calbindin, and substance P.[23]

Inputs

In conjunction with its ability to regulate circadian timing, the SCN is also positioned to receive information about environmental and behavioral states of the animal to ensure proper alignment of the circadian clock. This information is conveyed to the SCN by projections from a variety of different brain regions.

One of the most extensively studied inputs to the SCN comes from a subpopulation of retinal ganglion cells, the central projections of which form the retinohypothalamic tract (RHT). Lesions of the SCN disrupt the development of these neurons,[24] and disruption of the RHT results in an inability to respond to resetting light signals.[25,26] The class of retinal ganglion cells that comprise the RHT contain a blue-light photopigment, melanopsin.[27] These melanopsin-containing cells are photosensitive at the same wavelengths that are most effective for circadian resetting.[28] In addition, the terminals of the melanopsin-positive retinal ganglion cells colocalize glutamate (GLU) and pituitary adenylate cyclase-activating polypeptide (PACAP),[29] the neurotransmitters of the RHT.[30,31]

The RHT also sends projections to the thalamic intergeniculate leaflet (IGL), which, in turn, sends projections back to the SCN through the geniculohypothalamic tract (GHT). The GHT contains neuropeptide Y (NPY) and GABA. NPY is believed to be involved in activity-induced phase shifts during the daytime in nocturnal animals but also seems to be able to modulate light-induced phase shifts.[32-34] However, although the GHT pathway can transmit photic signals, disruption of this pathway does not prevent entrainment.[35]

The SCN also receives serotonergic input, primarily from the median raphe, which is primarily involved in activity-induced phase shifts during the daytime. Activation of the median raphe results in an increase in serotonin (5-HT) release at the SCN.[36-38] 5-HT release also shows a strong circadian release pattern in the SCN, with 5-HT release peaking at CT 14, and 5-hydroxyindole acetic acid, the major metabolite of 5-HT, peaking at CT 16.[39]

Cholinergic projections to the SCN originate both in the brainstem and basal forebrain in brain nuclei with identified roles in sleep and arousal[40] and were recently shown to also be present in diurnal animals.[41] Within the brainstem, these cholinergic projections arise from 3 nuclei. The parabigeminal nucleus is considered a satellite region of the superior colliculus, which seems to play a role in generating target-location information as part of saccadic eye movements.[42] The laterodorsal tegmental (LDTg) and pedunculopontine tegmental (PPTg) nuclei are both important for regulating the sleep-wake cycle.[43] In the basal forebrain, the substantia innominata within the nucleus basalis magnocellularis (NBM) in the basal forebrain contributes to arousal and focused attention.[44] The LDTg, PPTg, and NBM are interconnected, and all play roles in regulating the sleep and arousal states of the animal. This finding suggests that the cholinergic input to the SCN is providing a signal regarding the sleep and arousal states of the animal, and may provide a link between the sleep-wake cycle and circadian rhythms.

Additional sleep-wake input to the SCN may come from the tuberomammillary nucleus (TMN). Studies have shown histaminergic input to the SCN from the TMN.[45] Histamine is a regulator of the sleep-wake cycle, primarily providing a signal of wakefulness.

Outputs

The SCN exerts its influence on the body primarily at the level of the hypothalamus. Neurons from the ventral regions of the SCN project to the lateral region of the hypothalamic subparaventricular zone (sPVHz), the perisuprachiasmatic area, and the ventral tuberal area. The dorsal region of the SCN projects to the medial preoptic area (MPOA), medial sPVHz, dorsal parvocellular paraventricular nucleus (dPVN), and the dorsal medial hypothalamus (DMH), also all within the hypothalamus.[46] The targets of efferents to the dPVN consist of endocrine neurons, autonomic neurons, or intermediate neurons, which potentially serve to integrate several hypothalamic signals.[47]

Many SCN projection sites are regulators of sleep and arousal. The DMH projections are especially interesting, because many of these neurons seem to project to neurons containing hypocretin/orexin, a peptide well known for its role in arousal.[48,49] In addition, evidence exists for a multisynaptic pathway between the SCN and locus coeruleus, an important arousal center in the brain, mediated by orexin,[50] with the DMH as a relay.[51] A minor set of SCN efferents project to the ventrolateral preoptic nucleus, a region that, if lesioned, produces prolonged reduction in sleep duration and amplitude.[52] The SCN projects to the paraventricular nucleus (PVN) and IGL of the thalamus.

Both nuclei project back to the SCN. The PVN loop is proposed to provide assessment of sleep/arousal states and SCN modulation, whereas the IGL loop is believed to provide the SCN with information from higher, integrative visual centers.[53–55] The PVN seems to act as a relay between the SCN and the amygdala, which may provide a link between the circadian system and affective disorders.[56] Overall, the SCN seems to be uniquely situated within a network that allows it to interact closely with the regions controlling sleep and arousal states.

CIRCADIAN RESETTING

Despite the circuit-based organization of neural function, there is a consensus that timekeeping is a cellular process.[57] Indeed, the expression of independently phased circadian firing rhythms from individual neurons dissociated from neonatal rat SCN cultured on an electrode array provides compelling evidence for the cellular nature of this clock.[58] It follows that gating of sensitivity to resetting stimuli and phase resetting must be cellular properties. Moreover, the clock must be able to restrict the range of responses in the cellular repertoire so that activation of select signaling pathways can occur only at the appropriate time in the circadian cycle.[59] We have endeavored to determine how the clock temporally regulates the responsiveness of specific signaling pathways.

In an attempt to define and understand the underlying control mechanisms subserving clock-gated windows of sensitivity, SCN-bearing brain slices are exposed in vitro to treatments that activate elements of specific signaling pathways. Treatments are administered at various discrete points in the circadian cycle, and effects on the time-of-peak in the spontaneous rhythm of neuronal activity assessed over the next 1 or 2 circadian cycles in vitro. If the time-of-peak appears earlier during cycle(s) after treatment compared with controls, the phase of the rhythm is advanced. If the time-of-peak appears later than in controls, then the phase is delayed by the treatment. By assessing the changing relationship between the circadian time of treatment and its effect on phase, a phase-response curve can be generated. This relationship graphically presents the temporal pattern of SCN sensitivity to activation of specific signaling pathways and defines the window of sensitivity to phase resetting via this pathway. The permanence of the phase shift is examined by evaluating the time of the peak in neuronal activity over 1 or 2 days after a treatment. Timing of the peak after experimental reagents are

administered at the maximal point of sensitivity is compared with the time of the peak in media-treated controls.

Temporal spheres identified as sensitive to phase resetting via specific first and second messenger pathways coincide with discrete portions of the circadian cycle. In terms of these temporal restrictions, the circadian cycle can be divided into several discrete temporal states, or domains, of the clock: day, night, dusk, and dawn.[59,60] These studies not only contribute to defining the properties of the temporal domains of the clock, they emphasize the complexity of control that the clock exerts over signal integration and phase resetting within the SCN. These properties have been incorporated into putative clock-gated regulatory pathways. Each is discussed in the context of the clock domain that is regulated.

Subjective day and night are distinct with respect to their sensitivities and response characteristics. Furthermore, each correlates with discrete periods of sensitivity to specific neurotransmitter systems that are shown to impinge on this hypothalamic site, as shown by a large body of neuroanatomic studies.[61] This finding permits speculation regarding the nature of pathways that gain access to and regulate the biologic clock at different points in the circadian cycle. The major identified domains of clock sensitivity are now considered in turn.

Circadian Clock Regulators

Daytime
Several signaling molecules seem to be important in resetting circadian rhythms during the daytime, including 5-HT, PACAP, NPY, and GABA (**Fig. 2**). Most of these experiments have been performed in nocturnal rodents, so daytime is defined as the time during which the lights are on or the animal is inactive. As a result, the functional context of this regulation seems to be tied to arousal-induced resetting, often referred to as nonphotic resetting.[62,63] Nonphotic signals cover a wide variety of phenomena, including sleep deprivation, activity associated with exposure to a novel wheel, or even cage changes. The unifying factor in nonphotic signals is that they involve arousal during a time when the animal would normally be inactive.

5-HT is believed to play a role in nonphotic, activity-induced phase shifts during the day. Increasing 5-HT in the SCN during subjective day induces an advance in peak electrical firing rate in vitro or onset of wheel-running in vivo.[36,64] In vivo, 5-HT levels in the SCN are increased by electrical stimulation of the dorsal or median raphe.[36,65] Forced wheel-running or sleep deprivation during

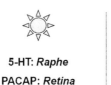 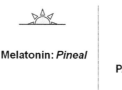

5-HT: *Raphe*	Melatonin: *Pineal*	Glutamate, PACAP: *Retina*
PACAP: *Retina*		ACh: *Brain stem (PBg, LDTg, PPTg) Basal forebrain (NBM)*
NPY, GABA: *Thalamic Intergeniculate Leaflet*		

Fig. 2. Circadian organization of temporal windows of SCN sensitivity to phase-resetting signals transmitted from various brain sites. Time-of-day–specific signals are presented together with the major sources of SCN innervation by projections bearing these neurotransmitters and neuropeptides. Daytime is marked by sensitivity to 5-HT, pituitary adenylate cyclase-activating peptide (PACAP), NPY, and GABA. During dusk and dawn, the pineal hormone melatonin can stimulate resetting of the SCN clock. At night, the SCN is sensitive to phase adjustment by GLU and PACAP from the eye, as well as by cholinergic inputs from brain regions that regulate sleep and wakefulness.

the day also increases 5-HT in the SCN,[66,67] which suggests a role for 5-HT in nonphotic phase-shifting. However, depleting 5-HT from raphe projections does not prevent this nonphotic daytime shift,[68] and serotonergic antagonists are not able to attenuate this phase shift,[69] providing mixed evidence for the role of 5-HT. This finding suggests modulation by additional messengers, possibly neuropeptides.

A second daytime modulator of the SCN clock is the peptide, PACAP. PACAP is not intrinsic to the SCN, but instead is released from the RHT, where it colocalizes with GLU.[70] Levels of PACAP have been found to oscillate throughout the day in SCN samples, which include synaptic terminals of the RHT, but not in other brain regions.[71] If PACAP is applied to the SCN brain slice in micromolar quantities, it elicits an advance in peak neuronal firing during the day, but has little effect during night.[29] However, in vivo findings conflict with this finding, because the long-term effect of PACAP injection into the SCN seems to be a delay in onset of wheel-running.[72] These conflicting data suggest that further study of the effects of PACAP on the clock during the day are warranted.

A third daytime regulator of the clock, NPY, also seems to play a dual role in the SCN, resetting the circadian clock both during the daytime and at night. NPY is released from the GHT, the projection from the IGL to the SCN. When NPY was applied during the daytime either to an SCN brain slice in vitro[32] or directly to the SCN in vivo,[73,74] it induced a phase advance. Additional in vivo studies stimulated the IGL, presumably inducing the release of NPY at the SCN. These stimulations also produced advances in wheel-running behavior during the daytime.[75] Exposing an animal to light[76] or applying GLU to the brain slice[77] are both capable of blocking the response to daytime

application of NPY. The addition of the GABA$_A$ antagonist, bicuculline, is also capable of inhibiting the effects of NPY,[78] suggesting that the effects of NPY are linked to GABAergic signaling.

One factor that daytime signaling pathways have in common is that they all may be mediated by cyclic adenosine monophosphate (cAMP). In the hypothalamic brain slice, cAMP or cAMP analogues applied during the daytime induce phase advances in the circadian clock, whereas at night they have little effect.[79,80] In addition, endogenous cAMP is high during late day and late night,[81] suggesting a role for cAMP in the transition periods between day and night. It can be hypothesized that by increasing cAMP, these daytime resetting signals are moving the animal to a state that resembles late day, thus resetting the clock.

Dawn and dusk
The primary resetting signal associated with dawn and dusk is melatonin (see **Fig. 2**). This hormone of darkness is produced at night in the absence of light, providing a means by which the animal can measure night length. Photoperiod is an important measure for animals, such as hamsters and sheep, which are seasonally reproductive. Melatonin is produced by the pineal gland, and in lower vertebrates, such as fish, lizards, and some birds, the pineal is the primary regulator of circadian rhythms, rather than the SCN. However, in mammals, this timekeeping mechanism has moved to the SCN, as shown by the fact that removal of the pineal does not significantly disrupt circadian rhythms of rats.[82]

Although the pineal is not necessary for maintenance of mammalian circadian rhythms, it is possible to entrain free-running rats with daily injections of melatonin. Entrainment seems to work best if the melatonin injections are timed to occur shortly before the onset of the animal's active period. This entrainment seems to work through the SCN, because lesioning the SCN, but not the pineal, abolishes the ability of a rat to entrain to melatonin injections.[83]

Evidence that melatonin can entrain circadian rhythms led to several studies looking at the direct effect of melatonin on the SCN. Melatonin application immediately before dusk in rat or hamster tissue in vitro decreases SCN activity, measured by 2-deoxy-[1-^{14}C]glucose uptake or neuronal firing rate.[84–86] In addition, melatonin applied to SCN brain slices at either dawn or dusk advances the peak in neuronal firing. Melatonin is ineffective when applied at other times of day.[87,88] This resetting pattern is reproduced by direct activation of protein kinase C (PKC), and can be blocked by inhibitors of PKC, suggesting that PKC is a downstream component of this resetting pathway.[88] In addition, melatonergic resetting is inhibited with antagonists specific for the MT-2 type melatonin receptor.[89] In humans, circadian sensitivity to melatonin also occurs at dawn and dusk, but the effect is to advance the circadian system at dusk and to delay it at dawn, opposite to the effects of light at night.

Nighttime

In the nighttime domain, there are 2 known key players, GLU and acetylcholine (ACh), as well as several modulatory substances associated with these signals (see **Fig. 2**). As discussed earlier, considerable evidence supports GLU as the neurochemical signal transmitting photic stimuli from the retina to the SCN, but the functional context of the cholinergic resetting signal is still unknown.

The GLU signaling pathway is similar to many of the pathways that have already been discussed in that it resets the circadian clock at a discrete time of day and in a specific direction. The GLU signaling pathway can either advance or delay the clock, depending on what time of day the signal is presented.[30,90] The GLU resetting pathway has been shown both in vitro and in vivo to be mediated through an N-methyl-D-aspartate (NMDA) receptor-mediated increase in intracellular calcium, followed by nitric oxide (NO) synthase induction and resultant production of NO.[30,91–94] Beyond this point, the early and late night pathways diverge. During the early night, GLU induces delays in the circadian clock through ryanodine receptor-mediated calcium release.[95] However, GLU exposure during the late night advances the circadian clock through a cyclic guanosine monophosphate/protein kinase G signaling cascade followed by cAMP response element-binding protein-activated transcription.[95–97]

Although GLU alone is capable of resetting circadian rhythms, there are many substances that modulate this resetting. These substances can be divided into 2 categories: those that decrease the amplitude of the phase-resetting effect of GLU during both the early and the late night, which include NPY and GABA,[33,64] and those that have differing effects on GLU-induced phase shifts, depending on what time of night they are applied.

This second category of time-dependent modulators include 5-HT and PACAP. If animals are depleted of 5-HT, they show increased phase delays in response to light.[98,99] However, coapplication of a PACAP antagonist, either in vitro or in vivo, decreases the phase delay seen with application in early night, and when applied during late night, increases the amplitude of the phase advance in both rat and hamster.[100,101] When PACAP is administered in conjunction with GLU in early night, it increases the delays, but in late night it decreases phase advances. This finding is similar to the effects seen after application of cAMP analogues to the hypothalamic brain slice, suggesting that the effects of PACAP may be mediated via a cAMP pathway.[102]

The role of ACh in resetting circadian rhythms has been unclear, with much of the confusion arising from the fact that its effects vary depending on the site of application. The first evidence that ACh might play a role in resetting the circadian clock came in 1979, when Zatz and Brownstein[103] examined whether pharmacologic manipulation of the SCN could affect circadian rhythms. Injections of the ACh agonist carbachol into the lateral ventricle of Sprague-Dawley rats at CT 15 caused phase delays that were similar to, but not as large as, the phase delays produced by light. Carbachol injections into the lateral ventricle were also later repeated in mice[104] and hamsters,[105] where administration of carbachol during early night caused phase delays, whereas late night administration caused phase advances.

This pattern of sensitivity and response is similar to that previously shown in response to light or GLU. Support for the involvement of ACh in the light response came from studies looking at ACh levels in the rat SCN using a radioimmunoassay.[106] Using this technique, no significant oscillation in ACh levels was found under constant conditions, but light pulses administered at CT 14 were found to increase ACh levels in the SCN. However, only 1 time point was examined, so it is not known whether this increase was a response to exposure to light or if there was a circadian pattern to the light-stimulated release. However, the implication of these studies is that ACh might be the primary neurotransmitter providing the signal of light to the clock.

However, significant evidence began to emerge indicating that ACh was not likely to be the primary signal of light. First, whereas it had previously been determined that the RHT transmitted the signal of light from the eye to the SCN, choline acetyltransferase (ChAT) was not present in this projection,[107] making it anatomically unlikely that ACh was the primary neurotransmitter involved in this signal. However, this evidence might warrant reconsideration, because recent studies have found an alternative splice variant of ChAT present in ganglion cells that was not picked up using previous antibodies.[108]

Additional evidence against ACh being the signal of light came from experiments that found intracerebroventricular injections of hemicholinium, which significantly depletes ACh stores in the brain, did not block the ability of the animal to phase shift in response to light.[109] There was also evidence that injecting NMDA receptor antagonists could block carbachol-induced phaseshifts, suggesting that although ACh may play a role in the light response, it must be upstream of a glutamatergic signal.[110] Liu and Gillette,[111] using extracellular recording in vitro, found that microdrop applications of carbachol directly to the SCN caused only phase advances, regardless of whether the carbachol was applied early or late in the night.

In an attempt to explain these contradicting data, it was hypothesized by our laboratory that the dual response pattern of the SCN to cholinergic stimulation was a result of the location of application. In the initial in vivo studies, carbachol was injected into the lateral or third ventricle, where the drug could have a diffuse effect, whereas in the in vitro studies carbachol was applied in microdrops directly to the SCN. As was predicted, if the in vivo experiments were performed by injecting carbachol directly into the SCN rather than into the ventricle, a phaseresponse pattern similar to that observed in the in vitro experiments using microdrop applications resulted.[112] This evidence suggests that ACh has at least 2 different effects on the circadian clock, depending on the site of application. There is an indirect response, working through ventricular pathways, that is likely upstream of a glutamatergic signal, and a direct response, which is mediated by the M_1AChR.[113] Based on the anatomic studies looking at cholinergic projections to the SCN that originate in the LDTg and PPTg, as well as the NBM, the current hypothesis is that this cholinergic signal may be involved in linking the sleep-wake and circadian cycles together.

GENETICS OF CIRCADIAN RHYTHMS

Much research effort has focused on determining how a biologic system keeps 24-hour time. With the discovery that single, dispersed cells can show circadian rhythms,[114] the focus turned toward understanding cellular processes that generate a near 24-hour time base. A molecular clockwork generates a ~24-hour rhythm through a feedback cycle involving a set of core clock genes, their mRNAs, and proteins.[115,116] This cycle consists of a set of interconnected positive and negative feedback loops, and their regulatory elements. Positive elements, which include *Clock* and *Bmal1*, are transcribed into mRNA, which is then translated into proteins that heterodimerize and are translocated into the nucleus. In the nucleus, they activate continued transcription of their own genes, as well as activating transcription of negative elements. The negative elements, which include *Period*, *Cryptochrome* and *Rev-erbα*, are then transcribed and translated. Proteins of the negative elements also associate in complexes and are translocated to the nucleus, where they feed back to inhibit transcription of the positive elements.[115,116] Additional genes that have been proposed to be involved in the circadian clock include *Rorα*,[117] *Timeless (Tim)*,[118] *Dec1*, and *Dec2*,[119] and more recently, *SIRT1*.[37,120,121] These feedback loops are further affected by regulatory enzymes, including casein kinase 1 epsilon (CKIε) and glycogen synthase kinase,[122–124] and small intracellular regulatory molecules, such as calcium and cAMP with established roles in signal transduction.[37,125] The cycle of these feedback loops takes approximately 24 hours to complete, providing a means by which cells can maintain a circadian rhythm.

Core clock elements have been found to play a critical role in human sleep disorders. For example, inherited forms of advanced sleep phase syndrome have been associated with a mutation in the *Per2* gene that interferes with a normal phosphorylation site of CKIδ/ε[126] or with a mutation in CKIδ.[127] Delayed sleep phase syndrome, on the other hand, has been found in some cases to be associated with a specific polymorphism of hPER3.[37,128,129] PER3 expression patterns in human leukocytes correlate with sleep-wake timing, particularly in those individuals with a preference for morningness.[130] Morningness or eveningness preferences have been associated with polymorphisms of the human *Clock* gene.[37,131,132]

The clock genes have proved useful for studying rhythms as well. Several of these genes, including *Bmal1* and 2 *Per* genes, have been fused to reporter molecules, such as green fluorescent protein and firefly luciferase, which enables study of the reporter as a marker of the transcription or translation of the gene. Both by transfecting cell cultures with a construct containing one of these fusion genes[133–136] and by creating transgenic rodents that express these fusion products,[137–140] new insights in clock dynamics have emerged. Among the most surprising is that all cells express them in a circadian pattern, even in dispersed cell culture. This finding established that circadian clocks are components of nearly all cells.

MOLECULAR CLOCKS IN DIVERSE MAMMALIAN CELLS

Although the SCN is necessary as the central circadian pacemaker, the discovery of autonomous clocks driven by oscillations in clock genes focused attention on extra-SCN clocks. Some non-SCN tissue, such as the mammalian pineal gland[141] and retina,[142] express circadian oscillations in metabolites or melatonin when cultured independently. The first oscillations of clock genes outside the SCN were found using a Rat-1 fibroblast cell line. These immortalized cells express clock gene mRNAs, such as *rev-erbα*, *per1*, and *per2*, which oscillate in cell culture with a period near 24 hours.[143] When primary mouse embryonic fibroblasts also showed clock gene oscillation, the possibility was raised that individual cells throughout the body might express the molecular components of a clock.[135,144–147]

With the advent of clock gene reporter systems, studies emerged supporting the evidence that peripheral, non-SCN tissues in the body contain functional clocks. The olfactory bulb oscillates in a transgenic rat that contains the promoter sequence for *mPer1* linked to luciferase.[139] The olfactory bulb maintains rhythmic luciferase expression when the SCN is surgically ablated,[148] the rat is made arrhythmic by placing it in constant light,[149] or when the olfactory bulb is isolated in tissue culture.[148,150] Many brain regions[150,151] and peripheral tissues, including skeletal muscle, liver, and lung, also show oscillations in clock genes, which remain rhythmic in culture for up to a week.[139,151,152]

Further technical advancements lead to the creation of a mouse containing a reporter of the PER2 protein fused to luciferase (PER2::LUC). This knock-in approach, which enabled direct assessment of PER2 protein expression, is more physiologic than transcriptional reporters and allows for study of peripheral tissues in culture for longer periods.[140] Many tissues from this mouse, including cornea, kidney, liver, lung, pituitary, and tail, show clear, robust oscillations in PER2::LUC for up to 1 week in vitro, although SCN, liver, and lung tissues continue to show circadian rhythms for up to 3 weeks. Unexpectedly, tissue taken from SCN-lesioned mice 3 to 5 weeks after surgery still showed robust near 24-hour rhythms in cellular luciferase luminescence, although the phasing of the rhythms were widely dispersed amongst the various tissues.[140] Individual fibroblasts from these PER2::LUC mice also maintain an oscillation in culture.[135] Experiments performed with these reporter animals, along with those performed using the transcriptional reporters, show that nearly all peripheral cells in the body and some in the brain contain the molecular machinery of a functional circadian clock.

COUPLING OF CENTRAL AND PERIPHERAL CLOCKS

This discussion emphasizes the myriad individual oscillating clocks in the body. In animals with a functional SCN, these clocks are aligned so that each individual tissue maintains a stable phase relationship to the SCN so that clock genes are expressed at the same time each day. When SCN rhythmicity is removed or the phase is shifted, the various tissues maintain their individual circadian rhythms, but they quickly fall out of phase with each other.[139,140,153] This finding indicates a hierarchical relationship in which the SCN is the master regulator that synchronizes and aligns the rest of the body's clocks. Much study of the coupling of extra-SCN clocks to the central pacemaker has been undertaken, and several examples are highlighted in the following discussion.

The earliest SCN isolation studies established the role of the SCN as the master clock, but these studies also hint at the various means by which this clock exerts control over peripheral structures. When the SCN is surgically isolated from the rest of the hypothalamus in rats, serum corticosterone oscillations continue, whereas locomotor rhythms are lost.[154] In addition, surgical cuts to rodent brains between the SCN and PVN abolish reproductive rhythms in hamsters, but rhythmic locomotor activity is maintained in hamsters[155,156] and rats.[157] These findings provide early evidence for both synaptic coupling of SCN to output tissues, as well as the possibility that humoral signals entrain peripheral tissues. This idea was furthered by transplant studies in which an encapsulated fetal SCN is transplanted into an animal with an SCN lesion. Fenestrations in the encapsulating polymer were too small to permit neurite passage, and no neural connectivity to the recipient brain could be found. The transplant restores locomotor, feeding, drinking, body temperature, and sleep/wake, but not endocrine, rhythms to the lesioned animal.[158] Clearly, some non-SCN rhythms require physical connections and some do not.

Many rhythm-generating tissues are coupled to the SCN by synaptic connections. Anatomic studies have shown SCN projections that extend to several hypothalamic nuclei, including the organum vasculosum of lamina terminalis, MPOA, and PVN, seemingly forming direct synapses with gonadotropin-releasing hormone (GnRH) and corticotropin-releasing hormone (CRH) neurons in these regions.[159–161] In addition, the neuronal networks connecting the SCN to the IGL and PVN of the thalamus provide the SCN and these sleep/arousal modulatory regions with bidirectional communication.[53–55]

The SCN is one of many regulators of opposing sympathetic and parasympathetic autonomic signals to peripheral organs. Anatomic studies using retrograde tracers injected into peripheral organs, such as liver, adrenal gland, pancreas, and adipose tissue, show a multisynaptic pathway connecting these tissues to autonomic centers in the spinal cord, brain stem, PVN, and DMH, and finally, to the SCN and other hypothalamic regions.[162–165] Discriminative tracing of either sympathetic or parasympathetic tracts identifies SCN neurons in overlapping areas of the nucleus, but these neurons seem to be involved in signaling to one or the other of these pathways.[163,164] Light from the external environment can affect these 2 pathways through SCN-mediated control. For example, exposure of rats to light at night results in increased sympathetic activity, but suppression of parasympathetic activity. When the SCN is abolished, this effect is lost.[166] Also, heart rate decreases after light exposure at night in a nocturnal rodent, whereas SCN-lesioned animals do not show this response.[167] Clearly, the SCN plays a role in modulating autonomic signals to the periphery, but it works in concert with many other regions of the brain, including those regulating body temperature, metabolism, reproductive state, and other physiologic functions.

A growing body of evidence supports a role for humoral signaling in the coupling of rhythms between the SCN and other regions. In brain-slice cultures containing PVN tissue, an electrical rhythm emerges in the PVN only after coculture with an SCN brain slice. The lack of neuronal connections between the 2 slices in vitro strongly supports a diffusible factor as cause of the electrical oscillation of the PVN.[168] In addition, parabiosis connecting the circulatory system of an intact mouse to that of an SCN-lesioned mouse indicates that diffusible signals from the intact animal can entrain peripheral tissue in the lesioned recipient. Peripheral rhythms of clock gene expression are restored after parabiosis in kidney and liver.[169] Coculturing functional SCN tissue with peripheral cells or tissue induces rhythms in these cells that follow the SCN under culture conditions that prevent synaptic connections.[146,170,171]

These studies indicate that diffusible signals can modulate rhythms between tissues. Neuropeptides are abundant in the SCN, and are good candidates for humoral signals. As described earlier, major neuropeptides found in the SCN include VIP, GRP, little SAAS, and AVP. These peptides are released from the SCN in a circadian fashion,[20,172,173] and each has been implicated in a physiologic role in some aspect of circadian biology.[20,172,174–180] Identification of the diffusible signals that couple other tissues to the SCN is the subject of intense study, with high therapeutic potential.

Another role for diffusible factors from the SCN seems to be to provide a signal inhibitory to activity. Two candidate factors for communicating such signals include transforming growth factor α (TGF-α) and prokineticin 2 (PK2). Under normal conditions, TGF-α peptide is expressed rhythmically in the SCN with a peak during the animal's inactive period, and a trough during the active period. When infused continuously into the ventricles, TGF-α fully inhibits locomotor activity. Conversely, mice lacking the cognate receptor, epidermal growth factor receptor, are unable to respond to TGF-α and show an excessive amount of daytime activity.[181] PK2 also is expressed rhythmically in the SCN, again showing peak expression during the animal's inactive period, and can inhibit locomotor activity when infused continuously.[182] This finding suggests a role for output signals from the SCN in promoting an inactive state that would be permissive for sleep.

Some tissues seem to require both synaptic and humoral signals to synchronize to the SCN. When autonomic nerve connections to the liver are severed, plasma insulin and corticosterone levels remain rhythmic, but plasma glucose levels do not.[183] However, liver tissue from an SCN-lesioned mouse with surgical parabiosis to an intact animal recovers and continues to maintain rhythmicity from that point onward.[169] This finding suggests that control of liver timing requires both neuronal and diffusible signals that coordinate separate physiologic functions. Dissecting the intricacies of circadian regulation among peripheral tissues requires careful study.

Coupling of the SCN to peripheral targets, regardless of the manner of this connection, has important implications for health. This interaction allows for synchronization of internal systems to environmental light signals, both on a day-by-day basis and to adjust the animal to seasonal changes. Modern human activities, such as shift work and transcontinental flight, result in significant desynchronization of the central internal clock and various body tissues. This circadian disarray can have dire consequences for human health, including increased risks of various cancers, reproductive health, stroke, metabolic syndrome, cardiovascular disease,[184–186] and overall mortality in aged individuals.[187]

SUMMARY

Circadian rhythms, the near 24-hour oscillations in brain and body functions, such as core body temperature, hormone release, and the sleep-wake cycle, are embedded in the physiology of cells and tissues. The master pacemaker regulating these rhythms, the SCN in the hypothalamus, is optimally situated to receive input about environmental light, sleep-wake state, and activity status. It can be reset in response to changes in environmental conditions and internal state. These stimuli, in turn, provide output signals to regulate the timing of rest/activity and behavioral cycles. The core mechanisms providing this timekeeping property are provided through transcription/translation feedback loops, consisting of both positive and negative elements, coupled with other intracellular elements associated with signaling events. Clock gene proteins are now being used as molecular tools to further study clocks in all tissues and how the SCN synchronizes and aligns these various body clocks to environmental cycles and imposed work schedules. Circadian rhythm sleep disorders as well as sleep phenotypes are correlated with abnormalities in the genes regulating circadian rhythms. Internal desynchrony of peripheral tissues and the SCN can have negative consequences for human health and longevity. Research to date has revealed surprising complexity in the ordering of body functions. Much remains to be discovered regarding the roles of the SCN and peripheral clocks in coordinating the brain and body in health and disease.

REFERENCES

1. Van Cauter E. Diurnal and ultradian rhythms in human endocrine function: a minireview. Horm Res 1990;34:45–53.

2. Schwartz WJ. A clinician's primer on the circadian clock: its localization, function, and resetting. Adv Intern Med 1993;38:81–106.

3. Arendt J, Minors DS, Waterhouse JM, editors. Biological rhythms in clinical practice. Bristol (England): John Wright; 1989. p. 299.

4. Van Cauter E, Turek FW. Endocrine and other biological rhythms. In: DeGroot JL, editor. Textbook of endocrinology. Philadelphia: WB Saunders; 1995. p. 2487–548.

5. Takahashi Y, Kipnis DM, Daughaday WH. Growth hormone secretion during sleep. J Clin Invest 1968;47:2079–90.

6. Van Cauter E, L'Hermite M, Copinschi G, et al. Quantitative analysis of spontaneous variations of plasma prolactin in normal man. Am J Physiol 1981;241:E355–63.

7. van Coevorden A, Laurent E, Decoster C, et al. Decreased basal and stimulated thyrotropin secretion in healthy elderly men. J Clin Endocrinol Metab 1989;69:177–85.

8. Kapen S, Boyar R, Hellman L, et al. The relationship of luteinizing hormone secretion to sleep in women during the early follicular phase: effects of sleep reversal and a prolonged three-hour sleep-wake schedule. J Clin Endocrinol Metab 1976;42:1031–40.

9. Licinio J, Mantzoros C, Negrao AB, et al. Human leptin levels are pulsatile and inversely related to pituitary-adrenal function. Nat Med 1997;3:575–9.

10. Licinio J, Negrao AB, Mantzoros C, et al. Synchronicity of frequently sampled, 24-h concentrations of circulating leptin, luteinizing hormone, and estradiol in healthy women. Proc Natl Acad Sci U S A 1998;95:2541–6.

11. Sinha MK, Ohannesian JP, Heiman ML, et al. Nocturnal rise of leptin in lean, obese, and non-insulin-dependent diabetes mellitus subjects. J Clin Invest 1996;97:1344–7.

12. Lejeune-Lenain C, Van Cauter E, Desir D, et al. Control of circadian and episodic variations of adrenal androgens secretion in man. J Endocrinol Invest 1987;10:267–76.

13. Weitzman ED, Zimmerman JC, Czeisler CA, et al. Cortisol secretion is inhibited during sleep in normal man. J Clin Endocrinol Metab 1983;56:352–8.

14. Moore RY, Eichler VB. Loss of a circadian adrenal corticosterone rhythm following suprachiasmatic lesions in the rat. Brain Res 1972;42:201–6.

15. Stephan FK, Zucker I. Circadian rhythms in drinking behavior and locomotor activity of rats are eliminated by hypothalamic lesions. Proc Natl Acad Sci U S A 1972;69:1583–6.

16. Drucker-Colin R, Aguilar-Roblero R, Garcia-Hernandez F, et al. Fetal suprachiasmatic nucleus

transplants: diurnal rhythm recovery of lesioned rats. Brain Res 1984;311:353–7.

17. Ralph MR, Foster RG, Davis FC, et al. Transplanted suprachiasmatic nucleus determines circadian period. Science 1990;247:975–8.

18. Abrahamson EE, Moore RY. Suprachiasmatic nucleus in the mouse: retinal innervation, intrinsic organization and efferent projections. Brain Res 2001;916:172–91.

19. Antle MC, Silver R. Orchestrating time: arrangements of the brain circadian clock. Trends Neurosci 2005;28:145–51.

20. Atkins N Jr, Mitchell JW, Romanova EV, et al. Circadian integration of glutamatergic signals by little SAAS in novel suprachiasmatic circuits. PLoS One 2010;5:e12612.

21. Morin LP. SCN organization reconsidered. J Biol Rhythms 2007;22:3–13.

22. Moore RY, Speh JC, Leak RK. Suprachiasmatic nucleus organization. Cell Tissue Res 2002;309: 89–98.

23. Mai JK, Kedziora O, Teckhaus L, et al. Evidence for subdivisions in the human suprachiasmatic nucleus. J Comp Neurol 1991;305:508–25.

24. Mosko S, Moore RY. Retinohypothalamic tract development: alteration by suprachiasmatic lesions in the neonatal rat. Brain Res 1979;164:1–15.

25. Johnson RF, Moore RY, Morin LP. Loss of entrainment and anatomical plasticity after lesions of the hamster retinohypothalamic tract. Brain Res 1988; 460:297–313.

26. Rusak B. Neural mechanisms for entrainment and generation of mammalian circadian rhythms. Fed Proc 1979;38:2589–95.

27. Hattar S, Lucas RJ, Mrosovsky N, et al. Melanopsin and rod-cone photoreceptive systems account for all major accessory visual functions in mice. Nature 2003;424:76–81.

28. Berson DM, Dunn FA, Takao M. Phototransduction by retinal ganglion cells that set the circadian clock. Science 2002;295:1070–3.

29. Hannibal J, Ding JM, Chen D, et al. Pituitary adenylate cyclase-activating peptide (PACAP) in the retinohypothalamic tract: a potential daytime regulator of the biological clock. J Neurosci 1997;17: 2637–44.

30. Ding JM, Chen D, Weber ET, et al. Resetting the biological clock: mediation of nocturnal circadian shifts by glutamate and NO. Science 1994;266: 1713–7.

31. Mintz EM, Marvel CL, Gillespie CF, et al. Activation of NMDA receptors in the suprachiasmatic nucleus produces light-like phase shifts of the circadian clock in vivo. J Neurosci 1999;19: 5124–30.

32. Medanic M, Gillette MU. Suprachiasmatic circadian pacemaker of rat shows two windows of sensitivity to neuropeptide Y in vitro. Brain Res 1993;620:281–6.

33. Yannielli PC, Harrington ME. Neuropeptide Y applied in vitro can block the phase shifts induced by light in vivo. Neuroreport 2000;11:1587–91.

34. Yannielli PC, Harrington ME. The neuropeptide Y Y5 receptor mediates the blockade of "Photic-like" NMDA-induced phase shifts in the golden hamster. J Neurosci 2001;21:5367–73.

35. Reghunandanan V, Reghunandanan R, Singh PI. Neurotransmitters of the suprachiasmatic nucleus: role in the regulation of circadian rhythms. Prog Neurobiol 1993;41:647–55.

36. Glass JD, DiNardo LA, Ehlen JC. Dorsal raphe nuclear stimulation of SCN serotonin release and circadian phase-resetting. Brain Res 2000;859: 224–32.

37. Imaizumi T, Kay SA, Schroeder JI. Circadian rhythms. Daily watch on metabolism. Science 2007;318:1730–1.

38. van den Pol AN, Tsujimoto KL. Neurotransmitters of the hypothalamic suprachiasmatic nucleus: immunocytochemical analysis of 25 neuronal antigens. Neuroscience 1985;15:1049–86.

39. Barassin S, Raison S, Saboureau M, et al. Circadian tryptophan hydroxylase levels and serotonin release in the suprachiasmatic nucleus of the rat. Eur J Neurosci 2002;15:833–40.

40. Bina KG, Rusak B, Semba K. Localization of cholinergic neurons in the forebrain and brainstem that project to the suprachiasmatic nucleus of the hypothalamus in rat. J Comp Neurol 1993;335: 295–307.

41. Castillo-Ruiz A, Nunez AA. Cholinergic projections to the suprachiasmatic nucleus and lower subparaventricular zone of diurnal and nocturnal rodents. Brain Res 2007;1151:91–101.

42. Cui H, Malpeli JG. Activity in the parabigeminal nucleus during eye movements directed at moving and stationary targets. J Neurophysiol 2003;89: 3128–42.

43. Deurveilher S, Hennevin E. Lesions of the pedunculopontine tegmental nucleus reduce paradoxical sleep (PS) propensity: evidence from a short-term PS deprivation study in rats. Eur J Neurosci 2001; 13:1963–76.

44. Semba K. Multiple output pathways of the basal forebrain: organization, chemical heterogeneity, and roles in vigilance. Behav Brain Res 2000;115: 117–41.

45. Michelsen KA, Lozada A, Kaslin J, et al. Histamine-immunoreactive neurons in the mouse and rat suprachiasmatic nucleus. Eur J Neurosci 2005; 22:1997–2004.

46. Leak RK, Moore RY. Topographic organization of suprachiasmatic nucleus projection neurons. J Comp Neurol 2001;433:312–34.

47. Kalsbeek A, Buijs RM. Output pathways of the mammalian suprachiasmatic nucleus: coding circadian time by transmitter selection and specific targeting. Cell Tissue Res 2002;309:109–18.

48. Abrahamson EE, Leak RK, Moore RY. The suprachiasmatic nucleus projects to posterior hypothalamic arousal systems. Neuroreport 2001;12: 435–40.

49. de Lecea L, Kilduff TS, Peyron C, et al. The hypocretins: hypothalamus-specific peptides with neuroexcitatory activity. Proc Natl Acad Sci U S A 1998;95:322–7.

50. Gompf HS, Aston-Jones G. Role of orexin input in the diurnal rhythm of locus coeruleus impulse activity. Brain Res 2008;1224:43–52.

51. Aston-Jones G, Chen S, Zhu Y, et al. A neural circuit for circadian regulation of arousal. Nat Neurosci 2001;4:732–8.

52. Chou TC, Bjorkum AA, Gaus SE, et al. Afferents to the ventrolateral preoptic nucleus. J Neurosci 2002;22:977–90.

53. Buijs RM, Hou YX, Shinn S, et al. Ultrastructural evidence for intra- and extranuclear projections of GABAergic neurons of the suprachiasmatic nucleus. J Comp Neurol 1994;340:381–91.

54. Moga MM, Weis RP, Moore RY. Efferent projections of the paraventricular thalamic nucleus in the rat. J Comp Neurol 1995;359:221–38.

55. Morin LP. The circadian visual system. Brain Res Brain Res Rev 1994;19:102–27.

56. Peng ZC, Bentivoglio M. The thalamic paraventricular nucleus relays information from the suprachiasmatic nucleus to the amygdala: a combined anterograde and retrograde tracing study in the rat at the light and electron microscopic levels. J Neurocytol 2004;33:101–16.

57. Welsh DK, Takahashi JS, Kay SA. Suprachiasmatic nucleus: cell autonomy and network properties. Annu Rev Physiol 2010;72:551–77.

58. Walsh IB, van den Berg RJ, Rietveld WJ. Ionic currents in cultured rat suprachiasmatic neurons. Neuroscience 1995;69:915–29.

59. Gillette MU. Regulation of entrainment pathways by the suprachiasmatic circadian clock: sensitivities to second messengers. Prog Brain Res 1996;111: 121–32.

60. Gillette MU, Mitchell JW. Signaling in the suprachiasmatic nucleus: selectively responsive and integrative. Cell Tissue Res 2002;309:99–107.

61. Moga MM, Moore RY. Putative excitatory amino acid projections to the suprachiasmatic nucleus in the rat. Brain Res 1996;743:171–7.

62. Antle MC, Mistlberger RE. Circadian clock resetting by sleep deprivation without exercise in the Syrian hamster. J Neurosci 2000;20:9326–32.

63. Reebs SG, Mrosovsky N. Effects of induced wheel running on the circadian activity rhythms of Syrian hamsters: entrainment and phase response curve. J Biol Rhythms 1989;4:39–48.

64. Medanic M, Gillette MU. Serotonin regulates the phase of the rat suprachiasmatic circadian pacemaker in vitro only during the subjective day. J Physiol 1992;450:629–42.

65. Dudley TE, Dinardo LA, Glass JD. In vivo assessment of the midbrain raphe nuclear regulation of serotonin release in the hamster suprachiasmatic nucleus. J Neurophysiol 1999;81:1469–77.

66. Dudley TE, DiNardo LA, Glass JD. Endogenous regulation of serotonin release in the hamster suprachiasmatic nucleus. J Neurosci 1998;18: 5045–52.

67. Grossman GH, Mistlberger RE, Antle MC, et al. Sleep deprivation stimulates serotonin release in the suprachiasmatic nucleus. Neuroreport 2000; 11:1929–32.

68. Bobrzynska KJ, Vrang N, Mrosovsky N. Persistence of nonphotic phase shifts in hamsters after serotonin depletion in the suprachiasmatic nucleus. Brain Res 1996;741:205–14.

69. Antle MC, Marchant EG, Niel L, et al. Serotonin antagonists do not attenuate activity-induced phase shifts of circadian rhythms in the Syrian hamster. Brain Res 1998;813:139–49.

70. Hannibal J, Moller M, Ottersen OP, et al. PACAP and glutamate are co-stored in the retinohypothalamic tract. J Comp Neurol 2000;418:147–55.

71. Fukuhara C, Suzuki N, Matsumoto Y, et al. Day-night variation of pituitary adenylate cyclase-activating polypeptide (PACAP) level in the rat suprachiasmatic nucleus. Neurosci Lett 1997;229:49–52.

72. Piggins HD, Marchant EG, Goguen D, et al. Phase-shifting effects of pituitary adenylate cyclase activating polypeptide on hamster wheel-running rhythms. Neurosci Lett 2001;305:25–8.

73. Albers HE, Ferris CF. Neuropeptide Y: role in light-dark cycle entrainment of hamster circadian rhythms. Neurosci Lett 1984;50:163–8.

74. Huhman KL, Albers HE. Neuropeptide Y microinjected into the suprachiasmatic region phase shifts circadian rhythms in constant darkness. Peptides 1994;15:1475–8.

75. Rusak B, Meijer JH, Harrington ME. Hamster circadian rhythms are phase-shifted by electrical stimulation of the geniculo-hypothalamic tract. Brain Res 1989;493:283–91.

76. Biello SM, Mrosovsky N. Blocking the phase-shifting effect of neuropeptide Y with light. Proc Biol Sci 1995;259:179–87.

77. Biello SM, Golombek DA, Harrington ME. Neuropeptide Y and glutamate block each other's phase shifts in the suprachiasmatic nucleus in vitro. Neuroscience 1997;77:1049–57.

78. Huhman KL, Babagbemi TO, Albers HE. Bicuculline blocks neuropeptide Y-induced phase advances

when microinjected in the suprachiasmatic nucleus of Syrian hamsters. Brain Res 1995;675:333–6.

79. Gillette MU, Prosser RA. Circadian rhythm of the rat suprachiasmatic brain slice is rapidly reset by daytime application of cAMP analogs. Brain Res 1988;474:348–52.

80. Prosser RA, Gillette MU. The mammalian circadian clock in the suprachiasmatic nuclei is reset in vitro by cAMP. J Neurosci 1989;9:1073–81.

81. Prosser RA, Gillette MU. Cyclic changes in cAMP concentration and phosphodiesterase activity in a mammalian circadian clock studied in vitro. Brain Res 1991;568:185–92.

82. Cheung PW, McCormack CE. Failure of pinealectomy or melatonin to alter circadian activity rhythm of the rat. Am J Physiol 1982;242:R261–4.

83. Cassone VM, Chesworth MJ, Armstrong SM. Entrainment of rat circadian rhythms by daily injection of melatonin depends upon the hypothalamic suprachiasmatic nuclei. Physiol Behav 1986;36:1111–21.

84. Cassone VM, Roberts MH, Moore RY. Effects of melatonin on 2-deoxy-[1-14C]glucose uptake within rat suprachiasmatic nucleus. Am J Physiol 1988;255:R332–7.

85. Margraf RR, Lynch GR. An in vitro circadian rhythm of melatonin sensitivity in the suprachiasmatic nucleus of the djungarian hamster, *Phodopus sungorus*. Brain Res 1993;609:45–50.

86. Shibata S, Cassone VM, Moore RY. Effects of melatonin on neuronal activity in the rat suprachiasmatic nucleus in vitro. Neurosci Lett 1989;97:140–4.

87. McArthur AJ, Gillette MU, Prosser RA. Melatonin directly resets the rat suprachiasmatic circadian clock in vitro. Brain Res 1991;565:158–61.

88. McArthur AJ, Hunt AE, Gillette MU. Melatonin action and signal transduction in the rat suprachiasmatic circadian clock: activation of protein kinase C at dusk and dawn. Endocrinology 1997;138:627–34.

89. Hunt AE, Al-Ghoul WM, Gillette MU, et al. Activation of MT(2) melatonin receptors in rat suprachiasmatic nucleus phase advances the circadian clock. Am J Physiol Cell Physiol 2001;280:C110–8.

90. Shirakawa T, Moore RY. Glutamate shifts the phase of the circadian neuronal firing rhythm in the rat suprachiasmatic nucleus in vitro. Neurosci Lett 1994;178:47–50.

91. Shibata S, Watanabe A, Hamada T, et al. N-Methyl-D-aspartate induces phase shifts in circadian rhythm of neuronal activity of rat SCN in vitro. Am J Physiol 1994;267:R360–4.

92. Watanabe A, Hamada T, Shibata S, et al. Effects of nitric oxide synthase inhibitors on N-methyl-D-aspartate-induced phase delay of circadian rhythm of neuronal activity in the rat suprachiasmatic nucleus in vitro. Brain Res 1994;646:161–4.

93. Watanabe A, Ono M, Shibata S, et al. Effect of a nitric oxide synthase inhibitor, N-nitro-L-arginine methylester, on light-induced phase delay of circadian rhythm of wheel-running activity in golden hamsters. Neurosci Lett 1995;192:25–8.

94. Weber ET, Gannon RL, Michel AM, et al. Nitric oxide synthase inhibitor blocks light-induced phase shifts of the circadian activity rhythm, but not c-fos expression in the suprachiasmatic nucleus of the Syrian hamster. Brain Res 1995;692:137–42.

95. Ding JM, Buchanan GF, Tischkau SA, et al. A neuronal ryanodine receptor mediates light-induced phase delays of the circadian clock. Nature 1998;394:381–4.

96. Ding JM, Faiman LE, Hurst WJ, et al. Resetting the biological clock: mediation of nocturnal CREB phosphorylation via light, glutamate, and nitric oxide. J Neurosci 1997;17:667–75.

97. Tischkau SA, Mitchell JW, Tyan SH, et al. Ca2+/cAMP response element-binding protein (CREB)-dependent activation of Per1 is required for light-induced signaling in the suprachiasmatic nucleus circadian clock. J Biol Chem 2003;278:718–23.

98. Bradbury MJ, Dement WC, Edgar DM. Serotonin-containing fibers in the suprachiasmatic hypothalamus attenuate light-induced phase delays in mice. Brain Res 1997;768:125–34.

99. Mintz EM, Jasnow AM, Gillespie CF, et al. GABA interacts with photic signaling in the suprachiasmatic nucleus to regulate circadian phase shifts. Neuroscience 2002;109:773–8.

100. Bergstrom AL, Hannibal J, Hindersson P, et al. Light-induced phase shift in the Syrian hamster (*Mesocricetus auratus*) is attenuated by the PACAP receptor antagonist PACAP6-38 or PACAP immunoneutralization. Eur J Neurosci 2003;18:2552–62.

101. Chen D, Buchanan GF, Ding JM, et al. Pituitary adenylyl cyclase-activating peptide: a pivotal modulator of glutamatergic regulation of the suprachiasmatic circadian clock. Proc Natl Acad Sci U S A 1999;96:13468–73.

102. Tischkau SA, Gallman EA, Buchanan GF, et al. Differential cAMP gating of glutamatergic signaling regulates long-term state changes in the suprachiasmatic circadian clock. J Neurosci 2000;20:7830–7.

103. Zatz M, Brownstein MJ. Intraventricular carbachol mimics the effects of light on the circadian rhythm in the rat pineal gland. Science 1979;203:358–61.

104. Zatz M, Herkenham MA. Intraventricular carbachol mimics the phase-shifting effect of light on the circadian rhythm of wheel-running activity. Brain Res 1981;212:234–8.

105. Earnest DJ, Turek FW. Role for acetylcholine in mediating effects of light on reproduction. Science 1983;219:77–9.

106. Murakami N, Takahashi K, Kawashima K. Effect of light on the acetylcholine concentrations of the suprachiasmatic nucleus in the rat. Brain Res 1984;311:358–60.

107. Wenthold RJ. Glutamate and aspartate as neuro-transmitters for the auditory nerve. In: DiChiara G, Gessa GL, editors. Glutamate as a neurotransmitter. New York: Raven Press; 1981. p. 69–78.

108. Yasuhara O, Tooyama I, Aimi Y, et al. Demonstration of cholinergic ganglion cells in rat retina: expression of an alternative splice variant of choline acetyltransferase. J Neurosci 2003;23: 2872–81.

109. Pauly JR, Horseman ND. Anticholinergic agents do not block light-induced circadian phase shifts. Brain Res 1985;348:163–7.

110. Colwell CS, Kaufman CM, Menaker M. Phase-shifting mechanisms in the mammalian circadian system: new light on the carbachol paradox. J Neurosci 1993;13:1454–9.

111. Liu C, Gillette MU. Cholinergic regulation of the suprachiasmatic nucleus circadian rhythm via a muscarinic mechanism at night. J Neurosci 1996;16:744–51.

112. Buchanan GF, Gillette MU. New light on an old paradox: site-dependent effects of carbachol on circadian rhythms. Exp Neurol 2005;193:489–96.

113. Gillette MU, Buchanan GF, Artinian L, et al. Role of the M1 receptor in regulating circadian rhythms. Life Sci 2001;68:2467–72.

114. Welsh DK, Logothetis DE, Meister M, et al. Individual neurons dissociated from rat suprachiasmatic nucleus express independently phased circadian firing rhythms. Neuron 1995;14:697–706.

115. Gallego M, Virshup DM. Post-translational modifications regulate the ticking of the circadian clock. Nat Rev Mol Cell Biol 2007;8:139–48.

116. Ko CH, Takahashi JS. Molecular components of the mammalian circadian clock. Hum Mol Genet 2006; 15(2):R271–7.

117. Sato TK, Panda S, Miraglia LJ, et al. A functional genomics strategy reveals Rora as a component of the mammalian circadian clock. Neuron 2004; 43:527–37.

118. Barnes JW, Tischkau SA, Barnes JA, et al. Requirement of mammalian Timeless for circadian rhythmicity. Science 2003;302:439–42.

119. Honma S, Kawamoto T, Takagi Y, et al. Dec1 and Dec2 are regulators of the mammalian molecular clock. Nature 2002;419:841–4.

120. Asher G, Gatfield D, Stratmann M, et al. SIRT1 regulates circadian clock gene expression through PER2 deacetylation. Cell 2008;134:317–28.

121. Nakahata Y, Kaluzova M, Grimaldi B, et al. The NAD+-dependent deacetylase SIRT1 modulates CLOCK-mediated chromatin remodeling and circadian control. Cell 2008;134:329–40.

122. Harms E, Young MW, Saez L. CK1 and GSK3 in the Drosophila and mammalian circadian clock. Novartis Found Symp 2003;253:267–77 [discussion: 102–9, 277–84].

123. Martinek S, Inonog S, Manoukian AS, et al. A role for the segment polarity gene shaggy/GSK-3 in the Drosophila circadian clock. Cell 2001;105: 769–79.

124. Virshup DM, Eide EJ, Forger DB, et al. Reversible protein phosphorylation regulates circadian rhythms. Cold Spring Harb Symp Quant Biol 2007;72:413–20.

125. Harrisingh MC, Nitabach MN. Circadian rhythms. Integrating circadian timekeeping with cellular physiology. Science 2008;320:879–80.

126. Toh KL, Jones CR, He Y, et al. An hPer2 phosphorylation site mutation in familial advanced sleep phase syndrome. Science 2001;291:1040–3.

127. Xu Y, Padiath QS, Shapiro RE, et al. Functional consequences of a CKIdelta mutation causing familial advanced sleep phase syndrome. Nature 2005;434:640–4.

128. Archer SN, Robilliard DL, Skene DJ, et al. A length polymorphism in the circadian clock gene Per3 is linked to delayed sleep phase syndrome and extreme diurnal preference. Sleep 2003;26: 413–5.

129. Ebisawa T, Uchiyama M, Kajimura N, et al. Association of structural polymorphisms in the human period3 gene with delayed sleep phase syndrome. EMBO Rep 2001;2:342–6.

130. Archer SN, Viola AU, Kyriakopoulou V, et al. Interindividual differences in habitual sleep timing and entrained phase of endogenous circadian rhythms of BMAL1, PER2 and PER3 mRNA in human leukocytes. Sleep 2008;31:608–17.

131. Katzenberg D, Young T, Finn L, et al. A clock polymorphism associated with human diurnal preference. Sleep 1998;21:569–76.

132. Mishima K, Tozawa T, Satoh K, et al. The 3111T/C polymorphism of hClock is associated with evening preference and delayed sleep timing in a Japanese population sample. Am J Med Genet B Neuropsychiatr Genet 2005;133:101–4.

133. Izumo M, Johnson CH, Yamazaki S. Circadian gene expression in mammalian fibroblasts revealed by real-time luminescence reporting: temperature compensation and damping. Proc Natl Acad Sci U S A 2003;100:16089–94.

134. Ueda HR, Chen W, Adachi A, et al. A transcription factor response element for gene expression during circadian night. Nature 2002;418:534–9.

135. Welsh DK, Yoo SH, Liu AC, et al. Bioluminescence imaging of individual fibroblasts reveals persistent, independently phased circadian rhythms of clock gene expression. Curr Biol 2004;14:2289–95.

136. Yamaguchi S, Mitsui S, Miyake S, et al. The 5' upstream region of mPer1 gene contains two promoters and is responsible for circadian oscillation. Curr Biol 2000;10:873–6.

137. Kuhlman SJ, Quintero JE, McMahon DG. GFP fluorescence reports Period 1 circadian gene regulation in the mammalian biological clock. Neuroreport 2000;11:1479–82.

138. Wilsbacher LD, Yamazaki S, Herzog ED, et al. Photic and circadian expression of luciferase in mPeriod1-luc transgenic mice invivo. Proc Natl Acad Sci U S A 2002;99:489–94.

139. Yamazaki S, Numano R, Abe M, et al. Resetting central and peripheral circadian oscillators in transgenic rats. Science 2000;288:682–5.

140. Yoo SH, Yamazaki S, Lowrey PL, et al. PERIOD2::-LUCIFERASE real-time reporting of circadian dynamics reveals persistent circadian oscillations in mouse peripheral tissues. Proc Natl Acad Sci U S A 2004;101:5339–46.

141. Klein DC, Weller JL. Indole metabolism in the pineal gland: a circadian rhythm in N-acetyltransferase. Science 1970;169:1093–5.

142. Tosini G, Menaker M. Circadian rhythms in cultured mammalian retina. Science 1996;272:419–21.

143. Balsalobre A, Damiola F, Schibler U. A serum shock induces circadian gene expression in mammalian tissue culture cells. Cell 1998;93:929–37.

144. Balsalobre A, Marcacci L, Schibler U. Multiple signaling pathways elicit circadian gene expression in cultured Rat-1 fibroblasts. Curr Biol 2000; 10:1291–4.

145. Brown SA, Zumbrunn G, Fleury-Olela F, et al. Rhythms of mammalian body temperature can sustain peripheral circadian clocks. Curr Biol 2002;12:1574–83.

146. Pando MP, Morse D, Cermakian N, et al. Phenotypic rescue of a peripheral clock genetic defect via SCN hierarchical dominance. Cell 2002;110: 107–17.

147. Yagita K, Tamanini F, van Der Horst GT, et al. Molecular mechanisms of the biological clock in cultured fibroblasts. Science 2001;292:278–81.

148. Abraham U, Prior JL, Granados-Fuentes D, et al. Independent circadian oscillations of Period1 in specific brain areas in vivo and in vitro. J Neurosci 2005;25:8620–6.

149. Granados-Fuentes D, Prolo LM, Abraham U, et al. The suprachiasmatic nucleus entrains, but does not sustain, circadian rhythmicity in the olfactory bulb. J Neurosci 2004;24:615–9.

150. Abe M, Herzog ED, Yamazaki S, et al. Circadian rhythms in isolated brain regions. J Neurosci 2002;22:350–6.

151. Yamazaki S, Straume M, Tei H, et al. Effects of aging on central and peripheral mammalian clocks. Proc Natl Acad Sci U S A 2002;99:10801–6.

152. Stokkan KA, Yamazaki S, Tei H, et al. Entrainment of the circadian clock in the liver by feeding. Science 2001;291:490–3.

153. Davidson AJ, Castanon-Cervantes O, Leise TL, et al. Visualizing jet lag in the mouse suprachiasmatic nucleus and peripheral circadian timing system. Eur J Neurosci 2009;29:171–80.

154. Honma S, Honma K, Hiroshige T. Dissociation of circadian rhythms in rats with a hypothalamic island. Am J Physiol 1984;246:R949–54.

155. Eskes GA, Rusak B. Horizontal knife cuts in the suprachiasmatic area prevent hamster gonadal responses to photoperiod. Neurosci Lett 1985;61: 261–6.

156. Nunez AA, Brown MH, Youngstrom TG. Hypothalamic circuits involved in the regulation of seasonal and circadian rhythms in male golden hamsters. Brain Res Bull 1985;15:149–53.

157. Brown MH, Nunez AA. Hypothalamic circuits and circadian rhythms: effects of knife cuts vary with their placement within the suprachiasmatic area. Brain Res Bull 1986;16:705–11.

158. Silver R, LeSauter J, Tresco PA, et al. A diffusible coupling signal from the transplanted suprachiasmatic nucleus controlling circadian locomotor rhythms. Nature 1996;382:810–3.

159. Buijs RM, Markman M, Nunes-Cardoso B, et al. Projections of the suprachiasmatic nucleus to stress-related areas in the rat hypothalamus: a light and electron microscopic study. J Comp Neurol 1993;335:42–54.

160. Van der Beek EM, Horvath TL, Wiegant VM, et al. Evidence for a direct neuronal pathway from the suprachiasmatic nucleus to the gonadotropin-releasing hormone system: combined tracing and light and electron microscopic immunocytochemical studies. J Comp Neurol 1997;384:569–79.

161. Vrang N, Larsen PJ, Mikkelsen JD. Direct projection from the suprachiasmatic nucleus to hypophysiotrophic corticotropin-releasing factor immunoreactive cells in the paraventricular nucleus of the hypothalamus demonstrated by means of Phaseolus vulgaris-leucoagglutinin tract tracing. Brain Res 1995;684:61–9.

162. Bamshad M, Aoki VT, Adkison MG, et al. Central nervous system origins of the sympathetic nervous system outflow to white adipose tissue. Am J Physiol 1998;275:R291–9.

163. Buijs RM, Chun SJ, Niijima A, et al. Parasympathetic and sympathetic control of the pancreas: a role for the suprachiasmatic nucleus and other hypothalamic centers that are involved in the regulation of food intake. J Comp Neurol 2001; 431:405–23.

164. Buijs RM, la Fleur SE, Wortel J, et al. The suprachiasmatic nucleus balances sympathetic and parasympathetic output to peripheral organs

through separate preautonomic neurons. J Comp Neurol 2003;464:36–48.

165. la Fleur SE, Kalsbeek A, Wortel J, et al. Polysynaptic neural pathways between the hypothalamus, including the suprachiasmatic nucleus, and the liver. Brain Res 2000;871:50–6.

166. Niijima A, Nagai K, Nagai N, et al. Light enhances sympathetic and suppresses vagal outflows and lesions including the suprachiasmatic nucleus eliminate these changes in rats. J Auton Nerv Syst 1992;40:155–60.

167. Scheer FA, Ter Horst GJ, van Der Vliet J, et al. Physiological and anatomic evidence for regulation of the heart by suprachiasmatic nucleus in rats. Am J Physiol Heart Circ Physiol 2001;280: H1391–9.

168. Tousson E, Meissl H. Suprachiasmatic nuclei grafts restore the circadian rhythm in the paraventricular nucleus of the hypothalamus. J Neurosci 2004;24: 2983–8.

169. Guo H, Brewer JM, Champhekar A, et al. Differential control of peripheral circadian rhythms by suprachiasmatic-dependent neural signals. Proc Natl Acad Sci U S A 2005;102:3111–6.

170. Allen G, Rappe J, Earnest DJ, et al. Oscillating on borrowed time: diffusible signals from immortalized suprachiasmatic nucleus cells regulate circadian rhythmicity in cultured fibroblasts. J Neurosci 2001;21:7937–43.

171. Guo H, Brewer JM, Lehman MN, et al. Suprachiasmatic regulation of circadian rhythms of gene expression in hamster peripheral organs: effects of transplanting the pacemaker. J Neurosci 2006; 26:6406–12.

172. Hatcher NG, Atkins N Jr, Annangudi SP, et al. Mass spectrometry-based discovery of circadian peptides. Proc Natl Acad Sci U S A 2008;105: 12527–32.

173. Lee JE, Atkins N Jr, Hatcher NG, et al. Endogenous peptide discovery of the rat circadian clock: a focused study of the suprachiasmatic nucleus by ultrahigh performance tandem mass spectrometry. Mol Cell Proteomics 2010;9:285–97.

174. Aton SJ, Colwell CS, Harmar AJ, et al. Vasoactive intestinal polypeptide mediates circadian rhythmicity and synchrony in mammalian clock neurons. Nat Neurosci 2005;8:476–83.

175. Brown TM, Colwell CS, Waschek JA, et al. Disrupted neuronal activity rhythms in the suprachiasmatic nuclei of vasoactive intestinal polypeptide-deficient mice. J Neurophysiol 2007; 97:2553–8.

176. Gillette MU, Reppert SM. The hypothalamic suprachiasmatic nuclei: circadian patterns of vasopressin secretion and neuronal activity in vitro. Brain Res Bull 1987;19:135–9.

177. Hatton GI. Emerging concepts of structure-function dynamics in adult brain: the hypothalamo-neurohypophysial system. Prog Neurobiol 1990; 34:437–504.

178. Piggins HD, Antle MC, Rusak B. Neuropeptides phase shift the mammalian circadian pacemaker. J Neurosci 1995;15:5612–22.

179. Reppert SM, Artman HG, Swaminathan S, et al. Vasopressin exhibits a rhythmic daily pattern in cerebrospinal fluid but not in blood. Science 1981;213:1256–7.

180. Reppert SM, Perlow MJ, Artman HG, et al. The circadian rhythm of oxytocin in primate cerebrospinal fluid: effects of destruction of the suprachiasmatic nuclei. Brain Res 1984;307:384–7.

181. Kramer A, Yang FC, Snodgrass P, et al. Regulation of daily locomotor activity and sleep by hypothalamic EGF receptor signaling. Science 2001;294: 2511–5.

182. Cheng MY, Bullock CM, Li C, et al. Prokineticin 2 transmits the behavioural circadian rhythm of the suprachiasmatic nucleus. Nature 2002;417: 405–10.

183. Cailotto C, La Fleur SE, Van Heijningen C, et al. The suprachiasmatic nucleus controls the daily variation of plasma glucose via the autonomic output to the liver: are the clock genes involved? Eur J Neurosci 2005;22:2531–40.

184. Knutsson A. Health disorders of shift workers. Occup Med (Lond) 2003;53:103–8.

185. Mahoney MM. Shift work, jet lag, and female reproduction. Int J Endocrinol 2010;2010:813764.

186. Megdal SP, Kroenke CH, Laden F, et al. Night work and breast cancer risk: a systematic review and meta-analysis. Eur J Cancer 2005;41:2023–32.

187. Davidson AJ, Sellix MT, Daniel J, et al. Chronic jetlag increases mortality in aged mice. Curr Biol 2006;16:R914–6.

Genetics of Sleep Timing, Duration, and Homeostasis in Humans

Namni Goel, PhD

KEYWORDS

- Genetics • Sleep duration • Sleep homeostasis • Sleep deprivation • Circadian timing
- Individual differences

KEY POINTS

- The circadian biological clock interacts with sleep homeostatic drive.
- Stable, trait-like (phenotypic) individual differences in circadian and sleep measures as well as in neurobehavioral performance have motivated recent studies using candidate gene approaches to predict baseline (fully rested conditions) responses as well as responses to sleep loss (acute total and chronic partial sleep deprivation).
- Results from this growing database point to several important circadian and noncircadian genetic biomarkers involved in differential vulnerability to sleep loss.
- Actively searching for other potential genetic biomarkers, using candidate gene and genome-wide association study approaches, will allow effective prediction of response and use of countermeasures in response to sleep loss.

Both sleep and wakefulness are modulated by an endogenous biological clock located in the supra-chiasmatic nuclei (SCN) of the anterior hypothalamus. Beyond driving the body to fall asleep and to wake up, the biologic clock also modulates waking behavior, as reflected in sleepiness and cognitive performance, generating circadian rhythmicity in almost all neurobehavioral variables investigated to date.[1,2] Theoretical conceptualizations of the daily temporal modulation of sleep and wakefulness (and, to a lesser extent, the modulation of waking cognitive functions) have been instantiated in the 2-process mathematical model of sleep regulation[3,4] and its mathematical variants.[5] The 2-process model of sleep regulation has been applied to the temporal profiles of sleep[4,6] and wakefulness.[7] The model consists of a sleep homeostatic process (S) and a circadian process (C), which interact to determine the timing of sleep onset and offset, as well as the stability of waking neurocognitive functions.[1,2,8] The homeostatic process represents the drive for sleep that increases during wakefulness (as can be observed when wakefulness is maintained beyond habitual bedtime into the night and subsequent day) and decreases during sleep (which represents

A version of this article originally appeared in *Sleep Medicine Clinics Volume 6, Issue 2.*
The writing of this article was supported by National Space Biomedical Research Institute through NASA NCC 9-58, NIH NR004281, and CTRC UL1RR024134, and by a grant from the Institute for Translational Medicine and Therapeutics' (ITMAT) Transdisciplinary Program in Translational Medicine and Therapeutics. The project described was supported in part by grant number UL1RR024134 from the National Center for Research Resources. The content is solely the responsibility of the authors and does not necessarily represent the official views of the National Center for Research Resources or the National Institutes of Health.
The author has nothing to disclose.

Division of Sleep and Chronobiology, Department of Psychiatry, University of Pennsylvania Perelman School of Medicine, Philadelphia, PA 19104-6021, USA
E-mail address: goel@mail.med.upenn.edu

Sleep Med Clin 7 (2012) 443–454
http://dx.doi.org/10.1016/j.jsmc.2012.06.013
1556-407X/12/$ – see front matter © 2012 Elsevier Inc. All rights reserved.

recuperation obtained from sleep). When this homeostatic drive increases beyond a certain threshold, sleep is triggered; when it decreases below a different threshold, wakefulness is invoked. The circadian process represents daily oscillatory modulation of these threshold levels. It has been suggested that the circadian system actively promotes wakefulness more than sleep,[9] although this hypothesis is not universally accepted. The circadian drive for wakefulness may be experienced as spontaneously enhanced alertness in the early evening, even after a sleepless night. Sleep deprivation, however, can elevate homeostatic pressure to the point that waking cognitive functions are degraded even at the time of the peak circadian drive for wakefulness.[10] There are robust individual differences in both the sleep homeostatic and circadian processes, pointing to genetic underpinnings.

This article begins with a discussion of the genetic basis of circadian rhythms and the timing of sleep. It next briefly discusses the genetic basis of sleep in healthy adults, including observed individual variability in sleep parameters. Next, it discusses individual differences in the context of the total absence of sleep and the restriction of sleep as phenotypes, and recent studies using candidate gene approaches to identify genes that may relate to such responses. Future areas of research are also discussed.

GENETICS OF INDIVIDUAL DIFFERENCES IN CIRCADIAN RHYTHMS AND THE TIMING OF SLEEP

There are genetic underpinnings of individual differences in the circadian system, which are important for the timing of sleep. Morningness-eveningness (ie, the tendency to be a early "lark" or a late "owl") is perhaps the most frequently used measure of interindividual variation in circadian rhythmicity. Morning-type and evening-type individuals differ endogenously in the circadian phase of their biological clocks.[11,12] Self-report measures, such as the Horne-Östberg Morningness-Eveningness Questionnaire (MEQ)[13] and its variants (eg, Smith and colleagues[14]), and more recent scales such as the Munich Chrono-Type Questionnaire,[15,16] which differentiates timing of activities on workdays versus free days, are the most commonly used measures of circadian phase preference, mainly because of their convenience and cost-effectiveness.

Age influences morningness-eveningness, as shown in laboratory studies[17] and more naturalistic population-based settings (see reviews in Refs.[16,18]). In addition, gender also affects morningness-eveningness, whereby women show a greater skew toward morningness than men.[16,19,20] This circadian phase preference difference is an enduring trait, with a significant genetic basis.[21–23] Thus, chronotype represents a circadian rhythmicity phenotype in humans.[24]

The genetic basis of morningness-eveningness in the general population has been investigated in several core circadian genes, with mixed results.[25] For example, the 3111C allele of the CLOCK (Circadian Locomotor Output Cycles Kaput) gene 5′-untranslated region (5′-UTR) has been associated with eveningness and delayed sleep timing in some studies[26,27] but not others.[28–30] The variable number tandem repeat (VNTR) polymorphism in PERIOD3 (PER3), another core clock gene, has similarly been linked to diurnal preference, but not uniformly so.[31–36] Both the 111G polymorphism in the 5′-UTR of PERIOD2 (PER2) and the T2434C polymorphism of PERIOD1 (PER1) also have been associated with morning preference.[37,38] Because morningness-eveningness represents a continuum, this trait is likely polygenic, influenced by several genes, each contributing to the determination of circadian phase preference. Thus, further studies investigating other clock genes, as well as replication of the PER and CLOCK findings, are needed to establish the molecular genetic components of behavioral circadian phase preference.

Individual differences in morningness-eveningness (chronotype) can manifest in extreme cases classified as primary circadian rhythm sleep disorders (CRSDs), with altered phase relationships of the biologic clock to the light-dark cycle, including alterations in sleep timing.[39,40] Thus, extreme eveningness is believed to result in CRSD, delayed sleep phase type (typically referred to as delayed sleep phase disorder [DSPD][40]), whereas extreme morningness can manifest as CRSD, advanced sleep phase type[39] (typically referred to as advanced sleep phase disorder [ASPD][40]). The extent to which these phase-displacement disorders reflect differences in endogenous circadian period, entrainment, amplitude, coupling, and other aspects of clock neurobiology has received recent attention.

The genetic basis of DSPD and ASPD has been investigated in recent years, with both disorders having links to core clock genes.[25] DSPD, the most common circadian rhythm sleep disorder in the general population, is characterized by an inability to fall asleep at the desired and "normal" time of day; the average onset of sleep in DSPD occurs in the early morning (3 AM–6 AM), and the average wake-up time occurs in the late morning to early afternoon (11 AM–2 PM).[40] DSPD also may be characterized by a longer than normal tau (25.38 hours).[41] The VNTR polymorphism in

PER3 is associated with DSPD in large-sample studies,[31,32,34] and the 3111C allele of the *CLOCK* gene 5′-UTR region also has been related to DSPD.[26] A specific haplotype of *PER3*, which includes the polymorphism G647, is also associated positively with DSPD,[34] whereas the N408 allele of casein kinase I ε (*CK1ε*) may protect against the development of DSPD.[42]

ASPD is a rare disorder characterized by advanced sleep onsets of 3 to 4 hours and wake times relative to desired, normal times.[40,43] It may be characterized by a shorter than normal tau (23.3 hours).[44] In 1 study, ASPD was associated with a mutation in *PER2*,[45] although this mutation is not found in all families with this disorder.[46] Another study has implicated mutations in casein kinase I δ (*CK1δ*) in ASPD.[47] Future studies on additional core clock genes are needed to determine other mutations that may underlie this disorder.

Morningness-eveningness and differences in circadian phase preference are reflected in the diurnal course of neurobehavioral variables (as reviewed by Kerkhof[48]); some people perform consistently better in the morning, whereas others are more alert and perform better in the evening. How genetic variants underlying morningness-eveningness and disorders of chronotype affect performance and alertness under normal and sleep-deprived conditions remains a new field of investigation. Recent studies[35,36,49] have shown that the longer, 5-repeat allele of the VNTR polymorphism in *PER3*, a clock gene linked to diurnal preference and DSPD, may be associated with higher sleep propensity both at baseline and after total sleep deprivation (TSD), and worse cognitive performance following TSD and higher sleep propensity during chronic partial sleep deprivation (PSD) (these studies are discussed in more detail later). The role of other clock gene polymorphisms, such as the 3111C allele of the *CLOCK* gene in response to TSD and to chronic PSD, remain unknown and are worthy of investigation.

Six core clock genes (*PER1*, *PER2*, *PER3*, *CLOCK*, *CK1δ*, and *CK1ε*) have thus far been associated with interindividual differences in diurnal preference or its extreme variants. This active area of research has promising implications for objectively detecting individual differences in circadian disorders and determining situations and lifestyles that adversely affect the timing of sleep and sleep homeostasis.

GENETICS OF SLEEP

Sleep is a highly complex trait that involves many genes and their interactions with environmental factors. In humans, research dating back to as early as the 1930s using twins has indicated a strong genetic basis underlying the regulation of normal sleep, including sleep duration, sleep onset, sleep quality, and sleep homeostasis (reviewed in Refs.[50–52]). In addition, in 2008, 2 studies in normal sleepers found strong heritability of the sleep electroencephalogram (EEG) power spectrum, underscoring prior studies indicating that, although the sleep EEG is consistent across nights in the same individual, it differs among individuals.[53,54] The genetic nature of sleep EEG is also observed across a variety of frequencies indicating trait-like features.[55–60] Moreover, waking EEG patterns are also highly heritable (reviewed by Tafti[52]). Of note, familial linkage studies on EEG traits are currently lacking (reviewed in Refs.[50,61]).

More recently, candidate gene studies have investigated the role of specific genes in the regulation of sleep. For example, a point mutation in the *DEC2* gene, believed to function in the circadian clock as a repressor of Clock/Bmal1, is associated with a short sleep duration phenotype (average 6.25 hours vs 8.06 hours of self-reported sleep) that is characterized by an earlier non-workday habitual sleep offset time, with normal onset time, in 2 adults.[62] Moreover, the insertion of this point mutation into mice also decreased sleep time without affecting tau. Future studies should determine the role of this *DEC2* mutation in individuals undergoing sleep deprivation and in studies using EEG and slow wave activity (SWA) physiologic sleep assessments for sleep duration, sleep homeostasis, and other related variables. By contrast, a recent study found that a polymorphism within intron 8 of the dopamine transporter 1 (*DAT1*) gene failed to correlate with the interindividual variability of basal polysomnographic sleep architecture, including slow wave sleep latency, rapid eye movement (REM) sleep latency, sleep efficiency, and sleep stage percentages (stages 1, 2, SWS, or REM) in a group of unrelated healthy men.[63]

CANDIDATE GENE STUDIES OF SLEEP DEPRIVATION

Beyond these studies, which assess habitual sleep or 1 night of baseline sleep, candidate gene studies have been used to study basal (fully rested) sleep and responses to sleep loss. This approach was motivated by the results of studies that indicated that there are stable phenotypic individual differences in response to sleep deprivation.

Subjects undergoing TSD display differential vulnerability to sleep loss, showing robust interindividual differences in response to the same laboratory conditions, as measured by various physiologic and subjective sleep measures and neurobehavioral tasks sensitive to sleep loss.[59,64–68] Approximately one third of healthy adults are highly vulnerable to the neurobehavioral effects of sleep deprivation, another third are vulnerable, and the remaining third are much less vulnerable. These stable (phenotypic) differences in neurobehavioral responses to sleep deprivation are not reliably accounted for by demographic factors (eg, age, sex, Intelligence quotient), by baseline functioning, by various aspects of habitual sleep timing, by circadian chronotype, or by any other investigated factor.[10,64,69,70]

Such differential vulnerability extends to chronic PSD—a condition associated with a wide range of serious health consequences and experienced by millions of people on a consecutive and daily basis[71,72]—in which sleep is restricted to 3 to 7 hours in bed per night.[49,70,73,74]

At present, it remains unknown whether the same individuals vulnerable to the adverse effects of acute TSD are also vulnerable to chronic PSD. The few reports comparing responses to both acute TSD and chronic PSD have used small sample sizes (9–13 subjects) and limited assessments,[70,75,76] and only 1[75] has systematically studied the same subjects in both types of sleep loss.

The stable, trait-like interindividual differences observed in response to TSD[64–67]—with intraclass correlations (which express the proportion of variance in the data that is explained by systematic interindividual variability) ranging from 58% to 92% for neurobehavioral measures[64,67]—strongly suggest an underlying genetic component. Despite this link, however, relatively little is known about the genetic basis of differential vulnerability in healthy subjects undergoing deprivation. Furthermore, as mentioned earlier, because of reported differences in sleep homeostatic, physiologic, and behavioral responses to chronic PSD and acute TSD,[70,75,76] it is likely that specific candidate genes play different roles in the degree of vulnerability and/or resilience to the sleep homeostatic and neurobehavioral effects of acute TSD and chronic PSD. These compelling questions have produced a rapidly emerging and promising field of scientific investigation; recent studies have thus far focused on several select candidate genes, which are reviewed later.

PERIOD3 VNTR Polymorphism

Three related studies investigated the role of the VNTR polymorphism of the circadian gene PERIOD3 (PER3)—which shows similar allelic frequencies in African Americans and white people[77,78] and is characterized by a 54-nucleotide coding region motif repeating in 4 or 5 units—in response to TSD using a small group of the same subjects specifically recruited for the homozygotic versions of this polymorphism. Compared with the 4-repeat allele (PER3$^{4/4}$; 14 subjects), the longer, 5-repeat allele (PER3$^{5/5}$; 10 subjects) was associated with higher sleep propensity including SWA in the sleep EEG both before and after TSD and worse cognitive performance, as assessed by a composite score of 12 tests, following TSD.[35] A subsequent report using the same 24 subjects clarified that the PER3$^{5/5}$ overall performance deficits were selective: they only occurred on certain executive function tests, and only at 2 to 4 hours following the melatonin rhythm peak, from approximately 6 to 8 AM.[36] Such performance differences were hypothesized to be mediated by sleep homeostasis.[35,36] Another publication using the same subjects showed that the PER3$^{5/5}$ subjects had more slow-wave sleep and elevated sympathetic predominance and a reduction of parasympathetic activity during baseline sleep.[79] These studies found no significant differences in the melatonin and cortisol circadian rhythms, PER3 mRNA levels, or in a self-report morningness-eveningness measure,[35,36] although another study using these same subjects found that PER3 expression and sleep timing were more strongly correlated in PER3$^{5/5}$ subjects.[80]

A recent neuroimaging study found that 27 healthy subjects categorized according to homozygosity for the PER3 VNTR genotype (15 PER3$^{4/4}$ subjects, 12 PER3$^{5/5}$ subjects) showed markedly different cerebral blood flow profiles using blood oxygenation level–dependent functional magnetic resonance imaging (BOLD fMRI) and corresponding differences in vulnerability of executive function performance in response to TSD.[81] More studies examining the relationship of the neural mechanisms mediating trait-like differential vulnerability to sleep deprivation with selective candidate genes (beyond the PER3 VNTR polymorphism) are warranted.

The PER3 findings in TSD may not generalize to responses to chronic PSD. My colleagues and I recently evaluated whether the PER3 VNTR polymorphism contributed to sleep homeostatic responses and cumulative neurobehavioral deficits during chronic PSD in PER3$^{4/4}$, PER3$^{4/5}$, and PER3$^{5/5}$ healthy adults.[49] During chronic PSD, PER3$^{5/5}$ subjects had slightly, but reliably, elevated sleep homeostatic pressure as measured by non-REM (NREM) slow wave energy (SWE) compared with one PER3$^{4/4}$ subjects (Fig. 1). The PER3$^{4/4}$,

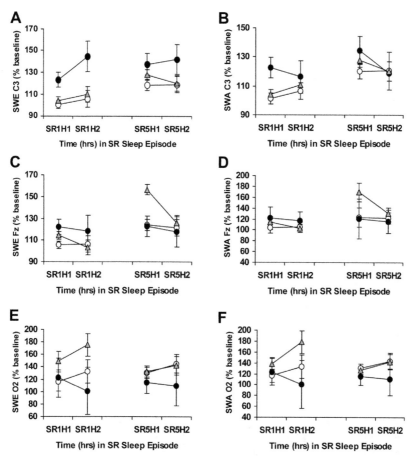

Fig. 1. SWE and SWA during chronic PSD for the *PER3* genotypes. Mean (± standard error of the mean [SEM]) hourly SWE and SWA as a percentage of baseline at the same corresponding hour derived from the C3 (*A, B*), Fz (*C, D*), or O2 (*E, F*) channels at PSD/restriction night 1 (SR1) and partial sleep deprivation/restriction night 5 (SR5) for hour 1 (H1) and hour 2 (H2) in *PER3*[4/4] (*open circles*), *PER3*[4/5] (*gray triangles*), and *PER3*[5/5] (*closed circles*) subjects. SWE derived from C3 (but not from Fz or O2) was significantly higher during chronic PSD in *PER3*[5/5] subjects compared with *PER3*[4/4] and *PER3*[4/5] subjects. (*From* Goel N, Banks S, Mignot E, et al. PER3 polymorphism predicts cumulative sleep homeostatic but not neurobehavioral changes to chronic partial sleep deprivation. PLoS ONE 2009;4:10; with permission.)

PER3[4/5] and *PER3*[5/5] genotypes also demonstrated large, but equivalent, cumulative increases in sleepiness and cumulative decreases in cognitive performance and physiologic alertness, with increasing daily intersubject variability in all genotypes. In contrast to the aforementioned data in TSD,[35,36] the *PER3* VNTR variants did not differ in baseline sleep measures or in their physiologic sleepiness, cognitive, executive functioning, or subjective responses to chronic PSD. Thus, the *PER3* VNTR polymorphism does not appear to be a genetic marker of differential vulnerability to the cumulative neurobehavioral effects of chronic PSD. It remains possible, however, that the *PER3*[5/5] genotype may contribute to differential neurobehavioral vulnerability to acute TSD because it involves wakefulness at a specific circadian time in the early morning

hours (6–8 AM), when subjects in the PSD study were asleep.[49]

DQB1*0602 Allele

The human leukocyte antigen *DQB1*0602* allele is closely associated with narcolepsy, a sleep disorder characterized by excessive daytime sleepiness, fragmented sleep, and shortened REM latency, although it is neither necessary nor sufficient for its development.[82,83]

In 1 large study, *DQB1*0602*-positive healthy sleepers showed shorter nighttime REM sleep latency, greater sleep continuity, and more REM sleep, but no differences in daytime sleepiness.[82] Positivity for *DQB1*0602* was also related to more sleep-onset REM sleep periods and greater REM sleep duration during naps.[84] Thus, *DQB1*0602*-positive subjects displayed subclinical presentations of some sleep features that were reminiscent of narcolepsy.

My colleagues and I recently evaluated whether *DQB1*0602* was a novel biomarker of differential vulnerability to homeostatic, sleepiness, and neurobehavioral deficits during chronic PSD in healthy sleepers positive and negative for *DQB1*0602*.[73] *DQB1*0602*-positive subjects showed decreased sleep homeostatic pressure with differentially steeper declines (**Fig. 2**), and greater sleepiness and fatigue during baseline.

During chronic PSD, positive subjects displayed SWE increases comparable with negative subjects (**Fig. 3**), despite higher sleepiness and fatigue. *DQB1*0602*-positive subjects also had more fragmented sleep during baseline and PSD and showed differentially greater REM sleep latency reductions and smaller stage 2 reductions, along with differentially greater increases in fatigue. Both groups showed comparable cumulative decreases in cognitive performance and increases in physiologic sleepiness to chronic PSD, and did not differ on executive function tasks.

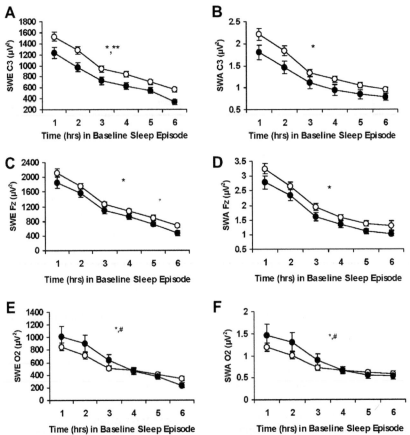

Fig. 2. Hourly SWE and SWA during baseline for the *DQB1*0602* groups. Mean (±SEM) hourly SWE and SWA derived from the C3 (*A, B*), Fz (*C, D*), or O2 (*E, F*) channels during baseline for *DQB1*0602* negative subjects (*open circles*) and *DQB1*0602* positive subjects (*closed circles*). SWE derived from C3 was lower in *DQB1*0602* positive subjects (denoted by **, $P<.05$); SWA derived from C3 and SWE and SWA derived from the Fz channel showed similar trends. As expected, SWE and SWA showed a typical pattern of dissipation across the baseline night in all 3 channels for both groups (denoted by *, $P<.05$); moreover, *DQB1*0602* positive subjects showed sharper declines in sleep pressure derived from the O2 channel during the first few hours of the night than *DQB1*0602* negative subjects (denoted by #, $P<.05$). In some records, EEG signal quality was insufficient or contained too much artifact for reliable power spectral analysis. Thus, the final sample sizes were: for C3, *DQB1*0602* negative (n = 68) and positive (n = 24) subjects; for Fz, *DQB1*0602* negative (n = 70) and positive (n = 28) subjects; for O2, *DQB1*0602* negative (n = 74) and positive (n = 27) subjects. (*From* Goel N, Banks S, Mignot E, et al. DQB1*0602 predicts interindividual differences in physiologic sleep, sleepiness and fatigue. Neurology 2010;75:1512; with permission.)

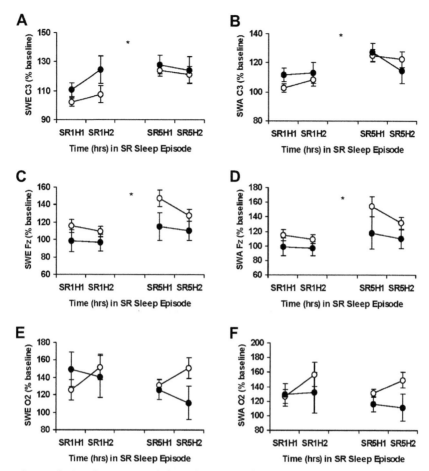

Fig. 3. SWE and SWA during chronic partial sleep deprivation for the *DQB1*0602* groups. Mean (±SEM) hourly SWE and SWA as a percentage of baseline at the same corresponding hour derived from the C3 (*A, B*), Fz (*C, D*), or O2 (*E, F*) channels at SR1 and SR5 for H1 and H2 for *DQB1*0602* negative subjects (*open circles*) and *DQB1*0602* positive subjects (*closed circles*). SWE and SWA increased from SR1 to SR5 for the C3 and Fz channels (denoted by *, *P*<.05). There were no group differences or differential changes across nights. In some records, EEG signal quality was insufficient or contained too much artifact for reliable power spectral analysis. Thus, the final sample sizes were: for SR1 and SR5 C3, *DQB1*0602* negative (n = 72) and positive (n = 28) subjects; for SR1 and SR5 Fz, *DQB1*0602* negative (n = 72) and positive (n = 27) subjects; for SR1 and SR5 O2, *DQB1*0602* negative (n = 72) and positive (n = 26) subjects. (*From* Goel N, Banks S, Mignot E, et al. DQB1*0602 predicts interindividual differences in physiologic sleep, sleepiness and fatigue. Neurology 2010;75:1513; with permission.)

Thus, *DQB1*0602* is associated with interindividual differences in sleep homeostasis, physiologic sleep, sleepiness and fatigue, but not cognitive responses, during baseline and PSD. *DQB1*0602* may be a genetic marker for predicting such individual differences in both basal (fully rested) and sleep loss conditions; moreover, its positivity in healthy subjects may represent a continuum of some sleep-wake features of narcolepsy. The influence of the *DQB1*0602* allele on sleep homeostatic and neurobehavioral responses has not yet been examined in healthy subjects undergoing acute TSD, or replicated in an independent sample of individuals undergoing chronic PSD.

Catechol O-Methyltransferase Val158Met Polymorphism

The valine158methionine (Val158Met) polymorphism of the catechol O-methyltransferase (*COMT* gene), replaces valine (*Val*) with methionine (*Met*) at codon 158 of the *COMT* protein. As a result of this common substitution, activity of the *COMT* enzyme, which modulates dopaminergic catabolism in the prefrontal cortex (PFC), is reduced 3- fold to-4-fold in *COMT Met* carriers compared with *Val* carriers, translating into more dopamine availability at the receptors and higher cortical dopamine concentrations.[85] This *COMT* polymorphism functionally predicts less efficient prefrontal cortex functioning and poor working memory performance in healthy subjects[86–89] who have the high-activity *Val* allele.

In sleep and neurodegenerative disorders, the *COMT* Val158Met polymorphism has been linked to daytime sleepiness. *Val/Val* female narcoleptic patients fell asleep 2 times faster than the *Val/Met* or *Met/Met* genotypes during the multiple sleep latency test (MSLT), whereas the opposite was true for men.[90] *Met/Met* narcoleptic patients also showed more sleep-onset REM periods during the MSLT, whereas *Val/Val* subjects showed less sleep paralysis[90] and were more responsive to modafinil's stimulating effects.[91] *Met/Met* and *Val/Met* Parkinson disease patients showed higher subjective daytime sleepiness than *Val/Val* subjects.[92]

In healthy men, the *COMT* Val158Met polymorphism is associated with sleep physiology. In acute TSD, the polymorphism predicted interindividual differences in brain α oscillations in wakefulness and 11-Hz to 13-Hz EEG activity in wakefulness, REM and non-REM sleep.[93] It also modulated the effects of the wake-promoting drug modafinil on subjective well-being, sustained vigilant attention and executive functioning, and on 3.0-Hz to 6.75-Hz and greater than 16.75-Hz activity in non-REM sleep, but was not associated with subjective sleepiness, SWA, or slow wave sleep changes in recovery sleep following TSD or at baseline.[94,95] Current studies are underway to investigate whether the *COMT* Val158Met polymorphism contributes to sleep homeostatic and cumulative neurobehavioral responses during basal (fully rested) conditions and during chronic PSD in *Met/Met*, *Val/Met*, and *Val/Val* healthy adult sleepers.

Adenosine-Related Polymorphisms

Other studies have investigated the role of select adenosine-related candidate genes in individual differences and in response to acute TSD. Rétey and colleagues[96] found that the 22G → A polymorphism of the adenosine deaminase gene (*ADA*) was associated with enhanced slow wave sleep and NREM SWA, contributing to interindividual variability in baseline sleep. Individuals with the *G/A* genotype (7 subjects) showed 30 minutes more slow wave sleep than subjects with the *G/G* genotype (7 subjects) and, consistent with this finding, SWA was higher in subjects with *G/A* than *G/G*. This study did not test responses of these individuals to sleep deprivation and thus it remains unknown whether these genotypes show differential sleep homeostatic responses under evoked phenotypic deprivation conditions. This

group also found that the c.1083T>C polymorphism of the adenosine A2A receptor gene (*ADORA2A*) related to objective and subjective differences in the effects of caffeine on NREM sleep after TSD[97] and associated with individual differences in various measures of baseline EEG during sleep and wakefulness.[96] Although promising, replication of these data in independent samples is needed; in addition, the role of these 2 genetic variants in response to chronic PSD has not yet been established.

Thus, several common genetic polymorphisms involved in circadian, sleep-wake, and cognitive regulation seem to underlie interindividual differences in basal (fully rested) sleep parameters and homeostatic regulation of sleep in response to sleep deprivation (both chronic restriction and acute TSD) in healthy adults.

GENOME-WIDE ASSOCIATION STUDIES OF HUMAN SLEEP

To date, only 1 study has used a genome-wide association approach to examine phenotypic-genotypic interactions in healthy human sleepers.[98] Moderate heritability estimates for self-rated sleepiness (29%; assessed by the Epworth Sleepiness Scale) and for habitual sleep duration (17%) and habitual bedtime (22%), assessed by a standard questionnaire used in the Sleep Heart Health Study, were found in 749 subjects. The genome-wide analysis revealed that habitual bedtime and sleep duration were modulated by genetic loci containing circadian clock–related genes including casein kinase 2A2 (*CSNK2A2*), prokineticin 2 (*PROK2*), and *CLOCK*. Furthermore, genes encoding *NPSRI* and *PDE4D* were identified as possible mediators of habitual bedtime and subjective sleepiness, respectively. Although intriguing, these data need to be replicated and extended to studies that include physiologic measures of sleep.

FUTURE DIRECTIONS

With the exception of 2 recent studies,[49,73] all candidate gene studies involving sleep physiologic and neurobehavioral responses to sleep loss have used small sample sizes (14–24 subjects) and have only examined homozygotic individuals.[35,36,93,94,96,97] Larger sample sizes and assessment of phenotype-genotype relationships in both homozygous and heterozygous individuals are needed to definitively determine whether such candidate genes involved in regulation of sleep-wake, circadian, and cognitive functions are associated with interindividual neurobehavioral responses to sleep loss across a population. This question is particularly critical because individuals are necessarily categorized into different genotypes, reducing sample sizes in each subgroup. Future candidate gene studies therefore must consistently use sample sizes in the hundreds, rather than tens, to detect statistically reliable differences across genotypes.

In addition, replication of findings in independent samples is needed to determine whether findings are genuine and not due to chance; ideally, studies should also be replicated in different ethnic groups to increase generalizability of the findings. Genome-wide association studies using physiologic sleep measures as outcomes are also needed to assess basal (fully rested) individual differences as well as responses to sleep deprivation; however, these will likely require data from several laboratories, given the expense, time, and effort needed to conduct such rigorous studies.

Searching for genetic markers of basal sleep measures and of sleep homeostatic and neurobehavioral differential vulnerability to sleep deprivation is an active and scientifically profitable area of research. Among other advantages, identification of such markers will provide a viable means to identify those individuals in the general population who may need more habitual sleep or who may need to prevent or mitigate sleep deprivation through lifestyle choices and effective interventions and countermeasures.

REFERENCES

1. Van Dongen HP, Dinges DF. Investigating the interaction between the homeostatic and circadian processes of sleep-wake regulation for the prediction of waking neurobehavioral performance. J Sleep Res 2003;12:181–7.
2. Goel N, Van Dongen HPA, Dinges DF. Circadian rhythms in sleepiness, alertness, and performance. In: Kryger MH, Dement WC, Roth T, editors. Principles and practice of sleep medicine. 5th edition. Philadelphia: Elsevier; 2011. p. 445–55.
3. Achermann P, Dijk DJ, Brunner DP, et al. A model of human sleep homeostasis based on EEG slow-wave activity; quantitative comparison of data and simulations. Brain Res Bull 1993;31:97–113.
4. Borbély AA. A two process model of sleep regulation. Hum Neurobiol 1982;1:195–204.
5. Mallis MM, Mejdal S, Nguyen TT, et al. Summary of the key features of seven biomathematical models of human fatigue and performance. Aviat Space Environ Med 2004;75:A4–14.
6. Daan S, Beersma DG, Borbély AA. Timing of human sleep: recovery process gated by a circadian pacemaker. Am J Physiol 1984;246:R161–78.
7. Achermann P, Borbély AA. Simulation of daytime vigilance by the additive interaction of a homeostatic and a circadian process. Biol Cybern 1994;71:115–21.
8. Khalsa SB, Jewett ME, Duffy JF, et al. The timing of the human circadian clock is accurately represented by the core body temperature rhythm following phase shifts to a three-cycle light stimulus near the critical zone. J Biol Rhythms 2000;15:524–30.
9. Edgar DM, Dement WC, Fuller CA. Effect of SCN lesions on sleep in squirrel monkeys: evidence for opponent processes in sleep-wake regulation. J Neurosci 1993;13:1065–79.
10. Doran SM, Van Dongen HP, Dinges DF. Sustained attention performance during sleep deprivation: evidence of state instability. Arch Ital Biol 2001; 139:253–67.
11. Kerkhof GA, Van Dongen HP. Morning-type and evening-type individuals differ in the phase position of their endogenous circadian oscillator. Neurosci Lett 1996;218:153–6.
12. Baehr EK, Revelle W, Eastman CI. Individual differences in the phase and amplitude of the human circadian temperature rhythm: with an emphasis on morningness-eveningness. J Sleep Res 2000;9: 117–27.
13. Horne JA, Östberg O. A self-assessment questionnaire to determine morningness–eveningness in human circadian rhythms. Int J Chronobiol 1976;4: 97–110.
14. Smith CS, Reilly D, Midkiff K. Evaluation of three circadian rhythm questionnaires with suggestions for an improved measure of morningness. J Appl Psychol 1989;74:728–38.
15. Roenneberg T, Wirz-Justice A, Merrow M. Life between clocks: daily temporal patterns of human chronotypes. J Biol Rhythms 2003;18:80–90.
16. Roenneberg T, Kuehnle T, Juda M, et al. Epidemiology of the human circadian clock. Sleep Med Rev 2007;11:429–38.
17. Duffy JF, Dijk DJ, Klerman EB, et al. Later endogenous circadian temperature nadir relative to an earlier wake time in older people. Am J Physiol 1998;275:R1478–87.
18. Foster RG, Roenneberg T. Human responses to the geophysical daily, annual and lunar cycles. Curr Biol 2008;18:R784–94.
19. Adan A, Natale V. Gender differences in morningness–eveningness preference. Chronobiol Int 2002; 19:709–20.
20. Randler C. Gender differences in morningness–eveningness assessed by self-report questionnaires: a meta-analysis. Pers Individ Dif 2007;43: 1667–75.
21. Hur YM. Stability of genetic influence on morningness-eveningness: a cross-sectional examination of South Korean twins from preadolescence to young adulthood. J Sleep Res 2007;16:17–23.

22. Hur YM, Bouchard TJ Jr, Lykken DT. Genetic and environmental influence on morningness–eveningness. Pers Individ Dif 1998;25:917–25.

23. Vink JM, Groot AS, Kerkhof GA, et al. Genetic analysis of morningness and eveningness. Chronobiol Int 2001;18:809–22.

24. Van Dongen HP, Kerkhof GA, Dinges DF. Human circadian rhythms. In: Sehgal A, editor. Molecular biology of circadian rhythms. New York: John Wiley; 2004. p. 255–69.

25. Takahashi JS, Hong HK, Ko CH, et al. The genetics of mammalian circadian order and disorder: implications for physiology and disease. Nat Rev Genet 2008;9:764–75.

26. Katzenberg D, Young T, Finn L, et al. A CLOCK polymorphism associated with human diurnal preference. Sleep 1998;21:569–76.

27. Mishima K, Tozawa T, Satoh K, et al. The 3111T/C polymorphism of hClock is associated with evening preference and delayed sleep timing in a Japanese population sample. Am J Med Genet B Neuropsychiatr Genet 2005;133:101–4.

28. Robilliard DL, Archer SN, Arendt J, et al. The 3111 Clock gene polymorphism is not associated with sleep and circadian rhythmicity in phenotypically characterized human subjects. J Sleep Res 2002; 11:305–12.

29. Iwase T, Kajimura N, Uchiyama M, et al. Mutation screening of the human Clock gene in circadian rhythm sleep disorders. Psychiatry Res 2002;109: 121–8.

30. Pedrazzoli M, Louzada FM, Pereira DS, et al. Clock polymorphisms and circadian rhythms phenotypes in a sample of the Brazilian population. Chronobiol Int 2007;24:1–8.

31. Archer SN, Robilliard DL, Skene DJ, et al. A length polymorphism in the circadian clock gene PER3 is linked to delayed sleep phase syndrome and extreme diurnal preference. Sleep 2003;26:413–5.

32. Pereira DS, Tufik S, Louzada FM, et al. Association of the length polymorphism in the human PER3 gene with the delayed sleep-phase syndrome: does latitude have an influence upon it? Sleep 2005;28:29–32.

33. Jones KH, Ellis J, von Schantz M, et al. Age-related change in the association between a polymorphism in the PER3 gene and preferred timing of sleep and waking activities. J Sleep Res 2007;16:12–6.

34. Ebisawa T, Uchiyama M, Kajimura N, et al. Association of structural polymorphisms in the human period3 gene with delayed sleep phase syndrome. EMBO Rep 2001;2:342–6.

35. Viola AU, Archer SN, James LM, et al. PER3 polymorphism predicts sleep structure and waking performance. Curr Biol 2007;17:613–8.

36. Groeger JA, Viola AU, Lo JC, et al. Early morning executive functioning during sleep deprivation is compromised by a PERIOD3 polymorphism. Sleep 2008;31:1159–67.

37. Carpen JD, Archer SN, Skene DJ, et al. A single-nucleotide polymorphism in the 5'-untranslated region of the hPER2 gene is associated with diurnal preference. J Sleep Res 2005;14:293–7.

38. Carpen JD, von Schantz M, Smits M, et al. A silent polymorphism in the PER1 gene associates with extreme diurnal preference in humans. J Hum Genet 2006;51:1122–5.

39. The International Classification of Sleep Disorders: diagnostic and coding manual. 2nd edition. Westchester (NY): American Academy of Sleep Medicine; 2005.

40. Sack RL, Auckley D, Auger RR, et al. Circadian rhythm sleep disorders: part II, advanced sleep phase disorder, delayed sleep phase disorder, free-running disorder, and irregular sleep-wake rhythm. An American Academy of Sleep Medicine review. Sleep 2007;30:1484–501.

41. Campbell SS, Murphy PJ. Delayed sleep phase disorder in temporal isolation. Sleep 2007;30:1225–8.

42. Takano A, Uchiyama M, Kajimura N, et al. A missense variation in human casein kinase I epsilon gene that induces functional alteration and shows an inverse association with circadian rhythm sleep disorders. Neuropsychopharmacology 2004; 29:1901–9.

43. Reid KJ, Chang AM, Dubocovich ML, et al. Familial advanced sleep phase syndrome. Arch Neurol 2001;58:1089–94.

44. Jones CR, Campbell SS, Zone SE, et al. Familial advanced sleep-phase syndrome: a short-period circadian rhythm variant in humans. Nat Med 1999; 5:1062–5.

45. Toh KL, Jones CR, He Y, et al. An hPer2 phosphorylation site mutation in familial advanced sleep phase syndrome. Science 2001;291:1040–3.

46. Satoh K, Mishima K, Inoue Y, et al. Two pedigrees of familial advanced sleep phase syndrome in Japan. Sleep 2003;26:416–7.

47. Xu Y, Padiath QS, Shapiro RE, et al. Functional consequences of a CKIdelta mutation causing familial advanced sleep phase syndrome. Nature 2005;434:640–4.

48. Kerkhof GA. Inter-individual differences in the human circadian system: a review. Biol Psychol 1985;20:83–112.

49. Goel N, Banks S, Mignot E, et al. PER3 polymorphism predicts cumulative sleep homeostatic but not neurobehavioral changes to chronic partial sleep deprivation. PLoS ONE 2009;4:e5874.

50. Dauvilliers Y, Maret S, Tafti M. Genetics of normal and pathological sleep in humans. Sleep Med Rev 2005;9:91–100.

51. Tafti M, Maret S, Dauvilliers Y. Genes for normal sleep and sleep disorders. Ann Med 2005;37:580–9.

52. Tafti M. Genetic aspects of normal and disturbed sleep. Sleep Med 2009;10(Suppl 1):S17–21.

53. Ambrosius U, Lietzenmaier S, Wehrle R, et al. Heritability of sleep electroencephalogram. Biol Psychiatry 2008;64:344–8.

54. De Gennaro L, Marzano C, Fratello F, et al. The electroencephalographic fingerprint of sleep is genetically determined: a twin study. Ann Neurol 2008; 64:455–60.

55. Werth E, Achermann P, Dijk DJ, et al. Spindle frequency activity in the sleep EEG: individual differences and topographic distribution. Electroencephalogr Clin Neurophysiol 1997;103:535–42.

56. Tan X, Campbell IG, Palagini L, et al. High internight reliability of computer-measured NREM delta, sigma, and beta: biological implications. Biol Psychiatry 2000;48:1010–9.

57. Finelli LA, Achermann P, Borbely AA. Individual 'fingerprints' in human sleep EEG topography. Neuropsychopharmacol 2001;25:S57–62.

58. De Gennaro L, Ferrara M, Vecchio F, et al. An electroencephalographic fingerprint of human sleep. Neuroimage 2005;26:114–22.

59. Tucker AM, Dinges DF, Van Dongen HP. Trait interindividual differences in the sleep physiology of healthy young adults. J Sleep Res 2007;16:170–80.

60. Buckelmuller J, Landolt HP, Stassen HH, et al. Trait-like individual differences in the human sleep electroencephalogram. Neuroscience 2006;138:351–6.

61. Andretic R, Franken P, Tafti M. Genetics of sleep. Annu Rev Genet 2008;42:361–88.

62. He Y, Jones CR, Fujiki N, et al. The transcriptional repressor DEC2 regulates sleep length in mammals. Science 2009;325:866–70.

63. Guindalini C, Martins RC, Andersen ML, et al. Influence of genotype on dopamine transporter availability in human striatum and sleep architecture. Psychiatry Res 2010;179:238–40.

64. Van Dongen HP, Baynard MD, Maislin G, et al. Systematic interindividual differences in neurobehavioral impairment from sleep loss: evidence of trait-like differential vulnerability. Sleep 2004;27:423–33.

65. Leproult R, Colecchia EF, Berardi AM, et al. Individual differences in subjective and objective alertness during sleep deprivation are stable and unrelated. Am J Physiol Regul Integr Comp Physiol 2003;284:R280–90.

66. Van Dongen HP, Dinges DF. Sleep, circadian rhythms, and psychomotor vigilance performance. Clin Sports Med 2005;24:237–49.

67. Van Dongen HP, Maislin G, Dinges DF. Dealing with interindividual differences in the temporal dynamics of fatigue and performance: importance and techniques. Aviat Space Environ Med 2004;75(3 Suppl):A147–54.

68. Frey DJ, Badia P, Wright KP Jr. Inter- and intra-individual variability in performance near the circadian nadir during sleep deprivation. J Sleep Res 2004;13:305–15.

69. Van Dongen HP, Dijkman MV, Maislin G, et al. Phenotypic aspect of vigilance decrement during sleep deprivation. Physiologist 1999;42:A-5.

70. Van Dongen HP, Maislin G, Mullington JM, et al. The cumulative cost of additional wakefulness: dose-response effects on neurobehavioral functions and sleep physiology from chronic sleep restriction and total sleep deprivation. Sleep 2003;26:117–26.

71. Banks S, Dinges DF. Behavioral and physiological consequences of sleep restriction in humans. J Clin Sleep Med 2007;3:519–28.

72. Goel N, Rao H, Durmer JS, et al. Neurocognitive consequences of sleep deprivation. Semin Neurol 2009;29:320–39.

73. Goel N, Banks S, Mignot E, et al. DQB1*0602 predicts interindividual differences in physiologic sleep, sleepiness and fatigue. Neurology 2010;75: 1509–19.

74. Bliese PD, Wesensten NJ, Balkin TJ. Age and individual variability in performance during sleep restriction. J Sleep Res 2006;15:376–85.

75. Drake CL, Roehrs TA, Burduvali E, et al. Effects of rapid versus slow accumulation of eight hours of sleep loss. Psychophysiology 2001;38:979–87.

76. Rowland LM, Thomas ML, Thorne DR, et al. Oculomotor responses during partial and total sleep deprivation. Aviat Space Environ Med 2005;76: C104–13.

77. Nadkarni NA, Weale ME, von Schantz M, et al. Evolution of a length polymorphism in the human PER3 gene, a component of the circadian system. J Biol Rhythms 2005;20:490–9.

78. Ciarleglio CM, Ryckman KK, Servick SV, et al. Genetic differences in human circadian clock genes among worldwide populations. J Biol Rhythms 2008; 23:330–40.

79. Viola AU, James LM, Archer SN, et al. PER3 polymorphism and cardiac autonomic control: effects of sleep debt and circadian phase. Am J Physiol Heart Circ Physiol 2008;295:H2156–63.

80. Archer SN, Viola AU, Kyriakopoulou V, et al. Interindividual differences in habitual sleep timing and entrained phase of endogenous circadian rhythms of BMAL1, PER2 and PER3 mRNA in human leukocytes. Sleep 2008;31:608–17.

81. Vandewalle G, Archer SN, Wuillaume C, et al. Functional magnetic resonance imaging-assessed brain responses during an executive task depend on interaction of sleep homeostasis, circadian phase, and PER3 genotype. J Neurosci 2009;29:7948–56.

82. Mignot E, Young T, Lin L, et al. Nocturnal sleep and daytime sleepiness in normal subjects with HLA-DQB1*0602. Sleep 1999;22:347–52.

83. Dauvilliers Y, Tafti M. Molecular genetics and treatment of narcolepsy. Ann Med 2006;38:252–62.

84. Mignot E, Lin L, Finn L, et al. Correlates of sleep-onset REM periods during the multiple sleep latency test in community adults. Brain 2006;129:1609–23.

85. Tunbridge EM, Harrison PJ, Weinberger DR. Catechol-O-methyltransferase, cognition, and psychosis: val158-Met and beyond. Biol Psychiatry 2006;60:141–51.

86. Savitz J, Solms M, Ramesar R. The molecular genetics of cognition: dopamine, COMT and BDNF. Genes Brain Behav 2006;5:311–28.

87. Egan MF, Goldberg TE, Kolachana BS, et al. Effect of COMT Val108/158 Met genotype on frontal lobe function and risk for schizophrenia. Proc Natl Acad Sci U S A 2001;98:6917–22.

88. Dickinson D, Elvevåg B. Genes, cognition and brain through a COMT lens. Neuroscience 2009;164:72–87.

89. Barnett JH, Jones PB, Robbins TW, et al. Effects of the catechol-O-methyltransferase Val158Met polymorphism on executive function: a meta-analysis of the Wisconsin Card Sort Test in schizophrenia and healthy controls. Mol Psychiatry 2007;12:502–9.

90. Dauvilliers Y, Neidhart E, Lecendreux M, et al. MAO-A and COMT polymorphisms and gene effects in narcolepsy. Mol Psychiatry 2001;6:367–72.

91. Dauvilliers Y, Neidhart E, Billiard M, et al. Sexual dimorphism of the catechol-O-methyltransferase gene in narcolepsy is associated with response to modafinil. Pharmacogenomics J 2002;2:65–8.

92. Frauscher B, Högl B, Maret S, et al. Association of daytime sleepiness with COMT polymorphism in patients with Parkinson disease: a pilot study. Sleep 2004;27:733–6.

93. Bodenmann S, Rusterholz T, Dürr R, et al. The functional Val158Met polymorphism of COMT predicts interindividual differences in brain α oscillations in young men. J Neurosci 2009;29:10855–62.

94. Bodenmann S, Xu S, Luhmann U, et al. Pharmacogenetics of modafinil after sleep loss: catechol-O-methyltransferase genotype modulates waking functions but not recovery sleep. Clin Pharmacol Ther 2009;85:296–304.

95. Bodenmann S, Landolt HP. Effects of modafinil on the sleep EEG depend on Val158Met genotype of COMT. Sleep 2010;33:1027–35.

96. Rétey JV, Adam M, Honegger E, et al. A functional genetic variation of adenosine deaminase affects the duration and intensity of deep sleep in humans. Proc Natl Acad Sci U S A 2005;102:15676–81.

97. Rétey JV, Adam M, Khatami R, et al. A genetic variation in the adenosine A2A receptor gene (ADORA2A) contributes to individual sensitivity to caffeine effects on sleep. Clin Pharmacol Ther 2007;81:692–8.

98. Gottlieb DJ, O'Connor GT, Wilk JB. Genome-wide association of sleep and circadian phenotypes. BMC Med Genet 2007;8(Suppl 1):S9.

Sleep States, Memory Processing, and Dreams

Carlyle Smith, PhD

KEYWORDS

- Sleep • Sleep states • Memory • Learning • Dreams

KEY POINTS

- Efficient memory consolidation is benefited by different stages of posttraining sleep, depending on the type or subtype of learning task involved.
- Because sleep is accompanied by dreams, it is possible that dreams are also involved with the memory consolidation of recently learned material.
- An examination of this hypothesis suggests that dreams may reflect the ongoing process of memory consolidation, but do not enhance this process.

INTRODUCTION

The fields of sleep and of memory have historically been studied in isolation from each other. However, in the last 40 years the understanding of the relationship between sleep states and memory processes has made considerable progress. The examination of dream activity as it relates to memory processing during sleep states is in its infancy. Despite this, there are some interesting studies that should form the basis for more research in this area. This article describes each of the concepts of memory, sleep states, and their relationship, followed by an examination of the nature of dream mentation during postlearning sleep.

MEMORY

Memory, from either a cognitive or neurophysiological perspective, is not a unitary phenomenon. The term should be used as a generic concept for information storage, and includes several specific subcategories.

There is believed to be a short-term memory that can last from seconds to minutes. At this stage, the newly acquired information is believed to be quite volatile and unstable. The learned material is then believed to be transformed into a more permanent long-term memory store. The information is believed to be converted into a more permanent, stable state that takes place over a period of hours, days, and possibly even years. This dynamic process is referred to as memory consolidation, which can be defined as the time-dependent process that converts labile memory traces into a more permanent form.

There are now understood to be several different memory systems that are relatively independent of each other. One of the models of memory suggests that there are 2 main memory systems, declarative and nondeclarative, which are served by different neural structures.[1]

Declarative material is easily accessible to verbal description, and both encoding and retrieval are usually performed explicitly. In other words, the subject is consciously aware of the information that is to be learned and also aware that it can be accessed when desired from the memory store. Declarative memory is further categorized into semantic and episodic components. Semantic memories comprise our factual knowledge of the world. For example, most individuals know that Paris is the capital city of France. However, they probably do not remember when or where they acquired

This article originally appeared in *Sleep Medicine Clinics, Volume 5, Issue 2.*
Department of Psychology, Trent University, 1600 West Bank Drive, Peterborough, Ontario K9J 7B8, Canada
E-mail address: csmith@trentu.ca

Sleep Med Clin 7 (2012) 455–467
http://dx.doi.org/10.1016/j.jsmc.2012.06.008
1556-407X/12/$ – see front matter © 2012 Elsevier Inc. All rights reserved.

this information; this distinguishes semantic memory from episodic memory. Episodic memories include the information of interest as well as their contextual location in time and space. Being able to recall what you ate for dinner as well as the fine details of where you were and who was with you is an example of an episodic memory.

By contrast, nondeclarative memories are not easily accessible to verbal description. Learning usually occurs implicitly or without conscious awareness, meaning that our behavior can be modified without our conscious awareness. Assessment that nondeclarative memories exist can best be done by observing behavior. If someone says that they have learned how to skate, the best way to be assured that this is so would be to ask the individual to put on a skating demonstration for you.

Within the category of nondeclarative types of learning there are several subtypes: procedural memory (the learning of skills and habits), priming, and simple classical conditioning (which includes both emotional responses and skeletal musculature responses). These learning subtypes are subtended by different neural substrates and are thus considered to be relatively independent learning systems.[1]

Sleep States

The states of sleep are now conventionally divided into two separate categories, rapid eye movement (REM) and non–rapid eye movement (NREM) sleep. NREM sleep is further divided into several categories. Sleep onset in humans is characterized by a light stage of sleep (Stage 1), which typically only lasts for a few minutes in healthy young adults. This stage gives way to Stage 2 sleep, a deeper stage of sleep with special electroencephalographic (EEG) features, including the spindle and K-complex. The most prominent background EEG is theta (5–7 Hz). This stage of sleep is more enduring and comprises about 50% of the sleep night. Deeper and more profound sleep is labeled Stage 3/4 sleep, and is characterized by slow (delta) waves (1–4 Hz). There are no rapid eye movements in NREM and while tension in the large muscle groups is much reduced, it is still present. By contrast, REM sleep is composed of faster EEG frequencies (7–10 Hz) and complete muscle atonia for all of the large muscle groups. Periodic rapid eye movements occur in this sleep state, which do not occur in any of the other states.

Throughout the sleep night there is an ultradian rhythm of 90 minutes, which is quite robust. The healthy young adult begins the night with a few minutes of Stage 1, but quickly drops to Stage 2. Stage 2 turns into Stage 3 (with between 20% and 50% delta waves) and then into Stage 4 (with more than 50% delta waves). Stages 3 and 4 are considered to be electrophysiologically similar and are often grouped together as a single stage called slow-wave sleep (SWS). After Stage 3/4, sleep then lightens and Stage 2 is again observed. In the first 90-minute sleep period of the night, Stage 2 is followed by the first episode of REM sleep, which is relatively short (approximately 10 minutes). Thus at the end of the first sleep cycle, the individual typically has had 80 minutes of NREM sleep and 10 minutes of REM sleep. As the cycles repeat, the time spent in Stages 3/4 declines while the amount of time spent in REM sleep increases. By the last cycle of the night, there is very little Stage 3/4 sleep, but the number of minutes of REM sleep has increased, and the final REM period can last 30 minutes or longer while NREM sleep is composed almost entirely of Stage 2 sleep.[2]

Sleep States and Memory Consolidation

Three main approaches have been used to examine the relationship between sleep and memory processes. The first method has been to look at the changes in sleep EEG following task acquisition in comparison with baseline values. More recently, the added use of brain imaging techniques such as positron emission tomography and functional magnetic resonance imaging (fMRI) has added to the understanding of postlearning brain changes during sleep. The second approach has been to examine the result of sleep deprivation following learning in comparison with normal postacquisition sleep. To avoid possible stress confounds, more recent studies have used a day-night design. The control group has a test-retest interval of 12 hours with no intervening sleep (such as 10 AM–10 PM). The test group also has a 12-hour test-retest interval, but for them the 12-hour interval includes a night of sleep (such as 10 PM–10 AM). The third approach has been to use various kinds of sensory stimulation during postlearning sleep to examine the possibility of memory enhancement.

Declarative Memory and Sleep

Using these various approaches, it seems clear that sleep states are beneficial for memory consolidation. However, different kinds of sleep are differentially beneficial for certain types of memory over other types. Declarative memory has been studied in both its semantic and episodic forms. For episodic memory, a large number of studies have examined the effect of sleep on verbal material such as paired-associate words and prose passages. Explicit encoding of landscapes, object locations and faces, or visuospatial memory and navigation within virtual or natural environments has also been studied. In general, it has been reported that SWS sleep is most beneficial for these kinds of memories.[3-7] Other studies have concluded that Stage 2 sleep is also important, with most observing an increase in Stage 2 sleep spindle activity.[8-12] Improvement in declarative memory has also been reported, either by directly enhancing SWS activity using direct current[13] or by directly boosting the level of slow oscillations following declarative learning.[14] One study has shown that while the improvements following sleep in explicit recall for word pairs in a paired-associate task is small, the ability to keep multiple lists separate is greatly improved.[15,16] Both SWS and Stage 2 have been reported to be involved in preliminary work using this retroactive interference paradigm.[17] A smaller number of studies have been involved in reporting that REM sleep was important for this type of memory. In one study, memory of the specific spatial and temporal features of the word pairs was impaired by REM sleep deprivation.[18] In a second study the power of both sigma and theta bands was observed to increase at very central brain sites during the REM sleep following paired-associate learning.[19]

There are far fewer studies that have looked at the role of sleep in semantic memory. Two studies have combined imaging with EEG to show that acquisition of paired associates[5] or pictures of landscapes[20] began with increased activity in the hippocampus but 6 months later, recall was associated with more activity in the medial prefrontal cortex (mPFC). Although the studies did not assess to what degree the memories had become semanticized, they did demonstrate that successful acquisition was positively correlated with amount of SWS and that the area where memories were stored had changed from the more temporary site of the hippocampus to the more permanent site of the mPFC over a period of months. For the paired-associate study, sleep deprivation resulted in a weaker mPFC activation than for a night of regular sleep when assessed 6 months later. This finding indicates that sleep deprivation leads to very long-lasting changes in degree of memory consolidation.[5]

Nondeclarative Memory and Sleep

These generally implicitly acquired memories may be relatively independent in terms of neural and cognitive substrates.[1] Skills and habits refer to acquisition of novel perceptual, motor, and cognitive abilities with repeated practice (such as perceptual discrimination, skating, and so

forth). For example, visual perceptual learning involving a texture discrimination task has shown that both REM and SWS should be involved for the most efficient acquisition of this task.[21-25]

For pure motor skill acquisition, such as the well-studied finger-tapping task, it is known that there is postsleep improvement that seems to be related to Stage 2 sleep.[26-28] For more complex perceptual-motor skills such as the rotary pursuit task, Stage 2[29-31] and REM[31] sleep have both been implicated. For a more cognitively demanding task such as the mirror-tracing task, REM sleep seemed to be the more important sleep state,[3,32,33] although improvement was also seen after NREM naps.[34] It has been proposed that these discrepancies can be explained by the initial skill levels of the individual participants. In one pursuit-rotor study, it was observed that participants with very low initial skill levels learned the task and showed corresponding increases in REM sleep. On the other hand, subjects who had high initial skill levels showed increases in Stage 2 sleep variables. It was proposed that individuals were using 1 of 2 overlapping consolidation systems depending on their previous experience. Subjects who found that the task required them to come up with a new cognitive strategy showed increases in REM sleep. Those individuals who already had some previous experience of the same type of task were simply refining and elaborating existing memories and showed Stage 2 sleep changes. This idea is consistent with REM sleep activity reported following acquisition of more complex perceptual motor[35,36] and cognitive[37-39] tasks. The idea that REM sleep is more important for consolidation of higher-order implicitly learned information is further supported by other studies reporting REM sleep changes.[33,40-42]

Emotional Memory

The role of sleep in consolidation of emotionally charged memories has only recently been examined.[43-49] In general, emotional memories were better consolidated after periods of REM sleep in comparison with NREM sleep.[44,49] Furthermore, emotional memories may be more resistant to total sleep deprivation.[43,46]

Hu and colleagues[45] studied the effects sleep on memory for neutral and emotionally arousing pictures, and found that if sleep intervened between training and retest, participants showed superior memory for the emotionally arousing pictures. In another study, it was reported that brief sleep after acquisition of emotional text was sufficient to keep those memories alive for 4 years when retesting was done. The neutral material, by contrast, was not well remembered. The investigators suggested that this process might well have relevance for the treatment of victims of posttraumatic sleep disorder, and proposed the idea that sleep deprivation following an emotional event might alleviate this problem.[50] However, in a brain imaging study (fMRI), participants were either allowed a night of sleep or were sleep deprived. It was observed that whereas positive emotional stimuli were impaired on retest in the sleep-deprived group compared with the rested group, negative emotional memories were not impaired. While hippocampal-cortical connections were weaker in the group that had been sleep deprived, they showed alternative amygdalocortical network activity. The investigators concluded that negative and potentially dangerous information was stored by means of an alternative brain network despite sleep deprivation. Such a result suggests that sleep deprivation alone will not allow negative emotional material to be forgotten as a result of sleep deprivation.

Sleep-Dependent Mechanisms of Memory Consolidation

Ponto-geniculo-occipital (PGO) waves have been extensively studied in animals. PGO waves consist of phasic bioelectric potentials, originating in the pons, that are closely related to the rapid eye movements of REM sleep. Increases in this PGO activity have been observed in rats following acquisition of an avoidance task.[51,52] Similar mechanisms are believed to exist in humans.[53–55] Several human studies have reported increases in REM density following procedural learning.[33,40,56]

One study presented sounds in the background while the subject was learning a complex logic task. Maximum memory enhancement was observed when the same sounds (below waking threshold) were again presented during REM sleep to coincide in time with the actual rapid eye movements. Presentations of the sound during tonic REM sleep did not produce any memory increases. Results further reinforce the idea that PGO activity is an important mechanism for efficient brain plasticity.[57]

Hippocampal theta rhythm (4–7 Hz) of the hippocampus is a prominent signature of REM sleep in both animals and humans.[58] It is theorized that cortical information activates the hippocampal CA3 system during learning associated with waking and REM sleep theta. During subsequent SWS, previously activated neurons are reactivated during sharp wave bursts. Memory transiently stored in the CA3 region can be transferred to cortical regions.[58] Several studies support the idea of hippocampal to cortical transfer.[5,20,59]

Sleep spindles have long been a distinctive characteristic of Stage 2 sleep, although they are also observed in SWS to a much lesser extent. The original 12- to 14-Hz spindle-shaped EEG burst lasting approximately 0.5 to 1.5 seconds has now been expanded to include frequencies of 11.5 to 16.5 Hz.[60] Spindle generation has been considered an ideal mechanism for synaptic plasticity, and involves thalamocortical connections. Several studies have reported an increase in spindle density following declarative memory task acquisition.[8,9,11,61] Similarly, for procedural memory, Stage 2 spindle increases were observed following acquisition of a simple motor task[27,28,62] and a perceptual-motor task.[19,30] As mentioned previously, one theory suggests that the spindle may represent a component of one memory-processing subsystem that is in use when individuals are already somewhat familiar with the material to be learned.[32]

Slow waves (<4 Hz) may regulate spindle oscillations that are thought to be important for memory consolidation.[63] Brain regional increases in SWS have been observed following motor task acquisition,[64] suggesting local homeostatic mechanisms for memory consolidation.[65] Memory enhancement was observed when slow oscillations (<1 Hz) were imposed on participants during post-learning sleep during normal SWS, also suggesting a facilitatory role for slow oscillatory EEG activity.

Summary of Sleep and Memory Literature

Different kinds of memory appear to involve different stages of sleep to further the process of memory consolidation. Declarative learning appears to invoke NREM (SWS and/or Stage 2) with less participation for REM sleep. For nondeclarative learning, SWS, Stage 2, or REM, or all of these, might be involved, depending on the type of task. It seems likely that implicit learning requiring new cognitive strategies might involve REM sleep more than NREM sleep. Tasks that are either explicit or for which the participant has had some previous experience seem to favor Stage 2 sleep. Emotionally charged memories favor recruitment of REM sleep processes.

DREAMS AND SLEEP STATES

For the purposes of this article, dreams are defined as mental activity reported on awakening from a sleep state.

Traditionally, dreams were considered to be occurring during REM sleep with very little mentation during other sleep states.[66] More recent work has indicated that dream reports can be obtained from subjects awakened from the other stages of sleep as well.[67] While some investigators have argued that REM- and NREM-derived dreams may not differ qualitatively,[68] awakenings from REM sleep still provide the highest frequency of dream reports.[69,70] Dream mentation from awakenings at sleep onset has been found to yield reports 35% of the time.[69] For NREM sleep, the rate has been reported to range from 43% to 60%[69,70] and for REM awakenings, percentage of recall was more than 80%.[69,70] REM reports are considered to be longer[68,71] as well as more vivid and bizarre in comparison with NREM dreams.[72,73]

Dreams and Memory in Children

It is well known that children in the lower age groups have different amounts of the stages of sleep than do adults. While the basic sleep-state architecture patterns observed in adults are also observed in children after about 3 years of age, the percentages of each sleep stage are different. In children, there are more hours of sleep and the percentage of SWS sleep is higher. The percentage of REM sleep is also higher than in adults Thus the sleep system, despite changes with age, is intact and functional from a very young age.[74]

There are only a few laboratory studies that have examined the relationship between sleep states and memory in young children.[75,76] It is interesting that sleep aids declarative memory consolidation but not procedural memory consolidation. Thus, the sleep-memory system appears to be active in young children but may not be mature.

The situation with respect to dreams in the very young also suggests some immaturity. Young children do not show the high level of dream reporting from REM awakenings seen in adults. In several careful dream-collection studies, children under the ages of 9 to 11 showed a median recall rate of 20% to 30%, much lower than the approximate 80% or more seen in adults. Similarly, recall from NREM awakenings was only 6% in the young, but rose to about 40% in young teenagers. Until ages 13 to 15, the dream reports had a different content. In the very young, REM dream reports were usually composed of single images that did not move. At ages 5 to 8, dream characters moved around, but dream narratives were not well developed compared with adult dreams. The maturity of dream reports seemed to parallel cognitive maturity and remained relatively immature until the development of good visuospatial skills.[77–79]

It is clear that children are learning many things at these young ages and are undoubtedly using

REM and NREM sleep. However, although no dreams have been collected in a sleep-memory experimental situation with young children, it seems unlikely at this point that their dreams are necessary for, or reflect the ongoing consolidation of memories during sleep.

Dream Delay: Do Relevant Dreams Always Occur the Night Following Task Acquisition?

The great majority of sleep-memory studies in both animals and humans have looked exclusively at the first few hours of sleep or the first night of sleep following task acquisition to examine the nature of the sleep consolidation mechanisms. However, a few studies have looked at sleep following acquisition for more than a single post-training day and have found sleep-state changes that continue for at least several days after the end of training. In rats, REM sleep increases have been observed to persist for up to a week after the end of avoidance-task acquisition.[80,81] Similarly, in humans, increases in REM sleep parameters have been observed 2 to 3 days after the end of the acquisition period.[40,82] Other laboratories have also noted the persistence of sleep-related consolidation several days after training.[83]

There is some evidence of a cyclic recurring dream content, for which a review has been done by Nielsen.[84] The results of several studies indicate that the events dreamed about on a given day were then not dreamed about for 5 to 7 days, when participants once more dreamed on the same topic as on day 1 (circaseptan rhythms). The dreams identified included self-selection of the most meaningful/significant events in their lives[85] or manipulation of an external stimulus, including the wearing of goggles with red filters[86] or an emotionally upsetting film.[87] It might be perceived that there was a longer-term sleep-state adjustment to the red goggles, for example, because it is known that wearing inverted prisms results in changes in REM sleep parameters[88] as well as dream incorporation.[89] It is premature to say that dreams are related to long-term post-learning increases. There do not appear to be any human studies that have recorded sleep states for a week after task acquisition and that have awakened their subjects to obtain dream reports under learning conditions. Such experiments might provide a fruitful avenue for future research. One group has reported qualitative differences in memory sources of recent versus delayed (about 1 week) dreams about significant life events,[85] suggesting an ongoing process of memory transfer from one brain site to another.

Examination of Dream Content Following Task Acquisition

If dreams reflect memory-processing activity, one might expect a correspondence between dreams from a given sleep state and the type of learning taking place. It has been suggested that there is a homology between dream content and memory type. REM dreams, being more hallucinatory, emotional, and bizarre,[72] would be present during emotional memory consolidation, whereas NREM dreams, being more thought-like and less hallucinatory,[69] would be involved in more neutral tasks such as memorization of word pairs, with REM sleep consolidating emotional memories.[90]

Given the number of tasks that have now been examined and the sleep states implicated in subsequent memory processing, it seems clear that a more precise examination of this idea has yet to be done. For example, while REM sleep seems involved with emotional memory consolidation,[44] it is also involved with tasks that require a new cognitive strategy,[33] including simple perceptual-motor tasks,[91] which are not particularly emotional.

Not many studies have looked at dream content following the task acquisition, and these few have examined REM dreams. In one study, the subjects were asked for their dreams after continuously wearing inverted prisms for 4 full days. REM dream reports were collected on nights 3 and 4. While subjects had few direct incorporations of the experience, they did exhibit indirect metaphorical content (eg, "...I wanted to know what it was. Then I looked at a word but it was upside down"). The dreams generally reflected increases in motor and visual difficulties, as well as misfortunes and dreamer confusion.[92]

In another study, the same laboratory[88] examined the changes in dream content during prolonged (several weeks) exposure to French-language learning. In terms of sleep states, the investigators found that progress in language learning was correlated with increases in percentage of REM sleep. For dream content, the more progress was made in learning, the more French incorporations and French communication were observed. Moreover, learning progress was significantly correlated with latency to first French-language incorporation into a dream. Those individuals who made little or no progress in learning the language did not report any French-language incorporations in their dreams. The results of this study suggest that a minimum level of learning must occur before the dream content is affected. There would also appear to be a gradient whereby more learning reflected more French content. At first glance, this task might

be considered declarative in type, but it is more probably a mix of both declarative and procedural, because language learning is much more complex than mere word memorization.

Another group has recently reported a correlation between learning progress and REM dream elements after the acquisition of a complex computer game. The number of game-related elements in dreams correlated with performance gains according to an inverted-U function.[93]

Examination of dream content from awakenings just after sleep onset was performed using the Tetris computer game,[94] which participants played for about 2 hours daily for 3 to 4 days. Subjects were novices, experts, and amnesics (temporal lobe damage). All participants saw very similar mental images from sleep-onset awakenings. The novices reported seeing the puzzle pieces falling, while the experts sometimes had the added experience of recognizing the pieces falling as being from their own games, years ago. The pieces were recognizable in terms of color and sound. The amnesics also reported falling pieces, but they were unable to remember having played the game or to recognize the experimenter from session to session. A second study[73,95] used a downhill skiing simulator (Alpine Racer) as the task. Subjects awakened at sleep onset reported visual and kinesthetic sensations of skiing down the hill. Those individuals who had previous skiing experience sometimes reported images from prior skiing experiences. The images usually had high emotional salience, such as places where the subjects tended to "crash."

Several interesting conclusions have been drawn from these data. First, the memories that were retrieved during the sleep-onset period were assessed as originating from a semantic memory source rather than from an episodic (hippocampal) source. There were virtually no reports of seeing the room where the experiment was held, the computer itself, the keyboard, or the desk holding the apparatus. Moreover, the amnesic subjects were unable to process episodic memories at any time, but could still recall the falling game pieces. This conclusion is consistent with that of another study, which examined the very small percentage of recalled home-report dreams that contained actual episodic replay of previous daytime events (1%–2%).[96] It is also consistent with the hypothesis, derived from animal studies, that there is no hippocampal outflow through the entorhinal cortex to the cerebral cortex during REM sleep.[97,98]

For the Tetris game, there was some evidence that this dream imagery was inversely related to task proficiency, for both novices and experts.

Lack of imagery seemed to predict better performance. These results were interesting in that they might provide an indicator of the initial skill level of the participant. In sleep-memory studies using the rotary pursuit task, individuals with high initial skill levels showed postsleep changes in Stage 2 sleep architecture, whereas subjects with low initial skill levels showed postlearning sleep changes in REM sleep. These results were consistent with a theory that there are least 2 sleep-memory subsystems, one subserved by Stage 2 sleep and the other by REM sleep mechanisms.[99] Could it be that the best performers (measured by initial Tetris performance) did not "direct" their memory processing to REM sleep–related mechanisms, but rather to the Stage 2 NREM sleep-memory system? Although the Tetris and Alpine Racer games are more complex than the rotary pursuit task, it seems possible that the participants might choose REM if they found the task novel, requiring a new cognitive strategy, and would alternatively choose the Stage 2 system if they already had done similar activities, and treated the task as one where mostly refinement was needed and no new cognitive strategy was required. Although the dreams were collected from dream onset, and there is no way of telling whether related dream mental activity might have appeared in either REM or Stage 2 sleep, it seems possible that the memory-processing system chosen might already be made at the time of sleep-onset imagery.

There was also some evidence that delayed incorporation (subject was allowed 2 hours of sleep before being awakened) resulted in more remote mental imagery, obviously related to the task, but modified. This phenomenon was also reported in delayed sleep mentation from the Alpine Racer task (eg, instead of skiing down the hill, they dreamed of "falling down a hill" or "moving through some kind of forest" with their "entire upper body-…incredibly straight"). It was concluded that the more directly related images had been replaced by more weakly associated images.[73,95]

In a study using declarative material, subjects were required to memorize nonsense sentences. Then during subsequent sleep they were awakened from REM sleep to provide dream reports. The content was judged to be related to the previously memorized sentences, although it manifested as words and phrases associated with the original words rather than the words themselves.[100] These results are consistent with the finding that associations made just after awakenings from REM sleep tend to be secondary, weaker associations than those made from the waking state. It has been argued that the participants

awakened from REM sleep are making their choices with a brain that is still, at least partially, a REM-sleep brain.[73,101,102]

In a memory enhancement study,[57] participants were trained in a cognitive procedural task (complex logic task). A clicking sound was present in the background during acquisition and acted as the conditioned stimulus (CS). During the post-learning sleep night, subjects were subjected to these CS clicks via a mini-earphone. The clicks were timed to coincide with the maximum deflection of the rapid eye movements of REM sleep. On retest, the experimental group showed memory for the task that was significantly better than that of the control group, with a 23% enhancement. The click cues were believed to have acted as reminders for the participants to remember to process the task. In a second, related study,[103] subjects were presented with a REM-dependent[94] cognitive procedural task (mirror trace) accompanied by the background CS clicks. The task required subjects to try and draw a pencil line inside the margins of complex figures by looking in a mirror. Subjects were then given subthreshold postacquisition CS clicks during REM sleep as before. However, they were then awakened after an estimated 50% to 80% of the REM period was over to obtain a dream report. Compared with control groups, the dream narratives of the test group were significantly longer. The groups did not differ on time spent in any sleep stage including REM sleep. Thus it is possible that the dreams of the test group were somehow more intense. There seemed to be many detailed references to cars and driving, so a detailed lexicon was developed and used to score the dreams in content-analysis fashion, taking care to control for dream length. The test group showed significantly more references to cars, driving, driving problems, and so forth. Thus, the most popular metaphor for keeping the pencil between the lines of the figures they traced in the mirror seemed to be about cars and driving. No one reported episodic types of dreams such as "trying to draw a figure while looking in a mirror," and so forth, supporting other research that has found very little episodic memory replay.[96]

The results are consistent with the idea that individuals use dream themes of previous experiences that are familiar to them to characterize more novel present problems.[95,104] In this experiment, they related the problem of trying to keep a pencil on track to a dream of trying to keep a vehicle on the road, and so forth. The mental representations were of a negative nature, despite the fact that learning occurred (eg, "…he started driving down the street and…he cut through a neighborhood and was going really fast and crashed into a house"). There were no positive or success dreams of being able to avoid driving mistakes and mishaps. These increases in negative outcomes and misfortunes were also reported by subjects adapting to the inverted prisms.[92]

Neural Structures Involved in Dream Generation

The original activation-synthesis hypothesis[105] suggested that dreams are produced primarily during REM sleep by mechanisms in the pons, which randomly bombard the visual cortex during REM sleep. More recent theory revisions include the possibility of REM intrusions into NREM sleep states and a more complete description of the mental states against the background of transmitter modulation. There is a strong emphasis on the role of the cholinergic transmitter system during REM dream generation. Also, it is assumed that there is a complex forebrain network that plays a major role in shaping dream content.[72] Stickgold and colleagues[101] have proposed an error-detection model of dream construction, based on the error-detection model of Cohen and colleagues.[106] In this model, the brain is presumed to evaluate the potential value of novel forms of behavior during REM sleep. Weak cortical associations are preferentially activated during REM,[101] in the absence of dorsolateral prefrontal cortex (DLPFC) input or hippocampal feedback.[97] There is an active error-detection system originating in the anterior cingulate cortex and including emotional evaluation by the amygdala and medial orbitofrontal cortex. All of the aforementioned theories are based on the original ideas of the activation-synthesis hypothesis, although many structures have now been added.

An alternative to activation-synthesis based models comes from the work of Solms.[107] His neuropsychological information was obtained from patients with brain lesions and suggested that several other brain structures are important for normal dream activity. Damage to medial prefrontal or parieto-temporal-occipital junction areas resulted in dream deficits while lesions of the temporal lobes resulted in an increase in nightmares. Increased intensity of dreaming involved damage to medial prefrontal, anterior cingulate, or basal forebrain areas. The model deemphasizes the role of the brainstem in dream generation. While sufficient brain activation is deemed necessary, it is argued that the dream-generation transmitter system is dopaminergic and originates in the ventral tegmentum, just above the pons. This system fans out to the amygdala, the anterior cingulate gyrus, and frontal cortex. A detailed critique of these theories is given by Domhoff.[108]

Despite some theoretical differences, it seems clear that the DLPFC is not active and that there is no hippocampus-to-cortex information flow during REM sleep; this is believed to account for the lack of attention to unusual incongruities that occur in the dream. An advantage might be that the weaker (but novel) associations made would result in creative new ways of solving problems. It has been reported that solutions to a novel math problem were solved much more quickly by students following a night of sleep in comparison with an equal time awake.[109] Unfortunately, no dreams were collected in this study. According to the error-detection model, the evaluation of the novel associations would be carried out by the amygdala and orbitofrontal cortex in the presence of the anterior cingulate cortex. The dream would be generated based on the relative activities of these brain structures.[95]

SOME GENERAL CONCLUSIONS

Despite the meager data at present to decide the relationship of the memory consolidation process during sleep and dream mentation, some tentative conclusions can be made. First, it is likely that dream generation is not episodic in nature and that the images generated use semantic memories that are somehow linked together, which would explain why learning new information often gives rise to dream images of related material. Very little sleep-memory work has been directed at this kind of memory.

The fact that the dreams of children are very primitive while many things that they learn are quite complex and sophisticated suggests that dreams are not absolutely necessary for sleep-related memory consolidation.

The fact that task experts produced relevant dream images of an earlier time in their lives (eg, the Tetris experiment) suggests that dreams are at least reflecting a cataloging process for storing similar experiences together (if we assume that sleep onset and later dream activity are part of the same dream-generating process).[73]

Dreams with negative outcomes do not necessarily mean lack of learning progress. This mental activity may simply be a "read-out" of the ongoing process.

Gauging learning progress from dreams later in the night was positively correlated with the French immersion study, but appeared to be inversely correlated in the Tetris and Alpine motor-skill studies. A critical factor may be the initial level of proficiency of a participant. One explanation, as previously mentioned, is that the subjects who found the task to be generally familiar used a memory consolidation system associated with Stage 2 sleep. It is possible that the mental activity associated with this system is different from that of the less proficient subjects, who needed a new cognitive strategy and were thus invoking the REM sleep system.

Overall, it would seem that dream mentation does reflect recent learning, although it would not appear necessary. In some complex tasks, the mentation might be helpful in creating new ways of looking at a problem.

FUTURE DIRECTIONS

It seems clear that there is differential involvement of different sleep states in the various types of memory tasks. However, the few studies done have only examined REM dreams and sleep-onset mental activity. We have no idea if tasks that use subsequent Stage 2 sleep, such as a perceptual-motor task, would provide dreams during this stage that are reflective of the task being learned. Furthermore, would the REM dreams from the same task also show this activity or would they be reflective of other problems of a more cognitive or emotional nature? Similarly, would a task known to involve REM sleep provide similar dream content from both REM and NREM dream awakenings? There is some information that REM dreams through the night have a similar theme and appear to be related to ongoing life problems.[110] However, there do not seem to be any instances of a learning situation whereby both REM and NREM dreams were collected. Studies that would examine dreams from awakenings through the night in both NREM and REM sleep, following task acquisition, would be invaluable in tracing the dream changes in parallel with memory-processing activity.

To find the answer to the question of whether dreams are related to memory processing, care must be taken to use objective techniques for collecting and scoring the dreams. Nielsen and Stenstrom[111] note that subjects should receive direction on how to recall dreams (self-observation) so that crucial information is not lost. The content-analysis methodology has provided a systematic way of scoring dreams that is reliable and has acceptable statistical procedures.[108] Although it can sometimes not be specific enough for the elements of a particular study, it does provide a general method that can be followed to ensure that dream elements are uniformly scored and reliably compared.

Virtually all of the studies on sleep and memory have assumed that the most important night is the first posttraining night. However, a substantial number of studies suggest that memory processing persists for days and weeks after the end of acquisition. Dream activity at these times has yet to be examined.

Dreaming in children appears to be immature for the early years of life, yet children obviously learn at a rapid pace. Developmental studies aimed at finding when mature dreams become associated with recently learned material have yet to be done.

The study of the change in dream characteristics following learning may well help us to understand the processes whereby dreams are generated. An examination of the dream mentation induced by a specific learning event may help us to gauge learning progress. A within-subject design comparing dream content before and after task acquisition, and using both EEG and brain imaging techniques, would provide valuable insights.

REFERENCES

1. Squire LR. Memory systems of the brain: a brief history and current perspective. Neurobiol Learn Mem 2004;82(3):171–7.
2. Carskadon M, Dement W. Normal human sleep: an overview. In: Kryger M, Roth T, Dement W, editors. Principles and practice of sleep medicine. 4th edition. Philadelphia: Elsevier; 2005. p. 13–23.
3. Plihal W, Born J. Effects of early and late nocturnal sleep on declarative and procedural memory. J Cogn Neurosci 1997;9(4):534–47.
4. Plihal W, Born J. Effects of early and late nocturnal sleep on priming and spatial memory. Psychophysiology 1999;36(5):571–82.
5. Gais S, Albouy G, Boly M, et al. Sleep transforms the cerebral trace of declarative memories. Proc Natl Acad Sci U S A 2007;104(47):18778–83.
6. Tucker MA, Hirota Y, Wamsley EJ, et al. A daytime nap containing solely non-REM sleep enhances declarative but not procedural memory. Neurobiol Learn Mem 2006;86(2):241–7.
7. Gais S, Born J. Low acetylcholine during slow-wave sleep is critical for declarative memory consolidation. Proc Natl Acad Sci U S A 2004;101(7):2140–4.
8. Gais S, Molle M, Helms K, et al. Learning-dependent increases in sleep spindle density. J Neurosci 2002;22(15):6830–4.
9. Schmidt C, Peigneux P, Muto V, et al. Encoding difficulty promotes postlearning changes in sleep spindle activity during napping. J Neurosci 2006;26(35):8976–82.

10. Clemens Z, Fabo D, Halasz P. Twenty-four hours retention of visuospatial memory correlates with the number of parietal sleep spindles. Neurosci Lett 2006;403(1–2):52–6.

11. Clemens Z, Fabo D, Halasz P. Overnight verbal memory retention correlates with the number of sleep spindles. Neuroscience 2005;132(2): 529–35.

12. Schabus M, Gruber G, Parapatics S, et al. Sleep spindles and their significance for declarative memory consolidation. Sleep 2004;27(8):1479–85.

13. Marshall L, Molle M, Hallschmid M, et al. Transcranial direct current stimulation during sleep improves declarative memory. J Neurosci 2004; 24(44):9985–92.

14. Marshall L, Helgadottir H, Molle M, et al. Boosting slow oscillations during sleep potentiates memory. Nature 2006;444(7119):610–3.

15. Ellenbogen JM, Hu PT, Payne JD, et al. Human relational memory requires time and sleep. Proc Natl Acad Sci U S A 2007;104(18):7723–8.

16. Ellenbogen JM, Hulbert JC, Stickgold R, et al. Interfering with theories of sleep and memory: sleep, declarative memory, and associative interference. Curr Biol 2006;16(13):1290–4.

17. Smith C, Moran CR, McGilvray MP, et al. Decreases in Stage 2 sleep, spindles and sigma power following acquisition of a declarative task. J Sleep Res 2008;17(Suppl 1):270.

18. Rauchs G, Bertran F, Guillery-Girard B, et al. Consolidation of strictly episodic memories mainly requires rapid eye movement sleep. Sleep 2004; 27(3):395–401.

19. Fogel SM, Smith CT, Cote KA. Dissociable learning-dependent changes in REM and non-REM sleep in declarative and procedural memory systems. Behav Brain Res 2007;180(1): 48–61.

20. Takashima A, Petersson KM, Rutters F, et al. Declarative memory consolidation in humans: a prospective functional magnetic resonance imaging study. Proc Natl Acad Sci U S A 2006; 103(3):756–61.

21. Gais S, Plihal W, Wagner U, et al. Early sleep triggers memory for early visual discrimination skills. Nat Neurosci 2000;3(12):1335–9.

22. Karni A, Sagi D. Where practice makes perfect in texture discrimination: evidence for primary visual cortex plasticity. Proc Natl Acad Sci U S A 1991; 88(11):4966–70.

23. Stickgold R, Whidbee D, Schirmer B, et al. Visual discrimination task improvement: a multi-step process occurring during sleep. J Cogn Neurosci 2000;12(2):246–54.

24. Mednick S, Nakayama K, Stickgold R. Sleep-dependent learning: a nap is as good as a night. Nat Neurosci 2003;6(7):697–8.

25. Mednick SC, Nakayama K, Cantero JL, et al. The restorative effect of naps on perceptual deterioration. Nat Neurosci 2002;5(7):677–81.

26. Nishida M, Walker MP. Daytime naps, motor memory consolidation and regionally specific sleep spindles. PLoS One 2007;2(4):e341.

27. Morin A, Doyon J, Dostie V, et al. Motor sequence learning increases sleep spindles and fast frequencies in post-training sleep. Sleep 2008;31(8):1149–56.

28. Walker MP, Brakefield T, Morgan A, et al. Practice with sleep makes perfect: sleep-dependent motor skill learning. Neuron 2002;35(1):205–11.

29. Smith C, MacNeill C. Impaired motor memory for a pursuit rotor task following stage 2 sleep loss in college students. J Sleep Res 1994;3(4):206–13.

30. Fogel SM, Smith CT. Learning-dependent changes in sleep spindles and stage 2 sleep. J Sleep Res 2006;15(3):250–5.

31. Peters KR, Smith V, Smith CT. Changes in sleep architecture following motor learning depend on initial skill level. J Cogn Neurosci 2007;19(5): 817–29.

32. Smith C, Aubrey J, Peters K. Different roles for REM and stage 2 sleep in motor learning: a proposed model. Psychologica Belgica 2004; 44(1/2):79–102.

33. Smith CT, Nixon MR, Nader RS. Posttraining increases in REM sleep intensity implicate REM sleep in memory processing and provide a biological marker of learning potential. Learn Mem 2004; 11(6):714–9.

34. Backhaus J, Junghanns K. Daytime naps improve procedural motor memory. Sleep Med 2006;7(6): 508–12.

35. Buchegger J, Fritsch R, Meier-Koll A, et al. Does trampolining and anaerobic physical fitness affect sleep? Percept Mot Skills 1991;73(1):243–52.

36. Buchegger J, Meier-Koll A. Motor learning and ultradian sleep cycle: an electroencephalographic study of trampoliners. Percept Mot Skills 1988; 67(2):635–45.

37. Maquet P. Functional neuroimaging of normal human sleep by positron emission tomography. J Sleep Res 2000;9(3):207–31.

38. Peigneux P, Laureys S, Fuchs S, et al. Learned material content and acquisition level modulate cerebral reactivation during posttraining rapid-eye-movements sleep. Neuroimage 2003;20(1): 125–34.

39. Laureys S, Peigneux P, Phillips C, et al. Experience-dependent changes in cerebral functional connectivity during human rapid eye movement sleep. Neurosci 2001;105(3):521–5.

40. Smith C, Smith D. Ingestion of ethanol just prior to sleep onset impairs memory for procedural but not declarative tasks. Sleep 2003;26(2):185–91.

41. Cajochen C, Knoblauch V, Wirz-Justice A, et al. Circadian modulation of sequence learning under high and low sleep pressure conditions. Behav Brain Res 2004;151(1–2):167–76.

42. De Koninck J, Lorrain D, Christ G, et al. Intensive language learning and increases in rapid eye movement sleep: evidence of a performance factor. Int J Psychophysiol 1989;8(1):43–7.

43. Wagner U, Degirmenci M, Drosopoulos S, et al. Effects of cortisol suppression on sleep-associated consolidation of neutral and emotional memory. Biol Psychiatry 2005;58(11):885–93.

44. Wagner U, Gais S, Born J. Emotional memory formation is enhanced across sleep intervals with high amounts of rapid eye movement sleep. Learn Mem 2001;8(2):112–9.

45. Hu P, Stylos-Allan M, Walker MP. Sleep facilitates consolidation of emotional declarative memory. Psychol Sci 2006;17(10):891–8.

46. Sterpenich V, Albouy G, Boly M, et al. Sleep-related hippocampo-cortical interplay during emotional memory recollection. PLoS Biol 2007;5(11):e282.

47. Atienza M, Cantero JL. Modulatory effects of emotion and sleep on recollection and familiarity. J Sleep Res 2008;17(3):285–94 [Epub 2008 May 22].

48. Payne JD, Stickgold R, Swanberg K, et al. Sleep preferentially enhances memory for emotional components of scenes. Psychol Sci 2008;19(8): 781–8.

49. Wagner U, Hallschmid M, Verleger R, et al. Signs of REM sleep dependent enhancement of implicit face memory: a repetition priming study. Biol Psychol 2003;62(3):197–210.

50. Wagner U, Hallschmid M, Rasch B, et al. Brief sleep after learning keeps emotional memories alive for years. Biol Psychiat 2006;60(7):788–90.

51. Datta S. Avoidance task training potentiates phasic pontine-wave density in the rat: a mechanism for sleep-dependent plasticity. J Neurosci 2000;20: 8607–13.

52. Datta S, Li G, Auerbach S. Activation of phasic pontine-wave generator in the rat: a mechanism for expression of plasticity-related genes and proteins in the dorsal hippocampus and amygdala. Eur J Neurosci 2008;27:1876–92.

53. Salzarulo P, Lairy GC, Bancaud J, et al. direct depth recording of the striate cortex during REM sleep in man: are there PGO potentials? EEG Clin Neurophysiol 1975;38:199–202.

54. Peigneux P, Laureys S, Fuchs S, et al. Generation of rapid eye movements during paradoxical sleep in humans. Neuroimage 2001;14(3):701–8.

55. Wehrle R, Czisch M, Kaufmann C, et al. Rapid eye movement-related brain activation in human sleep: a functional magnetic resonance imaging study. Neuroreport 2005;16(8):853–7.

56. Mandai O, Guerrien A, Sockeel P, et al. REM sleep modifications following a Morse code learning session in humans. Physiol Behav 1989;46(4): 639–42.

57. Smith C, Weeden K. Post training REMs co-incident auditory stimulation enhances memory in humans. Psychiatr J Univ Ott 1990;15(2): 85–90.

58. Buzsaki G. Theta oscillations in the hippocampus. Neuron 2002;33(3):325–40.

59. Poe GR, Nitz DA, Mcnaughton BL, et al. Experience-dependent phase-reversal of hippocampal neuron firing during REM sleep. Brain Res 2000; 855(1):176–80.

60. De Gennaro L, Ferrara M. Sleep spindles: an overview. Sleep Med Rev 2003;7:423–40.

61. Schabus M, Hoedlmoser K, Pecherstorfer T, et al. Interindividual sleep spindle differences and their relation to learning-related enhancements. Brain Res 2008;1191:127–35.

62. Walker MP, Brakefield T, Allan Hobson J, et al. Dissociable stages of human memory consolidation and reconsolidation. Nature 2003;425(6958): 616–20.

63. Molle M, Marshall L, Gais S, et al. Grouping of spindle activity during slow oscillations in human non-rapid eye movement sleep. J Neurosci 2002; 22(24):10941–7.

64. Huber R, Ghilardi MF, Massimini M, et al. Local sleep and learning. Nature 2004;430(6995): 78–81.

65. Tononi G, Cirelli C. Sleep function and synaptic homeostasis. Sleep Med Rev 2006;10(1):49–62.

66. Dement W, Kleitman N. The relation of eye movements during sleep to dream activity: an objective method for the study of dreaming. J Exp Psychol 1957;53:339–46.

67. Foulkes D. Dream reports from different stages of sleep. J Abnorm Soc Psychol 1962;65:14–25.

68. Antrobus JS. REM and NREM sleep reports: comparison of word frequencies by cognitive classes. Psychophysiology 1983;1983:562–8.

69. Fosse M, Stickgold R, Hobson A. Brain-mind states: reciprocal variation in thoughts and hallucinations. Psychol Sci 2001;12:30–6.

70. Nielsen TA. Mentation in REM and NREM sleep: a review and possible reconciliation of two models. Behav Brain Sci 2000;23:851–66.

71. Stickgold R, Pace-Schott E, Hobson JA. A new paradigm for dream research: mentation reports following spontaneous arousal from REM and NREM sleep recorded in a home setting. Conscious Cogn 1994;3:16–29.

72. Hobson JA, Pace-Schott EF, Stickgold R. Dreaming and the brain: toward a cognitive neuroscience of conscious states. Behav Brain Sci 2000; 23:793–842.

73. Stickgold R. Why we dream. In: Kryger M, Roth T, Dement W, editors. Principles and practice of sleep medicine. 4th edition. Philadelphia: Saunders; 2005. p. 579–87.

74. Ohayon MM, Carskadon M, Guilleminault C, et al. Meta-analysis of quantitative sleep parameters from childhood to old age in healthy individuals: developing normative sleep values across the human lifespan. Sleep 2004;27:1255–73.

75. Backhaus J, Hoecksesfeld R, Born J, et al. Immediate as well as delayed post learning sleep but not wakefulness enhances declarative memory consolidation in children. Neurobiol Learn Mem 2008;89:76–80.

76. Wilhelm I, Diekelmann S, Born J. Sleep in children improves memory performance on declarative but not procedural tasks. Learn Mern 2008; 15:373–7.

77. Foulkes D. Children's dreams. New York: Wiley; 1982.

78. Foulkes D. Children's dreaming and the development of consciousness. Cambridge (MA): Harvard University Press; 1999.

79. Foulkes D, Hollifield M, Sullivan B, et al. REM dreaming and cognitive skills at ages 5-8: a cross-sectional study. Internat J Behav Dev 1990;13: 447–65.

80. Smith C, Lapp L. Prolonged increases in both PS and number of REMS following a shuttle avoidance task. Physiol Behav 1986;36:1053–7.

81. Smith CT. The REM sleep window and memory processing. In: Maquet P, Smith C, Stickgold R, editors. Sleep and brain plasticity. Oxford (United Kingdom): Oxford Press; 2003. p. 117–33.

82. Smith C, Lapp L. Increases in number of REMs and REM density in humans following an intensive learning period. Sleep 1991;14:325–30.

83. Stickgold R, LaTanya J, Hobson JA. Visual discrimination learning requires sleep after training. Nat Neurosci 2000;3:1237–8.

84. Nielsen T. Chronobiology of dreaming. Philadelphia: Saunders; 2005.

85. Nielsen T, Kuiken D, Alain G, et al. Immediate and delayed incorporation of events into dreams: further replication and implications for dream function. J Sleep Res 2004;13:327–36.

86. Roffwarg H, Herman JH, Bowe-Anders C, et al. The effects of sustained alterations of waking visual input on dream content. In: Arkin A, Antrobus J, Ellman S, editors. The mind in sleep: psychology and psychophysiology. Hillsdale (NJ): Erlbaum; 1978. p. 295–350.

87. Nielsen T, Powell DA, Cheung JS. Temporal delays in incorporation of events into dreams. Percept Mot Skills 1995;81:95–104.

88. De Koninck J, Lorrain D, Christ G, et al. Intensive learning and increases in rapid eye movement sleep: evidence of a performance factor. Internat J Psychol 1989;8:43–7.

89. De Koninck J, Prevost F, Lortie-Lussier M. Vertical inversion of the visual field and REM sleep mentation. J Sleep Res 1996;5:16–20.

90. Stickgold R. Sleep-dependent memory consolidation. Nature 2005;437(7063):1272–8.

91. Peters KR, Smith V, Smith CT. The effect of initial skill level on the relationship between stage 2 sleep spindles, rapid eye movements and motor learning. J Cogn Neurosci 2006;19:817–29.

92. De Koninck J. Waking experiences and dreams. In: Kryger M, Roth T, Dement W, editors. Principles and practice of sleep medicine. 3rd edition. Philadelphia: Saunders; 2000. p. 502–10.

93. Pantoja AL, Faber J, Rocha LH, et al. Assessment of the adaptive value of dreams. Sleep 2009;32: A421.

94. Stickgold R, Malia A, Maguire D, et al. Replaying the game: hypnagogic images in normals and amnesics. Science 2000;290(5490):350–3.

95. Stickgold R. Memory, cognition, and dreams. In: Maquet P, Smith C, Stickgold R, editors. Sleep and brain plasticity. Oxford (United Kingdom): Oxford Press; 2003. p. 17–39.

96. Fosse M, Fosse R, Hobson A, et al. Dreaming and episodic memory: a functional dissociation? J Cogn Neurosci 2003;15:1–9.

97. Chrobak JJ, Buzsaki G. Selective activation of deep layer (V-VI) retrohippocampal cortical neurons during hippocampal sharp waves in the behaving rat. J Neurosci 1994;14(10):6160–70.

98. Chrobak JJ, Buzsaki G. High frequency oscillations in the output networks of the hippocampal-entorhinal axis of the freely behaving rat. J Neurosci 1996;16:3056–66.

99. Smith C, Aubrey JB, Peters KR. Different roles for REM and Stage 2 sleep in motor learning: a proposed model. Psychologica Belgica 2004;44:81–104.

100. Cipolli C, Bolzani R, Tuozzi G, et al. Active processing of declarative knowledge during REM sleep dreaming. J Sleep Res 2001;10:277–84.

101. Stickgold R, Scott L, Rittenhouse C, et al. Sleep-induced changes in associative memory. J Cogn Neurosci 1999;11(2):182–93.

102. Dinges DF. Are you awake? Cognitive performance and reverie during the hypnopompic state. In: Bootzin RR, Kihlstrom J, Schacter DL, editors. Sleep and cognition. Washington, DC: American Psychological Association; 1990. p. 159–78.

103. Smith C, Hanke J. Memory processing reflected in dreams from rapid eye movement sleep. Sleep 2004;27:A60.

104. Koukkou M, Lehmann D. Dreaming: the functional state shift hypothesis. Br J Psychiatry 1983;142:221–31.

105. Hobson JA, Stickgold R. The conscious state paradigm: a neurocognitive approach to waking,

sleeping, and dreaming. In: Gazzaniga M, editor. The cognitive neurosciences. Cambridge (MA): M.I.T. Press; 1994. p. 1373–89.

106. Cohen JD, Botvinick M, Carter CS. Anterior cingulate and prefrontal cortex: who's in control? Nat Neurosci 2000;3:421–3.

107. Solms M. The neuropsychology of dreams: a clinicoanatomical study. Mahwah (NJ): Lawrence Erlbaum; 1997.

108. Domhoff GW. The scientific study of dreams: neural networks, cognitive development and content

analysis. Washington, DC: American Psychological Association; 2003.

109. Wagner U, Gais S, Haider H, et al. Sleep inspires insight. Nature 2004;427:352–5.

110. Cartwright R. Dreams and adaption to divorce. In: Barrett D, editor. Trauma and dreams. Cambridge (MA): Harvard University Press; 1996. p. 179–85.

111. Nielsen TA, Stenstrom P. What are the memory sources of dreaming? Nature 2005;437: 1286–9.

Neuropharmacology of Sleep and Wakefulness: 2012 Update

Christopher J. Watson, PhD, Helen A. Baghdoyan, PhD,
Ralph Lydic, PhD*

KEYWORDS

- Neurotransmitters • Receptors • Translational research • Drug development

KEY POINTS

- Development of sedative/hypnotic molecules has been empiric rather than rational; the empiric approach has produced clinically useful drugs, but for no drug is the mechanism of action completely understood.
- All available sedative/hypnotic medications have unwanted side effects, and none of these medications creates a sleep architecture that is identical to the architecture of naturally occurring sleep.
- This article reviews recent advances in research aiming to elucidate the neurochemical mechanisms regulating sleep and wakefulness.

Sleep states comprise a constellation of physiologic and behavioral traits, and the mechanisms by which sedative/hypnotic medications alter these traits remain unclear. Drugs that enhance states of sleep also alter autonomic physiology, behavior, cognition, and affect. The complexities of brain neurochemistry and the extensive neural circuits regulating levels of behavioral arousal contribute to the present inability to understand exactly how sedative/hypnotics promote sleep. An additional complexity is that many sedative/hypnotic drugs have behavioral state-specific actions. For example, some sedative/hypnotic drugs promote the non–rapid eye movement (NREM) phase of sleep at the expense of decreasing the rapid eye movement (REM) phase of sleep. Despite the foregoing limitations, there has been progress in developing sleep medications that maximize desired actions such as rapid sleep onset, minimal next-day effect, low or no abuse

potential, and creation of a drug-induced state that is indistinguishable from physiologic sleep. To date, however, no sedative/hypnotic has produced all of these desired effects.

Rational drug design is an approach that has been successful in the development of antibiotic medications. Rational drug development of sedative/hypnotic medications is an approach based on understanding the receptor-binding properties of a molecule and how a molecule alters ligand binding, neurotransmitter synthesis, release, reuptake, and degradation. All of the foregoing cellular mechanisms can then be interpreted in the context of the overall drug effect. For sedative/hypnotic medications the desired action is, of course, promoting a safe and restorative sleeplike state. This article and **Fig. 1** provide an overview of neurotransmitters and brain regions currently known to modulate states of sleep and wakefulness. This overview of sleep neuropharmacology is an

A version of this article originally appeared in *Sleep Medicine Clinics, Volume 5, Issue 4.*
This work is supported by National Institutes of Health grants: HL40881, HL65272, MH45361; and the Department of Anesthesiology.
This work was not an industry-supported study and the authors have no financial conflicts of interest.
Department of Anesthesiology, University of Michigan, 7433 Medical Sciences Building I, 1150 West Medical Center Drive, Ann Arbor, MI 48109-5615, USA
* Corresponding author.
E-mail address: rlydic@umich.edu

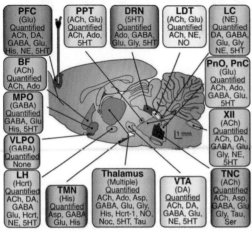

Fig. 1. Brain regions modulating sleep and wakefulness. Sagittal drawing of the rat brain schematizes the location, shape, and size of some brain regions that regulate sleep and wakefulness. The name of each brain region appears in bold print, the major neurotransmitters used for signaling to other brain regions are in parentheses, and neurochemical analytes relevant for arousal-state control that have been measured in that brain region are listed under the header "Quantified." The microdialysis probe is drawn to scale and is shown sampling from the prefrontal cortex. ACh, acetylcholine; Ado, adenosine; Asp, aspartate; BF, basal forebrain; DA, dopamine; DRN, dorsal raphé nucleus; GABA, γ-aminobutyric acid; Glu, glutamate; Gly, glycine; Hcrt, hypocretin; His, histamine; LC, locus coeruleus; LDT, laterodorsal tegmental nucleus; LH, lateral hypothalamus; MPO, medial preoptic area; NE, norepinephrine; NO, nitric oxide; Noc, nociceptin; PFC, prefrontal cortex; PnC, pontine reticular formation, caudal part; PnO, pontine reticular formation, oral part; PPT, pedunculopontine tegmental nucleus; Ser, serine; Tau, taurine; TMN, tuberomammillary nucleus; TNC, trigeminal nucleus complex; VLPO, ventrolateral preoptic area; VTA, ventral tegmental area; XII, hypoglossal nucleus; 5HT, serotonin. (*Modified from* Paxinos G, Watson C. The rat brain in stereotaxic coordinates. 6th edition. New York: Academic Press; 2007; and Watson CJ, Baghdoyan HA, Lydic R. A neurochemical perspective on states of consciousness. In: Hudetz AG, Pearce RA, editors. Suppressing the mind: anesthetic modulation of memory and consciousness. New York: Springer/Humana Press; 2010. p. 33–80; with permission.)

update of a précis[1] of a book chapter,[2] and interested readers are referred elsewhere for detailed reviews on sleep.[3–10]

γ-AMINOBUTYRIC ACID

γ-Aminobutyric acid (GABA) is the major inhibitory neurotransmitter in the brain. Although GABA transporters[11] and GABA$_B$[12] receptors can modulate sleep and wakefulness, most research into

GABAergic regulation of behavioral arousal focuses on the GABA$_A$ receptor. Activation of GABA$_A$ receptors causes neuronal inhibition by increasing chloride ion conductance. Because of their powerful inhibitory effects, GABA$_A$ receptors are the targets of most sedative/hypnotic and general anesthetic drugs. GABA$_A$ receptors exist as multiple subtypes (reviewed in Ref.[13]), and these subtypes are differentially located throughout the brain (reviewed in Ref.[14]). The differences in clinical effects caused by various benzodiazepine (eg, diazepam) and nonbenzodiazepine (eg, eszopiclone) sedative/hypnotics are attributed to the relative selectivity of these drugs for different GABA$_A$ receptor subtypes.[14] The complexity imparted by the numerous GABA$_A$ receptor subtypes is humbling. Although there is detailed knowledge about the many subunit isoforms that comprise GABA$_A$ receptor subtypes,[13] information is lacking about which of the many possible subtypes actually are expressed in specific brain regions,[15–17] and which subtypes are localized synaptically rather than extrasynaptically.[18] Extrasynaptically localized GABA$_A$ receptors possess a delta subunit and have particular relevance for sleep medicine.[19,20]

A better understanding of the in vivo characteristics and anatomic localization of GABA$_A$ receptor subtypes will contribute to rational drug development. The preclinical studies described in this section illustrate the complexity of the problem and provide examples of how the effects of GABAergic drugs on behavior vary as a function of brain region. For example, although systemic administration of GABA-mimetic drugs promotes sleep, sedation, or general anesthesia, enhancing GABAergic transmission within the pontine reticular formation actually increases wakefulness and decreases sleep. The pontine reticular formation is part of the ascending reticular activating system and contributes to the generation of REM sleep. Direct administration into the pontine reticular formation of drugs that increase GABAergic transmission increases wakefulness and inhibits sleep.[21–24] Similarly, pharmacologically increasing the concentration of endogenous GABA within the pontine reticular formation increases the time required for isoflurane to induce general anesthesia.[25] Consistent with this finding are data showing that endogenous GABA levels in the pontine reticular formation are higher during wakefulness than during REM sleep[26,27] (**Fig. 2**) or during the loss of wakefulness caused by isoflurane.[25] Inhibiting GABAergic signaling at GABA$_A$ receptors within the pontine reticular formation causes an increase in REM sleep and a decrease in wakefulness.[22,23,28,29] Likewise, decreasing

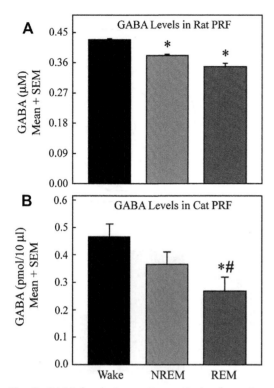

Fig. 2. GABA levels in pontine reticular formation (PRF) during wakefulness, NREM sleep, and REM sleep. These comparative data illustrate 2 key points. First, that in both rat (*A*) and cat (*B*) there are parallel, state-dependent changes in GABA levels. In rat and cat GABA levels are significantly lower in REM sleep than during wakefulness. Second, methodological differences in the collection of GABA preclude direct comparison of GABA levels between these 2 species. GABA levels shown in A and B reflect differences in microdialysis flow rate (0.4 μL/min for rat and 2.0 μL/min for cat), molecular weight cutoff of the microdialysis probe membrane (18,000 Da for rat and 6000 Da for cat), and possibly membrane material (regenerated cellulose for rat and cuprophane for cat). (*Modified from* Watson CJ, Lydic R, Baghdoyan HA. Sleep duration varies as a function of glutamate and GABA in rat pontine reticular formation. J Neurochem 2011;118(4):571–80; and Vanini G, Wathen BL, Lydic R, et al. Endogenous GABA levels in the pontine reticular formation are greater during wakefulness than during rapid eye movement sleep. J Neurosci 2011; 31(7):2649–56; with permission.)

extracellular GABA levels in the pontine reticular formation of rat decreases wakefulness and increases sleep,[24] and shortens the time required for isoflurane to induce loss of consciousness.[25] Furthermore, blocking GABA$_A$ receptors in the pontine reticular formation increases the time needed to regain wakefulness after isoflurane anesthesia.[22] Considered together, these data demonstrate a wakefulness-promoting role for GABA in the pontine reticular formation.

In brain regions containing neurons that promote wakefulness, GABAergic inhibition has been shown to cause an increase in sleep. These brain regions include the dorsal raphé nucleus, tuberomammillary nucleus of the posterior hypothalamus, medial preoptic area, and ventrolateral periaqueductal gray[30] (see **Fig. 1**) (for reviews see Refs.[8,31,32]).

ACETYLCHOLINE

Acetylcholine is distinguished as being the first identified neurotransmitter. Although the first neurochemical theory of sleep[33] correctly posited that acetylcholine plays a primary role in generating the brain-activated states of wakefulness and REM sleep, cholinergic drugs are not part of the standard pharmacologic armamentarium of sleep disorders medicine. Nonetheless, understanding the mechanisms by which cholinergic neurotransmission generates and maintains REM sleep is crucial, because acetylcholine interacts with other transmitter systems that are targets of sleep pharmacotherapy (eg, GABAergic and monoaminergic). Much of the research on the regulation of sleep by acetylcholine has focused on transmission mediated by muscarinic cholinergic receptors. Five subtypes (M1–M5) of the muscarinic receptor have been identified,[34] and the M2 subtype plays a key role in the generation of REM sleep.[35]

Cholinergic signaling originating from the laterodorsal tegmental and pedunculopontine tegmental nuclei (LDT/PPT) and the basal forebrain (see **Fig. 1**) promotes the cortically activated states of wakefulness and REM sleep (reviewed in Ref.[36]). LDT/PPT neurons can be divided into two populations based on discharge pattern. One population discharges maximally during wakefulness and REM sleep (referred to as Wake-On/REM-On) and another population fires only during wakefulness (Wake-On/REM-Off) (reviewed in Ref.[3]). This finding helps explain how acetylcholine can promote both wakefulness and REM sleep. LDT/PPT neurons project to numerous wakefulness-promoting brain regions.[3] Cholinergic terminals in the pontine reticular formation arise from the LDT/PPT,[3] and muscarinic receptors are present in the pontine reticular formation.[35,37,38] Many studies have administered cholinomimetics to the pontine reticular formation and have demonstrated that cholinergic transmission in the pontine reticular formation induces REM sleep (reviewed in Refs.[3,36]). Electrically stimulating the LDT/PPT increases acetylcholine release in the pontine reticular formation[39] and increases REM sleep.[40]

The release of endogenous acetylcholine in the pontine reticular formation is significantly greater during REM sleep than during wakefulness or NREM sleep.[41–43] Taken together, these data demonstrate that cholinergic projections from the LDT/PPT to the pontine reticular formation promote REM sleep.

Recent in vivo data obtained from normal rats demonstrate that the sedative/hypnotics zolpidem, diazepam, and eszopiclone differentially alter acetylcholine release in the pontine reticular formation.[44] Intravenous administration of eszopiclone prevented the REM phase of sleep, increased electroencephalograph (EEG) delta power, and decreased acetylcholine release in rat pontine reticular formation (**Fig. 3**).[44] These data provide the first functional evidence for a heterogeneous distribution of GABA$_A$ receptor subtypes within the pontine reticular formation. The different effects of GABA$_A$ receptor agonists on sleep have been attributed to brain-region–specific distributions of GABA$_A$ receptors and differences in sedative/hypnotic affinities for GABA$_A$ receptor subtypes.[45] These preclinical data can be contrasted with those of human psychopharmacology, where no study has convincingly demonstrated differential GABA$_A$ subtype binding among benzodiazepine and non-benzodiazepine sleeping medications.[45] To date, the nonbenzodiazepine, benzodiazepine-receptor agonist eszopiclone remains the only sleeping medication for which the long-term (6 months) effects have been characterized.[46,47]

Cholinergic neurons originating in the basal forebrain project throughout the entire cerebral cortex (reviewed in Ref.[48]). Acetylcholine release in the basal forebrain is highest during REM sleep, lower during quiet wakefulness, and lowest during NREM sleep.[49] Cortical acetylcholine release is increased during wakefulness[48,50,51] and REM sleep[50] in comparison with NREM sleep. These data support the interpretation that cholinergic transmission from the basal forebrain promotes cortical activation during wakefulness and REM sleep.

ADENOSINE

Adenosine is a breakdown product of adenosine triphosphate (ATP). Increases in endogenous adenosine levels in a specific brain region during a period of prolonged wakefulness indicate that the region has been metabolically active. Direct biochemical measures show that ATP levels increase during sleep in areas of the brain that are most active during wakefulness.[52] This finding provides direct support for the hypothesis that sleep serves a restorative function.[53]

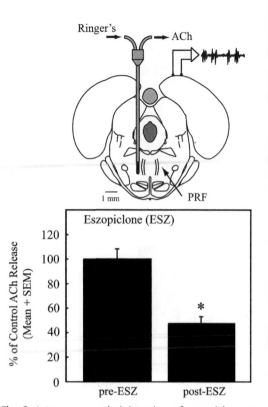

Fig. 3. Intravenous administration of eszopiclone to intact, behaving rats decreases acetylcholine (ACh) release in the pontine reticular formation (PRF). (*Top*) Schematic of coronal section of rat brain stem illustrates placement of a microdialysis probe in the PRF. Ringer's solution is pumped into the probe and samples are collected for quantification of ACh. At top right of the brain are electrodes and an amplifier for recording the cortical electroencephalogram (EEG), and a representative trace showing EEG activity after intravenous administration of eszopiclone. (*Bottom*) Histograms summarize the significant decrease in ACh release within the PRF caused by intravenous administration of eszopiclone. (*Reprinted from* Hambrecht-Wiedbusch VS, Gauthier EA, Baghdoyan HA, et al. Benzodiazepine receptor agonists cause drug-specific and state-specific alterations in EEG power and acetylcholine release in rat pontine reticular formation. Sleep 2010;33(7):911; with permission.)

Four subtypes of adenosine receptors, A$_1$, A$_{2A}$, A$_{2B}$, and A$_3$, have been identified and are distributed widely throughout the brain. Adenosine A$_1$ and A$_{2A}$ receptors are antagonized by caffeine, and the idea that adenosine promotes sleep is supported by the ubiquitous consumption of caffeine to maintain wakefulness and enhance alertness. In humans, oral administration of caffeine before nocturnal sleep increases sleep latency and reduces sleep efficiency.[54] Furthermore, morning caffeine ingestion has been shown to decrease sleep efficiency and overall sleep during the subsequent night.[55] No adenosine agonists are presently available to promote sleep. Adenosine, however, is relevant for sleep medicine, as insomnia can be caused by consumption of caffeine or by the respiratory stimulant theophylline. Of interest is that adenosine can have analgesic effects, and this action shows promise for clinical use.[56]

Adenosinergic transmission in brain regions that regulate sleep and wakefulness has been extensively investigated (reviewed in Refs.[3,57–60]). Activating adenosine A_1 receptors causes neuronal inhibition, and A_1 is the most abundant adenosine receptor subtype in the brain. This section highlights selected studies supporting the interpretation that adenosine promotes sleep, at least in part, by inhibiting neurons in several key wakeulness-promoting brain areas.

Prolonged wakefulness increases adenosine levels selectively in the basal forebrain and cortex (see **Fig. 1**),[61,62] and increases adenosine A_1 receptor binding in human[63] and rat[64] brain. Pharmacologically increasing adenosine levels in the basal forebrain[65] or administering adenosine A_1 receptor agonists to the basal forebrain[59] causes an increase in sleep. Intravenous administration of buprenorphine decreases adenosine levels in the basal forebrain and increases wakefulness.[66] Inactivating adenosine A_1 receptors in the basal forebrain decreases EEG delta power and NREM sleep time,[67] and immunohistochemical studies reveal that the basal forebrain contains A_1 receptors, but not A_{2A} receptors.[68] Cholinergic neurons in the basal forebrain project to the cortex and contribute to the EEG activation characteristic of wakefulness and REM sleep. Adenosine directly inhibits cholinergic neurons in the basal forebrain by activating A_1 receptors.[69] Adenosine indirectly inhibits wakefulness-promoting hypocretin (orexin)-containing neurons in the lateral hypothalamus by activating A_1 receptors.[70] Blocking adenosine A_1 receptors in the lateral hypothalamus causes an increase in wakefulness and a decrease in sleep.[71] Histaminergic neurons in the tuberomammillary nucleus (see **Fig. 1**) express adenosine A_1 receptors, and activating those receptors increases NREM sleep.[72] These complementary data suggest that adenosine promotes sleep by inhibiting wakefulness-promoting neurons localized to the basal forebrain, lateral hypothalamus, and tuberomammillary nucleus.

Adenosine also exerts sleep-promoting effects by actions at the level of the prefrontal cortex and the pontine reticular formation (see **Fig. 1**). In vivo microdialysis experiments in mouse[73] have shown that adenosine acting at A_1 receptors in the prefrontal cortex inhibits traits that characterize wakefulness (including acetylcholine release in the prefrontal cortex and activation of the EEG), as well as the state of wakefulness. Activation of adenosine A_1 receptors in the prefrontal cortex also causes a decrease in the release of acetylcholine in the pontine reticular formation. These findings demonstrate that in the prefrontal cortex, adenosine A_1 receptors mediate a descending inhibition of wakefulness-promoting systems. Within the pontine reticular formation, activation of adenosine A_{2A} receptors increases the time needed to recover from general anesthesia,[74] increases acetylcholine release,[74,75] and increases the amount of time spent in NREM sleep[75] and REM sleep.[75,76] The increase in REM sleep may be a result of the A_{2A}-mediated increase in acetylcholine release, because coadministration of a muscarinic receptor antagonist with the A_{2A} agonist blocks the REM sleep increase.[76] Studies examining the effects on sleep of adenosine receptor antagonists are required in order to conclude that endogenous adenosine within the pontine reticular formation modulates sleep. The finding that clinically used opioids, such as morphine, fentanyl, and buprenorphine, decrease adenosine levels in the pontine reticular formation[66,77] and disrupt REM sleep[66] (also reviewed in Ref.[78]) suggests the possibility that adenosinergic transmission within the pontine reticular formation participates in REM sleep generation.

BIOGENIC AMINES

The monoamines have long been known to promote wakefulness. Serotonin (5-hydroxytryptamine [5HT])-containing neurons of the dorsal raphé nucleus, norepinephrine-containing neurons of the locus coeruleus, and histamine-containing neurons of the tuberomammillary nucleus (see **Fig. 1**) discharge at their fastest rates during wakefulness, slow their firing in NREM sleep, cease discharging before and during REM sleep, and resume firing before the onset of wakefulness (reviewed in Ref.[3]). Dopaminergic neurons, by contrast, do not show major changes in firing rates across the sleep-wakefulness cycle.

Serotonin

Serotonin release in the dorsal raphé nucleus[79] and preoptic area[80] of the rat is highest during wakefulness. Furthermore, electrical stimulation of the dorsal raphé nucleus increases wakefulness.[81] Serotonin receptors are divided into 7 families ($5HT_1$–$5HT_7$).[82] Systemic administration of agonists for $5HT_{1A}$, $5HT_{1B}$, $5HT_{2A/2C}$, or $5HT_3$ receptors causes an increase in wakefulness and a decrease in sleep (reviewed in Ref.[7]). Local administration of a $5HT_{1A}$ receptor agonist to the dorsal raphé nucleus increases wakefulness in rats[83] but increases REM sleep in cats.[84] Microinjection of a $5HT_{2A/2C}$ receptor agonist into rat dorsal raphé nucleus also decreases REM sleep, with no significant effect on wakefulness.[85] These incongruent findings may be due to species differences, or may indicate that in addition to promoting wakefulness, serotonin plays a permissive role in the generation of REM sleep. Systemic administration of antagonists for the $5HT_{2A}$ receptor or the $5HT_6$ receptor to rat during the dark phase of the light/dark cycle (active period) decreases wakefulness, increases NREM sleep, and has no effect on REM sleep.[86] These data are consistent with the view that serotonin is wakefulness promoting. Genetically modified mice also have been used to explore the role of serotonin in sleep and wakefulness. Mice lacking the genes for the $5HT_{1A}$[87] or $5HT_{1B}$[88] receptor showed an increase in REM sleep. Administration of a $5HT_{1A}$,[87,89] a $5HT_{1B}$,[88] or a $5HT_{2A/2C}$[90] receptor agonist decreased REM sleep in rodent and human. These data indicate that serotonin acting at $5HT_{1A}$, $5HT_{1B}$, and $5HT_{2A/2C}$ receptors plays a role in suppressing REM sleep. The foregoing data underlie the fact that insomnia can be secondary to the use of selective serotonin reuptake inhibitors (SSRIs) or serotonin and norepinephrine reuptake inhibitors (SNRIs).

Norepinephrine

Noradrenergic cells of the locus coeruleus inhibit REM sleep, promote wakefulness, and project to a variety of other arousal-regulating brain regions (see **Fig. 1**) including the hypothalamus, thalamus, basal forebrain, and cortex (reviewed in Ref.[91]). Noradrenergic receptors include α_1-, α_2-, and β-adrenergic subtypes.[92] Administration of noradrenaline or α- and β-receptor agonists to the medial septal area[93,94] or the medial preoptic area[95,96] increases wakefulness. Stimulation of locus coeruleus neurons increases noradrenaline in the prefrontal cortex of anesthetized rat,[97,98] and contributes to cortical activation. These data are consistent with the view that noradrenaline promotes wakefulness. However, bilateral microinjection of an α_1-antagonist (prazosin), an α_2-agonist (clonidine), or a β-antagonist (propranolol) into the PPT increases REM sleep with little to no effect on NREM sleep or wakefulness.[99] The arousal-regulating effects of noradrenaline are brain-region specific. The treatment of hypertension with blockers of α- and/or β-adrenergic receptors can disrupt normal sleep.

Histamine

Histaminergic cell bodies, which are located in the tuberomammillary nucleus of the posterior hypothalamus, have diffuse projections throughout the brain (reviewed in Refs.[100,101]). Data from posterior hypothalamic lesion studies and from single-unit recordings indicate that the tuberomammillary nucleus promotes wakefulness.[100,101] Three histaminergic receptors, denoted H_1, H_2, and H_3, are present in the brain (for review see Ref.[102]). First-generation H_1 receptor antagonists, such as diphenhydramine, cause drowsiness (sedation) and impaired performance in humans[103] and rats.[104] Newer antagonists that are relatively selective for the H_1 histamine receptor, such as the potent antagonist doxepin, improve subjective and objective measures of sleep in insomnia patients without causing sedation or psychomotor impairments the next day.[105] Systemic administration of the H_1 receptor antagonists mepyramine[106] and cyproheptadine[107] caused a significant increase in NREM sleep in cat and rat, respectively. Decreasing brain histamine levels by inhibiting synthesis significantly decreases wakefulness and increases NREM sleep in rats[108,109] and cats.[106] These data suggest that histaminergic signaling via the H_1 receptor promotes wakefulness. New therapies for sleep disorders and for maintaining vigilance include H_3 receptor antagonists and inverse agonists.[110–114]

Dopamine

Stimulants such as amphetamine, cocaine, and methylphenidate increase wakefulness and counter hypersomnia by increasing levels of endogenous dopamine (reviewed in Ref.[115]). In vivo imaging studies suggest that sleep deprivation increases dopamine levels in human brain.[116] The cell bodies of dopaminergic neurons that regulate arousal reside in the ventral tegmental area and the substantia nigra pars compacta (see **Fig. 1**).[117] These dopaminergic neurons project to the dorsal raphé nucleus, basal forebrain, locus coeruleus, thalamus, and laterodorsal tegmental nucleus (reviewed in Ref.[118]). There are also dopaminergic neurons in the ventrolateral periaqueductal gray that are active during wakefulness and have reciprocal connections with sleep-regulating brain areas.[119]

Five dopaminergic receptors have been cloned (D1–D5). Dopaminergic neurons of the substantia nigra and ventral tegmental area do not change firing rates as a function of states of sleep and wakefulness (reviewed in Ref.[3]). Dopamine does promote wakefulness, and dopamine-transporter knockout mice display increased wakefulness and decreased NREM sleep compared with controls.[120] Systemic administration of D1 receptor agonists or antagonists causes an increase or decrease, respectively, in wakefulness.[121] Intracerebroventricular administration of a D1 or D2 receptor agonist to rat increases wakefulness.[122] Systemic administration of a D2 receptor agonist causes biphasic effects, with low doses decreasing wakefulness and high doses increasing wakefulness.[123,124] Systemic administration of D-amphetamine to rats increases wakefulness and decreases NREM sleep and REM sleep.[125] The mechanisms by which modafinil counters excessive daytime sleepiness remain to be specified. There is evidence that modafinil enhances synaptic release of dopamine and norepinephrine.[126]

GLUTAMATE

Glutamate is the main excitatory neurotransmitter in the brain, and acts at α-amino-3-hydroxy-5-methyl-4-isoxazole propionic acid (AMPA), kainate, and N-methyl-D-aspartate (NMDA) ionotropic receptors. Surprisingly little is known about glutamatergic regulation of sleep and wakefulness. Sleep state–dependent changes in levels of endogenous glutamate change differentially across the brain (see Table 8 of Ref.[127]). For example, glutamate levels in some areas of rat cortex show increases in concentration during wakefulness and REM sleep, and decreases during NREM sleep,[128] and glutamate concentrations in rat pontine reticular formation are higher during wakefulness than during NREM sleep and REM sleep.[27] Sleep deprivation increases glutamate concentrations in rat dorsal hippocampus and medial thalamus.[129] Microinjection and electrophysiological studies provide evidence that glutamate acts within the LDT/PPT,[130–132] the pontine reticular formation[31,133,134] (PnO, PnC; see **Fig. 1**), the medial preoptic area,[135] the insular cortex,[136] and medial portions of the medullary reticular formation[137,138] to modulate traits and states of arousal. Glutamatergic neurons are present in rat pontine reticular formation[139] and neurons in the pontine reticular formation are capable of synthesizing glutamate for use as a neurotransmitter.[140] Glutamate elicits excitatory responses from neurons of the pontine reticular formation,[141,142] and glutamatergic and cholinergic transmission in the pontine reticular formation interact synergistically to potentiate catalepsy.[143] Given individually, agonists for AMPA, kainate, and NMDA receptors evoke excitatory responses from neurons of the pontine reticular formation.[133] Dialysis delivery of the NMDA receptor antagonists ketamine or MK-801 to cat pontine reticular formation decreases acetylcholine release in the pontine reticular formation and disrupts breathing.[43]

PEPTIDES

Many peptides are known to modulate sleep (reviewed in Ref.[144]). This article focuses on hypocretin (orexin), leptin, and ghrelin, because of their relevance for sleep disorders medicine.

Hypocretin-1 and -2

Numerous lines of evidence support a role for hypocretin-1 and -2 (also called orexin A and B) in the maintenance of wakefulness. The cell bodies of hypocretin-producing neurons are localized to the dorsolateral hypothalamus[145,146] and send projections to all the major brain regions that regulate arousal.[147,148] Hypocretinergic neurons discharge with the highest frequency during active wakefulness and show almost no discharge activity during sleep.[149,150] Hypocretin-1 levels in the hypothalamus of the cat are greater during wakefulness and REM sleep than during NREM sleep.[151] Dogs displaying a narcoleptic phenotype have a mutation of the hypocretin receptor-2 gene,[152] and hypocretin mRNA and peptide levels are greatly reduced in human narcoleptic patients.[153,154] Patients presenting with narcolepsy-cataplexy also have greatly reduced levels of hypocretin in their cerebrospinal fluid compared with controls.[155] Preclinical studies have demonstrated that selective lesions of hypocretin-containing neurons[156,157] or genetic removal of the peptide[158] result in a narcoleptic phenotype. By what mechanisms might hypocretin enhance wakefulness?

Two receptors for the hypocretin peptides have been identified. Hypocretin-1 and -2 receptors have been localized to the LDT/PPT, pontine reticular formation, dorsal raphé nucleus, and locus coeruleus.[159–163] Electrophysiological studies demonstrate that hypocretin-1 and/or hypocretin-2 excite neurons in these same brain regions.[164–172] Hypocretin-1 and -2 also excite tuberomammillary neurons[173,174] and cholinergic neurons of the basal forebrain.[175] Studies using intracerebroventricular injection in wild-type and knockout mice ($OX_1R^{-/-}$, $OX_2R^{-/-}$, and $OX_1R^{-/-}$; $OX_2R^{-/-}$) suggest a differential regulation of arousal state via each hypocretin receptor subtype.[176]

Intracerebroventricular administration of hypocretin-1 increases wakefulness and decreases NREM sleep and REM sleep in rats.[177,178]

When administered into the lateral preoptic area,[179] LDT,[180] pontine reticular formation,[24,181] or basal forebrain,[182,183] hypocretin-1 causes an increase in wakefulness. In the cat, microinjection of hypocretin-1 into the pontine reticular formation increases REM sleep if delivered during NREM sleep,[166] but suppresses REM sleep if delivered during wakefulness.[181] The wakefulness-promoting effect of hypocretin in the pontine reticular formation is further supported by evidence that delivery of antisense oligonucleotides against the hypocretin-2 receptor to the pontine reticular formation of rats enhances REM sleep and induces cataplexy.[184]

Measuring the effect of hypocretin-1 on the release of other arousal-regulating transmitters may provide insight into how hypocretin-1 promotes wakefulness. Microinjection of hypocretin-1 into the basal forebrain of rats increases cortical acetylcholine release.[185] Intracerebroventricular delivery of hypocretin-1 increases histamine in rodent frontal cortex[186] and anterior hypothalamus.[187] Microinjection of hypocretin-1 into the ventricles or the ventral tegmental area increases dopamine release in rat prefrontal cortex.[178] Hypocretin-1 delivered to rat dorsal raphé nucleus increases serotonin release in the dorsal raphé nucleus,[188] and dialysis delivery of hypocretin-1 to rat pontine reticular formation increases acetylcholine release[189] and GABA levels[24] in the pontine reticular formation. The increase in wakefulness produced by microinjecting hypocretin-1 into the pontine reticular formation is prevented by blocking GABA$_A$ receptors.[190] This finding suggests that hypocretin may increase wakefulness, in part, by increasing GABA levels in the pontine reticular formation. Considered together, these data support the classification of hypocretin-1 as a wakefulness-promoting neuropeptide.

An alternative hypothesis is that a primary function of hypocretin is to enhance activity in motor systems, the increase in wakefulness being secondary. This hypothesis is supported by data showing that hypocretin-1 concentrations in the cerebrospinal fluid are significantly greater during active wakefulness with movement than during quiet wakefulness with no movement.[151] Hypocretinergic neurons also have very low firing rates during quiet wakefulness (without movement) than during active wakefulness.[149,150] Oral administration of the hypocretin-1 and -2 receptor antagonists ACT-078573, DORA-22, or MK-6096 increases NREM sleep and/or REM sleep in mouse,[191] rat,[191,192] dog,[191,192] and human,[192] suggesting a direct, wakefulness-promoting effect of endogenous hypocretin.

Leptin and Ghrelin

Because of the ongoing epidemic of obesity and the association between metabolic syndrome and sleep disorders, many studies aim to understand the sleep-related roles of leptin and ghrelin. Decreased levels of leptin (a hormone that suppresses appetite) and increased levels of ghrelin (a hormone that stimulates appetite) are associated with short sleep duration in humans.[193,194] Obese patients with obstructive sleep apnea syndrome (OSAS) have increased plasma levels of leptin[195] and ghrelin[196] compared with age-matched obese patients without OSAS. Obese patients with OSAS and excessive daytime sleepiness have significantly lower levels of ghrelin and a trend for lower plasma levels of leptin compared with obese patients with OSAS but without excessive daytime sleepiness.[197] These data suggest that there is a complex relationship between leptin, ghrelin, obesity, and sleep disruption that warrants further investigation.

Rodent models that may increase the understanding of the link between metabolic syndrome, leptin, and sleep disorders include *ob/ob* mice (obese mice with reduced levels of leptin) and *db/db* mice (which are also obese but are resistant to leptin). Leptin-deficient mice have attenuated responses to certain drug treatments when compared with control species. When dialyzed into the prefrontal cortex of mouse, the atypical antipsychotic olanzapine increases acetylcholine release in the prefrontal cortex.[198] The increase in acetylcholine release is significantly greater in C57BL/6J mice than in leptin-deficient mice. However, when leptin is restored to leptin-deficient mice, the olanzapine-induced increase in acetylcholine release is the same as that in the C57BL/6J mouse (**Fig. 4**). Similarly, leptin-deficient mice have a reduced antinociceptive response to supraspinal administration of neostigmine (an acetylcholinesterase inhibitor that increases levels of acetylcholine) when compared with C57BL/6J mice.[199] Leptin replacement restores the antinociceptive responses of the leptin-deficient mice to that of the C57BL/6J mice. These data indicate a possible link between leptin and cholinergic signaling within the prefrontal cortex and the pontine reticular formation, 2 brain areas that play a role in the regulation of sleep and wakefulness (see **Fig. 1**).

The sleep of *ob/ob* mice is characterized by an increase in number of arousals and a decrease in the duration of sleep bouts compared with wild-type controls.[200] The *ob/ob* mice also have an impaired response to the cholinergic enhancement of REM sleep.[201] Similarly, *db/db* mice have significant alterations in sleep architecture

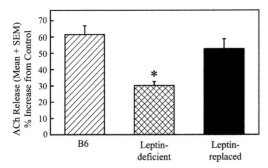

Fig. 4. Leptin replacement restores the olanzapine-induced increase of acetylcholine (ACh) release in the prefrontal cortex of leptin-deficient mice. Dialysis administration of olanzapine (100 μM) to the prefrontal cortex of C57BL/6J (B6), leptin-deficient, or leptin-replaced mice caused an increase in ACh release in the prefrontal cortex. The increase in ACh release was significantly smaller in leptin-deficient mice compared with B6 controls. The olanzapine-induced increase in ACh release was not significantly different between B6 controls and leptin-replaced mice. This result suggests that leptin modulates the release of ACh within the prefrontal cortex and may also play a role in the cortical activation that occurs during wakefulness and REM sleep. (*Reprinted from* Wathen AB, West EM, Lydic R, et al. Olanzapine causes a leptin-dependent increase in acetylcholine release in mouse prefrontal cortex. Sleep 2012;35(3):319; with permission.)

compared with wild-type control mice that include, but are not limited to, increases in NREM sleep and REM sleep during the dark phase and decreases in wakefulness and NREM sleep bout duration.[202] Local administration of ghrelin into rat lateral hypothalamus, medial preoptic area, or paraventricular nucleus increases wakefulness, decreases NREM sleep, and increases food intake.[203] Together these findings suggest that leptin and ghrelin, hormones that are important for appetite regulation, significantly influence sleep and are significantly modulated by sleep.

OPIOIDS

Opioids are the major class of drugs used to treat acute and chronic pain, and one side effect of opioids is sleep disruption. Sleep disruption, in turn, exacerbates pain[204–206] and increases the dose of opioids required for successful pain management (reviewed in Refs.[77,78,206]). Clinically relevant doses of opioids given to naïve rats[66] or to otherwise healthy humans (reviewed in Ref.[207]) disrupt sleep. For example, a single intravenous infusion of morphine in healthy volunteers decreases stages 3 and 4 NREM sleep, decreases

REM sleep, and increases stage 2 NREM sleep.[208] A nighttime dose of morphine or methadone also decreases stages 3 and 4 NREM sleep while increasing stage 2 NREM sleep.[209] Constant infusion of analgesic doses of remifentanil overnight decreases REM sleep in healthy volunteers.[210] Patients receiving methadone treatment for opioid dependence experience sleep disturbances including insomnia, decreases in total sleep time, slow-wave sleep, and sleep efficiency, as well as increases in the number of awakings.[211–213] The cycle of opioid-induced sleep disruption leading to increased pain and increased opioid requirement is recognized as a significant clinical problem that must be addressed at the mechanistic level.[214]

Opioid-induced disruption of REM sleep is mediated, at least in part, by decreasing acetylcholine release in the pontine reticular formation.[78] Opioids also decrease adenosine levels in the basal forebrain and pontine reticular formation,[77] 2 brain regions where adenosine has sleep-promoting effects. Local administration of morphine into the pontine reticular formation of cats[215] or rats[216] increases wakefulness and decreases REM sleep.

FUTURE DIRECTIONS

This selective overview was completed during the summer of 2010, a date also marking the 20th anniversary of the human genome project. The stunning successes—and unmet hopes—of genomic approaches to medicine were highlighted in the *The New York Times* June 12 and June 14 issues.[217,218] These two articles offer a sobering reminder that taking a molecule from preclinical discovery to commercially available drug typically requires 15 or more years. This time interval exists without any mandate to understand the mechanisms of drug action. As a former director of research and development at Wyeth noted,[218] "Genomics did not speed up drug development. It gave us more rapid access to new molecular targets." Potential molecular targets can be rapidly interrogated with high-throughput screening programs that use a cell line transfected to contain a reporter construct. But identifying potential molecular targets leaves unanswered the question of whether the candidate targets will be druggable in vivo. This complexity is exemplified by sedative/hypnotic medications commonly used in sleep medicine. GABA$_A$ receptors are drug targets that promote a sleeplike state by unknown actions[45] when they are activated in some brain regions, yet GABA$_A$ receptors enhance wakefulness when activated selectively in the posterior hypothalamus[219] or pontine reticular formation.[22,23,25] As busy as **Fig. 1** may seem, it barely hints at the complexity of data that must be logically integrated if we are to derive a coherent model of the endogenous neurochemical processes that regulate states of sleep and wakefulness.

Recent progress in understanding the basic neuropharmacology of sleep can be appreciated by comparing the 1990 and 2005 editions of *Brain Control of Wakefulness and Sleep.*[3] The incorporation of basic neuropharmacology into sleep disorders medicine is readily apparent by comparing the first and most recent editions of *Principles and Practice of Sleep Medicine.*[220] Future progress is most likely to come from a systems biology approach that seeks to integrate genomic, cellular, network, and behavioral levels of analysis.[221] The focus on sleep medications in the *Clinics of North America* series demonstrates the cross-cutting relevance of sleep for the practice of medicine. The pressing clinical problem of sleep disorders medicine will continue to stimulate advances in understanding the neurochemical regulation of sleep.

ACKNOWLEDGMENTS

The authors thank Mary A. Norat and Sarah L. Watson for critical comments on this article.

REFERENCES

1. Watson CJ, Baghdoyan HA, Lydic R. Neuropharmacology of sleep and wakefulness. Sleep Med Clin 2010;5(4):513–28.
2. Watson CJ, Baghdoyan HA, Lydic R. A neurochemical perspective on states of consciousness. In: Hudetz AG, Pearce RA, editors. Suppressing the mind: anesthetic modulation of memory and consciousness. New York: Springer/Humana Press; 2010. p. 33–80.
3. Steriade M, McCarley RW, editors. Brain control of wakefulness and sleep. New York: Kluwer Academic/Plenum Publishers; 2005.
4. Datta S, MacLean RR. Neurobiological mechanisms for the regulation of mammalian sleep-wake behavior: reinterpretation of historical evidence and inclusion of contemporary cellular and molecular evidence. Neurosci Biobehav Rev 2007;31(5):775–824.
5. McCarley RW. Neurobiology of REM and NREM sleep. Sleep Med 2007;8(4):302–30.
6. Stenberg D. Neuroanatomy and neurochemistry of sleep. Cell Mol Life Sci 2007;64(10):1187–204.
7. Monti JM, Pandi-Perumal SR, Sinton CM, editors. Neurochemistry of sleep and wakefulness. New York: Cambridge University Press; 2008.
8. Szymusiak R, McGinty D. Hypothalamic regulation of sleep and arousal. Ann N Y Acad Sci 2008;1129: 275–86.
9. Mallick BN, Pandi-Perumal SR, McCarley RW, et al. Rapid eye movement sleep: regulation and function. New York: Cambridge University Press; 2010.
10. Espana RA, Scammell TE. Sleep neurobiology from a clinical perspective. Sleep 2011;34(7):845–58.
11. Narita M, Niikura K, Nanjo-Niikura K, et al. Sleep disturbances in a neuropathic pain-like condition in the mouse are associated with altered GABAergic transmission in the cingulate cortex. Pain 2011;152(6):1358–72.
12. Vienne J, Bettler B, Franken P, et al. Differential effects of $GABA_B$ receptor subtypes, γ-hydroxybutyric acid, and baclofen on EEG activity and sleep regulation. J Neurosci 2010;30(42): 14194–204.
13. Olsen RW, Sieghart W. International Union of Pharmacology. LXX. Subtypes of γ-aminobutyric acid$_A$ receptors: classification on the basis of subunit composition, pharmacology, and function. Update. Pharmacol Rev 2008;60(3):243–60.
14. Winsky-Sommerer R. Role of $GABA_A$ receptors in the physiology and pharmacology of sleep. Eur J Neurosci 2009;29(9):1779–94.
15. Fritschy JM, Mohler H. $GABA_A$-receptor heterogeneity in the adult rat brain: differential regional and cellular distribution of seven major subunits. J Comp Neurol 1995;359(1):154–94.
16. Heldt SA, Ressler KJ. Forebrain and midbrain distribution of major benzodiazepine-sensitive $GABA_A$ receptor subunits in the adult C57 mouse as assessed with in situ hybridization. Neuroscience 2007;150(2):370–85.
17. Pirker S, Schwarzer C, Wieselthaler A, et al. $GABA_A$ receptors: immunocytochemical distribution of 13 subunits in the adult rat brain. Neuroscience 2000;101(4):815–50.
18. Farrant M, Nusser Z. Variations on an inhibitory theme: phasic and tonic activation of $GABA_A$ receptors. Nat Rev Neurosci 2005;6(3):215–29.
19. Orser BA. Extrasynaptic $GABA_A$ receptors are critical targets for sedative-hypnotic drugs. J Clin Sleep Med 2006;2(2):S12–8.
20. Walsh JK, Deacon S, Dijk DJ, et al. The selective extrasynaptic $GABA_A$ agonist, gaboxadol, improves traditional hypnotic efficacy measures and enhances slow wave activity in a model of transient insomnia. Sleep 2007;30(5):593–602.
21. Camacho-Arroyo I, Alvarado R, Manjarrez J, et al. Microinjections of muscimol and bicuculline into the pontine reticular formation modify the sleep-waking cycle in the rat. Neurosci Lett 1991; 129(1):95–7.
22. Flint RR, Chang T, Lydic R, et al. $GABA_A$ receptors in the pontine reticular formation of C57BL/6J

mouse modulate neurochemical, electrographic, and behavioral phenotypes of wakefulness. J Neurosci 2010;30(37):12301–9.

23. Xi MC, Morales FR, Chase MH. Evidence that wakefulness and REM sleep are controlled by a GABAergic pontine mechanism. J Neurophysiol 1999;82(4):2015–9.

24. Watson CJ, Soto-Calderon H, Lydic R, et al. Pontine reticular formation (PnO) administration of hypocretin-1 increases PnO GABA levels and wakefulness. Sleep 2008;31(4):453–64.

25. Vanini G, Watson CJ, Lydic R, et al. γ-aminobutyric acid-mediated neurotransmission in the pontine reticular formation modulates hypnosis, immobility, and breathing during isoflurane anesthesia. Anesthesiology 2008;109(6):978–88.

26. Vanini G, Wathen BL, Lydic R, et al. Endogenous GABA levels in the pontine reticular formation are greater during wakefulness than during rapid eye movement sleep. J Neurosci 2011;31(7):2649–56.

27. Watson CJ, Lydic R, Baghdoyan HA. Sleep duration varies as a function of glutamate and GABA in rat pontine reticular formation. J Neurochem 2011;118(4):571–80.

28. Sanford LD, Tang X, Xiao J, et al. GABAergic regulation of REM sleep in reticularis pontis oralis and caudalis in rats. J Neurophysiol 2003;90(2):938–45.

29. Marks GA, Sachs OW, Birabil CG. Blockade of GABA, type A, receptors in the rat pontine reticular formation induces rapid eye movement sleep that is dependent upon the cholinergic system. Neuroscience 2008;156(1):1–10.

30. Vanini G, Torterolo P, McGregor R, et al. GABAergic processes in the mesencephalic tegmentum modulate the occurrence of active (rapid eye movement) sleep in guinea pigs. Neuroscience 2007;145(3):1157–67.

31. Vanini G, Lydic R, Baghdoyan HA. GABAergic modulation of REM sleep. In: Mallick BN, Pandi-Perumal SR, McCarley RW, et al, editors. Rapid eye movement sleep: regulation and function. New York: Cambridge University Press; 2010. p. 206–13.

32. Vanini G, Baghdoyan HA, Lydic R. Relevance of sleep neurobiology for cognitive neuroscience and anesthesiology. In: Mashour GA, editor. Consciousness, awareness, and anesthesia. New York: Cambridge University Press; 2010. p. 1–23.

33. Jouvet M. The role of monoamines and acetylcholine-containing neurons in the regulation of the sleep-waking cycle. Ergeb Physiol 1972;64:166–307.

34. Ishii M, Kurachi Y. Muscarinic acetylcholine receptors. Curr Pharm Des 2006;12(28):3573–81.

35. Baghdoyan HA, Lydic R. M2 muscarinic receptor subtype in the feline medial pontine reticular formation modulates the amount of rapid eye movement sleep. Sleep 1999;22(7):835–47.

36. Lydic R, Baghdoyan HA. Acetylcholine modulates sleep and wakefulness: a synaptic perspective. In: Monti JM, Pandi-Perumal SR, Sinton CM, editors. Neurochemistry of sleep and wakefulness. Cambridge (UK): Cambridge University Press; 2008. p. 109–43.

37. Baghdoyan HA. Location and quantification of muscarinic receptor subtypes in rat pons: implications for REM sleep generation. Am J Physiol 1997;273(3 Pt 2):R896–904.

38. Demarco GJ, Baghdoyan HA, Lydic R. Differential cholinergic activation of G proteins in rat and mouse brainstem: relevance for sleep and nociception. J Comp Neurol 2003;457(2):175–84.

39. Lydic R, Baghdoyan HA. Pedunculopontine stimulation alters respiration and increases ACh release in the pontine reticular formation. Am J Physiol 1993;264(3 Pt 2):R544–54.

40. Thakkar M, Portas C, McCarley RW. Chronic low-amplitude electrical stimulation of the laterodorsal tegmental nucleus of freely moving cats increases REM sleep. Brain Res 1996;723(1–2):223–7.

41. Kodama T, Takahashi Y, Honda Y. Enhancement of acetylcholine release during paradoxical sleep in the dorsal tegmental field of the cat brain stem. Neurosci Lett 1990;114(3):277–82.

42. Leonard TO, Lydic R. Pontine nitric oxide modulates acetylcholine release, rapid eye movement sleep generation, and respiratory rate. J Neurosci 1997;17(2):774–85.

43. Lydic R, Baghdoyan HA. Ketamine and MK-801 decrease acetylcholine release in the pontine reticular formation, slow breathing, and disrupt sleep. Sleep 2002;25(5):617–22.

44. Hambrecht-Wiedbusch VS, Gauthier EA, Baghdoyan HA, et al. Benzodiazepine receptor agonists cause drug-specific and state-specific alterations in EEG power and acetylcholine release in rat pontine reticular formation. Sleep 2010;33(7):909–18.

45. Krystal AD. In vivo evidence of the specificity of effects of GABAA receptor modulating medications. Sleep 2010;33(7):859–60.

46. Krystal AD, Walsh JK, Laska E, et al. Sustained efficacy of eszopiclone over 6 months of nightly treatment: results of a randomized, double-blind, placebo-controlled study in adults with chronic insomnia. Sleep 2003;26(7):793–9.

47. Walsh JK, Krystal AD, Amato DA, et al. Nightly treatment of primary insomnia with eszopiclone for six months: effect on sleep, quality of life, and work limitations. Sleep 2007;30(8):959–68.

48. Sarter M, Bruno JP. Cortical cholinergic inputs mediating arousal, attentional processing and dreaming: differential afferent regulation of the

basal forebrain by telencephalic and brainstem afferents. Neuroscience 2000;95(4):933–52.

49. Vazquez J, Baghdoyan HA. Basal forebrain acetylcholine release during REM sleep is significantly greater than during waking. Am J Physiol Regul Integr Comp Physiol 2001;280(2):R598–601.

50. Marrosu F, Portas C, Mascia MS, et al. Microdialysis measurement of cortical and hippocampal acetylcholine release during sleep-wake cycle in freely moving cats. Brain Res 1995;671(2):329–32.

51. Materi LM, Rasmusson DD, Semba K. Inhibition of synaptically evoked cortical acetylcholine release by adenosine: an in vivo microdialysis study in the rat. Neuroscience 2000;97(2):219–26.

52. Dworak M, McCarley RW, Kim T, et al. Sleep and brain energy levels: ATP changes during sleep. J Neurosci 2010;30(26):9007–16.

53. Benington JH, Heller HC. Restoration of brain energy metabolism as the function of sleep. Prog Neurobiol 1995;45(4):347–60.

54. Landolt HP, Dijk DJ, Gaus SE, et al. Caffeine reduces low-frequency delta activity in the human sleep EEG. Neuropsychopharmacology 1995; 12(3):229–38.

55. Landolt HP, Werth E, Borbely AA, et al. Caffeine intake (200 mg) in the morning affects human sleep and EEG power spectra at night. Brain Res 1995; 675(1–2):67–74.

56. Gan TJ, Habib AS. Adenosine as a non-opioid analgesic in the perioperative setting. Anesth Analg 2007;105(2):487–94.

57. Radulovacki M. Adenosine sleep theory: how I postulated it. Neurol Res 2005;27(2):137–8.

58. Basheer R, Strecker RE, Thakkar MM, et al. Adenosine and sleep-wake regulation. Prog Neurobiol 2004;73(6):379–96.

59. Strecker RE, Morairty S, Thakkar MM, et al. Adenosinergic modulation of basal forebrain and preoptic/anterior hypothalamic neuronal activity in the control of behavioral state. Behav Brain Res 2000;115(2):183–204.

60. Porkka-Heiskanen T, Kalinchuk AV. Adenosine, energy metabolism and sleep homeostasis. Sleep Med Rev 2011;15(2):123–35.

61. Porkka-Heiskanen T, Strecker RE, McCarley RW. Brain site-specificity of extracellular adenosine concentration changes during sleep deprivation and spontaneous sleep: an in vivo microdialysis study. Neuroscience 2000;99(3):507–17.

62. Kalinchuk AV, McCarley RW, Porkka-Heiskanen T, et al. The time course of adenosine, nitric oxide (NO) and inducible NO synthase changes in the brain with sleep loss and their role in the non-rapid eye movement sleep homeostatic cascade. J Neurochem 2011;116(2):260–72.

63. Elmenhorst D, Meyer PT, Winz OH, et al. Sleep deprivation increases A$_1$ adenosine receptor binding in the human brain: a positron emission tomography study. J Neurosci 2007;27(9):2410–5.

64. Elmenhorst D, Basheer R, McCarley RW, et al. Sleep deprivation increases A$_1$ adenosine receptor density in the rat brain. Brain Res 2009;1258:53–8.

65. Porkka-Heiskanen T, Strecker RE, Thakkar M, et al. Adenosine: a mediator of the sleep-inducing effects of prolonged wakefulness. Science 1997; 276(5316):1265–8.

66. Gauthier EA, Guzick SE, Brummett CM, et al. Buprenorphine disrupts sleep and decreases adenosine concentrations in sleep-regulating brain regions of Sprague Dawley rat. Anesthesiology 2011;115(4):743–53.

67. Thakkar MM, Winston S, McCarley RW. A$_1$ receptor and adenosinergic homeostatic regulation of sleep-wakefulness: effects of antisense to the A$_1$ receptor in the cholinergic basal forebrain. J Neurosci 2003;23(10):4278–87.

68. Basheer R, Halldner L, Alanko L, et al. Opposite changes in adenosine A$_1$ and A$_{2A}$ receptor mRNA in the rat following sleep deprivation. Neuroreport 2001;12(8):1577–80.

69. Arrigoni E, Chamberlin NL, Saper CB, et al. Adenosine inhibits basal forebrain cholinergic and non-cholinergic neurons in vitro. Neuroscience 2006; 140(2):403–13.

70. Liu ZW, Gao XB. Adenosine inhibits activity of hypocretin/orexin neurons by the A1 receptor in the lateral hypothalamus: a possible sleep-promoting effect. J Neurophysiol 2007;97(1):837–48.

71. Thakkar MM, Engemann SC, Walsh KM, et al. Adenosine and the homeostatic control of sleep: effects of A1 receptor blockade in the perifornical lateral hypothalamus on sleep-wakefulness. Neuroscience 2008;153(4):875–80.

72. Oishi Y, Huang ZL, Fredholm BB, et al. Adenosine in the tuberomammillary nucleus inhibits the histaminergic system via A1 receptors and promotes non-rapid eye movement sleep. Proc Natl Acad Sci U S A 2008;105(50):19992–7.

73. Van Dort CJ, Baghdoyan HA, Lydic R. Adenosine A$_1$ and A$_{2A}$ receptors in mouse prefrontal cortex modulate acetylcholine release and behavioral arousal. J Neurosci 2009;29(3):871–81.

74. Tanase D, Baghdoyan HA, Lydic R. Dialysis delivery of an adenosine A$_1$ receptor agonist to the pontine reticular formation decreases acetylcholine release and increases anesthesia recovery time. Anesthesiology 2003;98(4):912–20.

75. Coleman CG, Baghdoyan HA, Lydic R. Dialysis delivery of an adenosine A$_{2A}$ agonist into the pontine reticular formation of C57BL/6J mouse increases pontine acetylcholine release and sleep. J Neurochem 2006;96(6):1750–9.

76. Marks GA, Shaffery JP, Speciale SG, et al. Enhancement of rapid eye movement sleep in the

rat by actions at A1 and A2a adenosine receptor subtypes with a differential sensitivity to atropine. Neuroscience 2003;116(3):913–20.

77. Nelson AM, Battersby AS, Baghdoyan HA, et al. Opioid-induced decreases in rat brain adenosine levels are reversed by inhibiting adenosine deaminase. Anesthesiology 2009;111(6):1327–33.

78. Lydic R, Baghdoyan HA. Neurochemical mechanisms mediating opioid-induced REM sleep disruption. In: Lavigne G, Sessle B, Choinière M, et al, editors. Sleep and pain. Seattle (WA): IASP Press; 2007. p. 99–122.

79. Portas CM, Bjorvatn B, Fagerland S, et al. On-line detection of extracellular levels of serotonin in dorsal raphé nucleus and frontal cortex over the sleep/wake cycle in the freely moving rat. Neuroscience 1998;83(3):807–14.

80. Python A, Steimer T, de Saint Hilaire Z, et al. Extracellular serotonin variations during vigilance states in the preoptic area of rats: a microdialysis study. Brain Res 2001;910(1–2):49–54.

81. Houdouin F, Cespuglio R, Jouvet M. Effects induced by the electrical stimulation of the nucleus raphé dorsalis upon hypothalamic release of 5-hydroxyindole compounds and sleep parameters in the rat. Brain Res 1991;565(1):48–56.

82. Fink KB, Gothert M. 5-HT receptor regulation of neurotransmitter release. Pharmacol Rev 2007; 59(4):360–417.

83. Monti JM, Jantos H. Dose-dependent effects of the 5-HT$_{1A}$ receptor agonist 8-OH-DPAT on sleep and wakefulness in the rat. J Sleep Res 1992;1(3):169–75.

84. Portas CM, Thakkar M, Rainnie D, et al. Microdialysis perfusion of 8-hydroxy-2-(di-n-propylamino) tetralin (8-OH-DPAT) in the dorsal raphé nucleus decreases serotonin release and increases rapid eye movement sleep in the freely moving cat. J Neurosci 1996;16(8):2820–8.

85. Monti JM, Jantos H. Effects of activation and blockade of 5-HT$_{2A/2C}$ receptors in the dorsal raphé nucleus on sleep and waking in the rat. Prog Neuropsychopharmacol Biol Psychiatry 2006;30(7):1189–95.

86. Morairty SR, Hedley L, Flores J, et al. Selective 5HT$_{2A}$ and 5HT$_6$ receptor antagonists promote sleep in rats. Sleep 2008;31(1):34–44.

87. Boutrel B, Monaca C, Hen R, et al. Involvement of 5-HT$_{1A}$ receptors in homeostatic and stress-induced adaptive regulations of paradoxical sleep: studies in 5-HT$_{1A}$ knock-out mice. J Neurosci 2002; 22(11):4686–92.

88. Boutrel B, Franc B, Hen R, et al. Key role of 5-HT$_{1B}$ receptors in the regulation of paradoxical sleep as evidenced in 5-HT$_{1B}$ knock-out mice. J Neurosci 1999;19(8):3204–12.

89. Wilson SJ, Bailey JE, Rich AS, et al. The use of sleep measures to compare a new 5HT$_{1A}$ agonist with buspirone in humans. J Psychopharmacol 2005;19(6):609–13.

90. Monti JM, Jantos H. Effects of the serotonin 5-HT$_{2A/2C}$ receptor agonist DOI and of the selective 5-HT$_{2A}$ or 5-HT$_{2C}$ receptor antagonists EMD 281014 and SB-243213, respectively, on sleep and waking in the rat. Eur J Pharmacol 2006; 553(1–3):163–70.

91. Berridge CW, Waterhouse BD. The locus coeruleus-noradrenergic system: modulation of behavioral state and state-dependent cognitive processes. Brain Res Brain Res Rev 2003;42(1): 33–84.

92. Hein L. Adrenoceptors and signal transduction in neurons. Cell Tissue Res 2006;326(2):541–51.

93. Berridge CW, Foote SL. Enhancement of behavioral and electroencephalographic indices of waking following stimulation of noradrenergic beta-receptors within the medial septal region of the basal forebrain. J Neurosci 1996;16(21): 6999–7009.

94. Berridge CW, Isaac SO, Espana RA. Additive wake-promoting actions of medial basal forebrain noradrenergic α1- and β-receptor stimulation. Behav Neurosci 2003;117(2):350–9.

95. Kumar VM, Datta S, Chhina GS, et al. Alpha adrenergic system in medial preoptic area involved in sleep-wakefulness in rats. Brain Res Bull 1986; 16(4):463–8.

96. Sood S, Dhawan JK, Ramesh V, et al. Role of medial preoptic area beta adrenoceptors in the regulation of sleep-wakefulness. Pharmacol Biochem Behav 1997;57(1–2):1–5.

97. Berridge CW, Abercrombie ED. Relationship between locus coeruleus discharge rates and rates of norepinephrine release within neocortex as assessed by in vivo microdialysis. Neuroscience 1999;93(4):1263–70.

98. Florin-Lechner SM, Druhan JP, Aston-Jones G, et al. Enhanced norepinephrine release in prefrontal cortex with burst stimulation of the locus coeruleus. Brain Res 1996;742(1–2):89–97.

99. Pal D, Mallick BN. Role of noradrenergic and GABA-ergic inputs in pedunculopontine tegmentum for regulation of rapid eye movement sleep in rats. Neuropharmacology 2006;51(1):1–11.

100. Haas HL, Sergeeva OA, Selbach O. Histamine in the nervous system. Physiol Rev 2008;88(3): 1183–241.

101. Thakkar MM. Histamine in the regulation of wakefulness. Sleep Med Rev 2011;15(1):65–74.

102. Haas H, Panula P. The role of histamine and the tuberomammillary nucleus in the nervous system. Nat Rev Neurosci 2003;4(2):121–30.

103. Nicholson AN, Stone BM. Antihistamines: impaired performance and the tendency to sleep. Eur J Clin Pharmacol 1986;30(1):27–32.

104. Kaneko Y, Shimada K, Saitou K, et al. The mechanism responsible for the drowsiness caused by first generation H1 antagonists on the EEG pattern. Methods Find Exp Clin Pharmacol 2000;22(3):163–8.

105. Roth T, Rogowski R, Hull S, et al. Efficacy and safety of doxepin 1 mg, 3 mg, and 6 mg in adults with primary insomnia. Sleep 2007;30(11):1555–61.

106. Lin JS, Sakai K, Jouvet M. Evidence for histaminergic arousal mechanisms in the hypothalamus of cat. Neuropharmacology 1988;27(2):111–22.

107. Tokunaga S, Takoda Y, Shinomiya K, et al. Effects of some H_1-antagonists on the sleep-wake cycle in sleep-disturbed rats. J Pharmacol Sci 2007;103(2):201–6.

108. Monti JM, D'Angelo L, Jantos H, et al. Effects of α-fluoromethylhistidine on sleep and wakefulness in the rat. Short note. J Neural Transm 1988;72(2):141–5.

109. Kiyono S, Seo ML, Shibagaki M, et al. Effects of α-fluoromethylhistidine on sleep-waking parameters in rats. Physiol Behav 1985;34(4):615–7.

110. Parmentier R, Anaclet C, Guhennec C, et al. The brain H_3-receptor as a novel therapeutic target for vigilance and sleep-wake disorders. Biochem Pharmacol 2007;73(8):1157–71.

111. Ligneau X, Perrin D, Landais L, et al. BF2.649 [1-{3-[3-(4-Chlorophenyl)propoxy]propyl}piperidine, hydrochloride], a nonimidazole inverse agonist/antagonist at the human histamine H_3 receptor: preclinical pharmacology. J Pharmacol Exp Ther 2007;320(1):365–75.

112. Le S, Gruner JA, Mathiasen JR, et al. Correlation between ex vivo receptor occupancy and wake-promoting activity of selective H_3 receptor antagonists. J Pharmacol Exp Ther 2008;325(3):902–9.

113. James LM, Iannone R, Palcza J, et al. Effect of a novel histamine subtype-3 receptor inverse agonist and modafinil on EEG power spectra during sleep deprivation and recovery sleep in male volunteers. Psychopharmacology (Berl) 2011;215(4):643–53.

114. Lin JS, Sergeeva OA, Haas HL. Histamine H3 receptors and sleep-wake regulation. J Pharmacol Exp Ther 2011;336(1):17–23.

115. Boutrel B, Koob GF. What keeps us awake: the neuropharmacology of stimulants and wakefulness-promoting medications. Sleep 2004;27(6):1181–94.

116. Volkow ND, Wang GJ, Telang F, et al. Sleep deprivation decreases binding of [^{11}C]raclopride to dopamine D2/D3 receptors in the human brain. J Neurosci 2008;28(34):8454–61.

117. Monti JM, Jantos H. The roles of dopamine and serotonin, and of their receptors, in regulating sleep and waking. Prog Brain Res 2008;172:625–46.

118. Monti JM, Monti D. The involvement of dopamine in the modulation of sleep and waking. Sleep Med Rev 2007;11(2):113–33.

119. Lu J, Jhou TC, Saper CB. Identification of wake-active dopaminergic neurons in the ventral periaqueductal gray matter. J Neurosci 2006;26(1):193–202.

120. Wisor JP, Nishino S, Sora I, et al. Dopaminergic role in stimulant-induced wakefulness. J Neurosci 2001;21(5):1787–94.

121. Monti JM, Fernandez M, Jantos H. Sleep during acute dopamine D1 agonist SKF 38393 or D1 antagonist SCH 23390 administration in rats. Neuropsychopharmacology 1990;3(3):153–62.

122. Isaac SO, Berridge CW. Wake-promoting actions of dopamine D1 and D2 receptor stimulation. J Pharmacol Exp Ther 2003;307(1):386–94.

123. Monti JM, Hawkins M, Jantos H, et al. Biphasic effects of dopamine D-2 receptor agonists on sleep and wakefulness in the rat. Psychopharmacology (Berl) 1988;95(3):395–400.

124. Monti JM, Jantos H, Fernandez M. Effects of the selective dopamine D-2 receptor agonist, quinpirole on sleep and wakefulness in the rat. Eur J Pharmacol 1989;169(1):61–6.

125. Andersen ML, Margis R, Frey BN, et al. Electrophysiological correlates of sleep disturbance induced by acute and chronic administration of D-amphetamine. Brain Res 2009;1249:162–72.

126. Minzenberg MJ, Carter CS. Modafinil: a review of neurochemical actions and effects on cognition. Neuropsychopharmacology 2008;33(7):1477–502.

127. Brevig HN, Baghdoyan HA. Neurotransmitters and neuromodulators regulating sleep and wakefulness. In: Koob GF, Le Moa M, Thompson RF, editors. Encyclopedia of behavioral neuroscience, vol. 3. Oxford (United Kingdom): Academic Press; 2010. p. 456–63.

128. Dash MB, Douglas CL, Vyazovskiy VV, et al. Long-term homeostasis of extracellular glutamate in the rat cerebral cortex across sleep and waking states. J Neurosci 2009;29(3):620–9.

129. Cortese BM, Mitchell TR, Galloway MP, et al. Region-specific alteration in brain glutamate: possible relationship to risk-taking behavior. Physiol Behav 2010;99(4):445–50.

130. Datta S, Patterson EH, Spoley EE. Excitation of the pedunculopontine tegmental NMDA receptors induces wakefulness and cortical activation in the rat. J Neurosci Res 2001;66(1):109–16.

131. Datta S, Spoley EE, Patterson EH. Microinjection of glutamate into the pedunculopontine tegmentum induces REM sleep and wakefulness in the rat. Am J Physiol Regul Integr Comp Physiol 2001;280(3):R752–9.

132. Datta S, Spoley EE, Mavanji VK, et al. A novel role of pedunculopontine tegmental kainate receptors: a mechanism of rapid eye movement sleep generation in the rat. Neuroscience 2002;114(1):157–64.

133. Stevens DR, McCarley RW, Greene RW. Excitatory amino acid-mediated responses and synaptic potentials in medial pontine reticular formation neurons of the rat in vitro. J Neurosci 1992; 12(11):4188–94.

134. Onoe H, Sakai K. Kainate receptors: a novel mechanism in paradoxical (REM) sleep generation. Neuroreport 1995;6(2):353–6.

135. Kaushik MK, Kumar VM, Mallick HN. Glutamate microinjection at the medial preoptic area enhances slow wave sleep in rats. Behav Brain Res 2011;217(1):240–3.

136. Cui L, Wang JH, Wang M, et al. Injection of L-glutamate into the insular cortex produces sleep apnea and serotonin reduction in rats. Sleep Breath 2011. Available at: http://dx.doi.org/10.1007/s11325-011-0586-x. [Epub ahead of print].

137. Lai YY, Siegel JM. Medullary regions mediating atonia. J Neurosci 1988;8(12):4790–6.

138. Lai YY, Siegel JM. Pontomedullary glutamate receptors mediating locomotion and muscle tone suppression. J Neurosci 1991;11(9):2931–7.

139. Kaneko T, Itoh K, Shigemoto R, et al. Glutaminase-like immunoreactivity in the lower brainstem and cerebellum of the adult rat. Neuroscience 1989; 32(1):79–98.

140. Jones BE. Arousal systems. Front Biosci 2003;8: s438–51.

141. Núñez A, Buño W, Reinoso-Suárez F. Neurotransmitter actions on oral pontine tegmental neurons of the rat: an in vitro study. Brain Res 1998; 804(1):144–8.

142. Greene RW, Carpenter DO. Actions of neurotransmitters on pontine medial reticular formation neurons of the cat. J Neurophysiol 1985;54(3):520–31.

143. Elazar Z, Berchanski A. Glutamatergic-cholinergic synergistic interaction in the pontine reticular formation. Effects on catalepsy. Naunyn Schmiedebergs Arch Pharmacol 2001;363(5):569–76.

144. de Lecea L. Neuropeptides and sleep-wake regulation. In: Monti JM, Pandi-Perumal SR, Sinton CM, editors. Neurochemistry of sleep and wakefulness. New York: Cambridge University Press; 2008. p. 387–401.

145. de Lecea L, Kilduff TS, Peyron C, et al. The hypocretins: hypothalamus-specific peptides with neuroexcitatory activity. Proc Natl Acad Sci U S A 1998;95(1):322–7.

146. Sakurai T, Amemiya A, Ishii M, et al. Orexins and orexin receptors: a family of hypothalamic neuropeptides and G protein-coupled receptors that regulate feeding behavior. Cell 1998;92(4): 573–85.

147. Peyron C, Tighe DK, van den Pol AN, et al. Neurons containing hypocretin (orexin) project to multiple neuronal systems. J Neurosci 1998;18(23): 9996–10015.

148. Zhang JH, Sampogna S, Morales FR, et al. Distribution of hypocretin (orexin) immunoreactivity in the feline pons and medulla. Brain Res 2004; 995(2):205–17.

149. Lee MG, Hassani OK, Jones BE. Discharge of identified orexin/hypocretin neurons across the sleep-waking cycle. J Neurosci 2005;25(28): 6716–20.

150. Mileykovskiy BY, Kiyashchenko LI, Siegel JM. Behavioral correlates of activity in identified hypocretin/orexin neurons. Neuron 2005;46(5): 787–98.

151. Kiyashchenko LI, Mileykovskiy BY, Maidment N, et al. Release of hypocretin (orexin) during waking and sleep states. J Neurosci 2002; 22(13):5282–6.

152. Lin L, Faraco J, Li R, et al. The sleep disorder canine narcolepsy is caused by a mutation in the hypocretin (orexin) receptor 2 gene. Cell 1999; 98(3):365–76.

153. Thannickal TC, Moore RY, Nienhuis R, et al. Reduced number of hypocretin neurons in human narcolepsy. Neuron 2000;27(3):469–74.

154. Peyron C, Faraco J, Rogers W, et al. A mutation in a case of early onset narcolepsy and a generalized absence of hypocretin peptides in human narcoleptic brains. Nat Med 2000;6(9):991–7.

155. Nishino S, Kanbayashi T. Symptomatic narcolepsy, cataplexy and hypersomnia, and their implications in the hypothalamic hypocretin/orexin system. Sleep Med Rev 2005;9(4):269–310.

156. Beuckmann CT, Sinton CM, Williams SC, et al. Expression of a poly-glutamine-ataxin-3 transgene in orexin neurons induces narcolepsy-cataplexy in the rat. J Neurosci 2004;24(18):4469–77.

157. Murillo-Rodriguez E, Liu M, Blanco-Centurion C, et al. Effects of hypocretin (orexin) neuronal loss on sleep and extracellular adenosine levels in the rat basal forebrain. Eur J Neurosci 2008;28(6): 1191–8.

158. Willie JT, Chemelli RM, Sinton CM, et al. Distinct narcolepsy syndromes in orexin receptor-2 and orexin null mice: molecular genetic dissection of non-REM and REM sleep regulatory processes. Neuron 2003;38(5):715–30.

159. Bernard R, Lydic R, Baghdoyan HA. Hypocretin-1 causes G protein activation and increases ACh release in rat pons. Eur J Neurosci 2003;18(7): 1775–85.

160. Greco MA, Shiromani PJ. Hypocretin receptor protein and mRNA expression in the dorsolateral pons of rats. Brain Res Mol Brain Res 2001;88 (1–2):176–82.

161. Hervieu GJ, Cluderay JE, Harrison DC, et al. Gene expression and protein distribution of the orexin-1 receptor in the rat brain and spinal cord. Neuroscience 2001;103(3):777–97.

162. Marcus JN, Aschkenasi CJ, Lee CE, et al. Differential expression of orexin receptors 1 and 2 in the rat brain. J Comp Neurol 2001;435(1):6–25.

163. Brischoux F, Mainville L, Jones BE. Muscarinic-2 and orexin-2 receptors on GABAergic and other neurons in the rat mesopontine tegmentum and their potential role in sleep-wake state control. J Comp Neurol 2008;510(6):607–30.

164. Burlet S, Tyler CJ, Leonard CS. Direct and indirect excitation of laterodorsal tegmental neurons by Hypocretin/Orexin peptides: implications for wakefulness and narcolepsy. J Neurosci 2002;22(7): 2862–72.

165. Takahashi K, Koyama Y, Kayama Y, et al. Effects of orexin on the laterodorsal tegmental neurones. Psychiatry Clin Neurosci 2002;56(3):335–6.

166. Xi MC, Fung SJ, Yamuy J, et al. Induction of active (REM) sleep and motor inhibition by hypocretin in the nucleus pontis oralis of the cat. J Neurophysiol 2002;87(6):2880–8.

167. Liu RJ, van den Pol AN, Aghajanian GK. Hypocretins (orexins) regulate serotonin neurons in the dorsal raphé nucleus by excitatory direct and inhibitory indirect actions. J Neurosci 2002; 22(21):9453–64.

168. Soffin EM, Gill CH, Brough SJ, et al. Pharmacological characterisation of the orexin receptor subtype mediating postsynaptic excitation in the rat dorsal raphé nucleus. Neuropharmacology 2004;46(8): 1168–76.

169. Brown RE, Sergeeva OA, Eriksson KS, et al. Convergent excitation of dorsal raphé serotonin neurons by multiple arousal systems (orexin/hypocretin, histamine and noradrenaline). J Neurosci 2002;22(20):8850–9.

170. Bourgin P, Huitron-Resendiz S, Spier AD, et al. Hypocretin-1 modulates rapid eye movement sleep through activation of locus coeruleus neurons. J Neurosci 2000;20(20):7760–5.

171. Hagan JJ, Leslie RA, Patel S, et al. Orexin A activates locus coeruleus cell firing and increases arousal in the rat. Proc Natl Acad Sci U S A 1999; 96(19):10911–6.

172. Horvath TL, Peyron C, Diano S, et al. Hypocretin (orexin) activation and synaptic innervation of the locus coeruleus noradrenergic system. J Comp Neurol 1999;415(2):145–59.

173. Eriksson KS, Sergeeva O, Brown RE, et al. Orexin/hypocretin excites the histaminergic neurons of the tuberomammillary nucleus. J Neurosci 2001; 21(23):9273–9.

174. Bayer L, Eggermann E, Serafin M, et al. Orexins (hypocretins) directly excite tuberomammillary neurons. Eur J Neurosci 2001;14(9):1571–5.

175. Eggermann E, Serafin M, Bayer L, et al. Orexins/hypocretins excite basal forebrain cholinergic neurones. Neuroscience 2001;108(2):177–81.

176. Mieda M, Hasegawa E, Kisanuki YY, et al. Differential roles of orexin receptor-1 and -2 in the regulation of non-REM and REM sleep. J Neurosci 2011;31(17):6518–26.

177. Piper DC, Upton N, Smith MI, et al. The novel brain neuropeptide, orexin-A, modulates the sleep-wake cycle of rats. Eur J Neurosci 2000; 12(2):726–30.

178. Vittoz NM, Berridge CW. Hypocretin/orexin selectively increases dopamine efflux within the prefrontal cortex: involvement of the ventral tegmental area. Neuropsychopharmacology 2006; 31(2):384–95.

179. Methippara MM, Alam MN, Szymusiak R, et al. Effects of lateral preoptic area application of orexin-A on sleep-wakefulness. Neuroreport 2000; 11(16):3423–6.

180. Xi MC, Morales FR, Chase MH. Effects on sleep and wakefulness of the injection of hypocretin-1 (orexin-A) into the laterodorsal tegmental nucleus of the cat. Brain Res 2001;901(1–2):259–64.

181. Moreno-Balandran E, Garzon M, Bodalo C, et al. Sleep-wakefulness effects after microinjections of hypocretin 1 (orexin A) in cholinoceptive areas of the cat oral pontine tegmentum. Eur J Neurosci 2008;28(2):331–41.

182. Espana RA, Baldo BA, Kelley AE, et al. Wake-promoting and sleep-suppressing actions of hypocretin (orexin): basal forebrain sites of action. Neuroscience 2001;106(4):699–715.

183. Thakkar MM, Ramesh V, Strecker RE, et al. Microdialysis perfusion of orexin-A in the basal forebrain increases wakefulness in freely behaving rats. Arch Ital Biol 2001;139(3):313–28.

184. Thakkar MM, Ramesh V, Cape EG, et al. REM sleep enhancement and behavioral cataplexy following orexin (hypocretin)-II receptor antisense perfusion in the pontine reticular formation. Sleep Res Online 1999;2(4):112–20.

185. Dong HL, Fukuda S, Murata E, et al. Orexins increase cortical acetylcholine release and electroencephalographic activation through orexin-1 receptor in the rat basal forebrain during isoflurane anesthesia. Anesthesiology 2006;104(5): 1023–32.

186. Hong ZY, Huang ZL, Qu WM, et al. Orexin A promotes histamine, but not norepinephrine or serotonin, release in frontal cortex of mice. Acta Pharmacol Sin 2005;26(2):155–9.

187. Ishizuka T, Yamamoto Y, Yamatodani A. The effect of orexin-A and -B on the histamine release in the anterior hypothalamus in rats. Neurosci Lett 2002; 323(2):93–6.

188. Tao R, Ma Z, McKenna JT, et al. Differential effect of orexins (hypocretins) on serotonin release in the dorsal and median raphé nuclei of freely behaving rats. Neuroscience 2006;141(3):1101–5.

189. Bernard R, Lydic R, Baghdoyan HA. Hypocretin (orexin) receptor subtypes differentially enhance acetylcholine release and activate g protein subtypes in rat pontine reticular formation. J Pharmacol Exp Ther 2006;317(1):163–71.

190. Brevig HN, Watson CJ, Lydic R, et al. Hypocretin and GABA interact in the pontine reticular formation to increase wakefulness. Sleep 2010;33(10):1285–93.

191. Winrow CJ, Gotter AL, Cox CD, et al. Pharmacological characterization of MK-6096 - a dual orexin receptor antagonist for insomnia. Neuropharmacology 2012;62(2):978–87.

192. Brisbare-Roch C, Dingemanse J, Koberstein R, et al. Promotion of sleep by targeting the orexin system in rats, dogs and humans. Nat Med 2007; 13(2):150–5.

193. Taheri S, Lin L, Austin D, et al. Short sleep duration is associated with reduced leptin, elevated ghrelin, and increased body mass index. PLoS Med 2004; 1(3):e62.

194. Spiegel K, Tasali E, Penev P, et al. Brief communication: sleep curtailment in healthy young men is associated with decreased leptin levels, elevated ghrelin levels, and increased hunger and appetite. Ann Intern Med 2004;141(11):846–50.

195. Basoglu OK, Sarac F, Sarac S, et al. Metabolic syndrome, insulin resistance, fibrinogen, homocysteine, leptin, and C-reactive protein in obese patients with obstructive sleep apnea syndrome. Ann Thorac Med 2011;6(3):120–5.

196. Ursavas A, Ilcol YO, Nalci N, et al. Ghrelin, leptin, adiponectin, and resistin levels in sleep apnea syndrome: role of obesity. Ann Thorac Med 2010; 5(3):161–5.

197. Sanchez-de-la-Torre M, Barcelo A, Pierola J, et al. Plasma levels of neuropeptides and metabolic hormones, and sleepiness in obstructive sleep apnea. Respir Med 2011;105(12):1954–60.

198. Wathen AB, West EM, Lydic R, et al. Olanzapine causes a leptin-dependent increase in acetylcholine release in mouse prefrontal cortex. Sleep 2012;35(3):315–23.

199. Wang W, Baghdoyan HA, Lydic R. Leptin replacement restores supraspinal cholinergic antinociception in leptin-deficient obese mice. J Pain 2009; 10(8):836–43.

200. Laposky AD, Shelton J, Bass J, et al. Altered sleep regulation in leptin-deficient mice. Am J Physiol Regul Integr Comp Physiol 2006;290(4): R894–903.

201. Douglas CL, Bowman GN, Baghdoyan HA, et al. C57BL/6J and B6.V-LEP[OB] mice differ in the cholinergic modulation of sleep and breathing. J Appl Physiol 2005;98(3):918–29.

202. Laposky AD, Bradley MA, Williams DL, et al. Sleep-wake regulation is altered in leptin-resistant (db/db) genetically obese and diabetic mice. Am J Physiol Regul Integr Comp Physiol 2008;295(6): R2059–66.

203. Szentirmai E, Kapas L, Krueger JM. Ghrelin micro-injection into forebrain sites induces wakefulness and feeding in rats. Am J Physiol Regul Integr Comp Physiol 2007;292(1):R575–85.

204. Roehrs T, Hyde M, Blaisdell B, et al. Sleep loss and REM sleep loss are hyperalgesic. Sleep 2006; 29(2):145–51.

205. Chhangani BS, Roehrs TA, Harris EJ, et al. Pain sensitivity in sleepy pain-free normals. Sleep 2009;32(8):1011–7.

206. Mystakidou K, Clark AJ, Fischer J, et al. Treatment of chronic pain by long-acting opioids and the effects on sleep. Pain Pract 2011;11(3):282–9.

207. Lavigne G, Sessle BJ, Choinière M, et al, editors. Sleep and pain. Seattle (WA): International Association for the Study of Pain Press; 2007.

208. Shaw IR, Lavigne G, Mayer P, et al. Acute intravenous administration of morphine perturbs sleep architecture in healthy pain-free young adults: a preliminary study. Sleep 2005;28(6):677–82.

209. Dimsdale JE, Norman D, DeJardin D, et al. The effect of opioids on sleep architecture. J Clin Sleep Med 2007;3(1):33–6.

210. Bonafide CP, Aucutt-Walter N, Divittore N, et al. Remifentanil inhibits rapid eye movement sleep but not the nocturnal melatonin surge in humans. Anesthesiology 2008;108(4):627–33.

211. Sharkey KM, Kurth ME, Anderson BJ, et al. Assessing sleep in opioid dependence: a comparison of subjective ratings, sleep diaries, and home polysomnography in methadone maintenance patients. Drug Alcohol Depend 2011; 113(2–3):245–8.

212. Trksak GH, Jensen JE, Plante DT, et al. Effects of sleep deprivation on sleep homeostasis and restoration during methadone-maintenance: a ^{31}P MRS brain imaging study. Drug Alcohol Depend 2010;106(2–3):79–91.

213. Xiao L, Tang YL, Smith AK, et al. Nocturnal sleep architecture disturbances in early methadone treatment patients. Psychiatry Res 2010;179(1):91–5.

214. Moore JT, Kelz MB. Opiates, sleep, and pain: the adenosinergic link. Anesthesiology 2009;111(6): 1175–6.

215. Keifer JC, Baghdoyan HA, Lydic R. Sleep disruption and increased apneas after pontine micro-injection of morphine. Anesthesiology 1992;77(5): 973–82.

216. Watson CJ, Lydic R, Baghdoyan HA. Sleep and GABA levels in the oral part of rat pontine reticular formation are decreased by local and systemic administration of morphine. Neuroscience 2007; 144(1):375–86.

217. Wade N. A decade later, genetic map yields few new cures. New York Times 2010.

218. Pollack A. Awaiting the genome payoff. New York Times 2010.

219. Lin JS, Sakai K, Vanni-Mercier G, et al. A critical role of the posterior hypothalamus in the mechanisms of wakefulness determined by microinjection of muscimol in freely moving cats. Brain Res 1989; 479(2):225–40.

220. Kryger MH, Roth T, Dement WC, editors. Principles and practice of sleep medicine. 5th edition. Philadelphia: W.B. Saunders; 2010.

221. Klipp E, Herwig R, Kowald A, et al. Systems biology in practice: concepts, implementation, and application. Weinheim (Germany): Wiley-VCH; 2005.

Staging Sleep

Michael H. Silber, MBChB

KEYWORDS

- Sleep scoring • Sleep staging • AASM manual • Polysomnography • Non-REM sleep • REM sleep

KEY POINTS

- This article reviews the historical development of sleep staging, including the development of the new American Academy of Sleep Medicine (AASM) manual, with the scientific background underlying the choice of staging criteria.
- The rules for the different stages of wakefulness (stage W), non–rapid eye movement sleep (stages N1–N3) and rapid eye movement sleep (stage R) are described, as well as variations recommended for scoring sleep in children.
- Recent studies evaluating the AASM method are reviewed.

Although a sleeper may perceive a night's sleep as a continuous uniform experience, profound physiologic changes occur over the course of a night. Recognizing these alterations in state is essential for understanding the mechanisms of sleep, documenting the changes that occur with disease, and studying the consequences of experimental and clinical interventions. For more than 70 years, it has been recognized that the changes in cortical electrical activity during sleep do not occur randomly but follow in a particular order in repeated cycles during the night. Transitions between recognizably different states of sleep are not usually abrupt, sometimes lasting even minutes. However, quantitation of sleep stages requires clear, reliable definitions, even though these may be arbitrary, especially at the start and end of each stage.

This article reviews the historical development of human visual sleep staging and describes the current recommended American Academy of Sleep Medicine (AASM) classification of 4 sleep stages: N1, N2, N3, and R. The theoretic basis for the selection of specific staging criteria is discussed, with particular emphasis on their biologic substrates and the evidence on which they are based. The only authoritative sources for the rules of sleep staging are the official manuals published as freestanding monographs,[1,2] and physicians,

scientists, and technologists learning sleep staging should consult these sources. A discussion of computerized analysis of sleep stages is beyond the scope of this article.

HISTORICAL SURVEY

Barely 8 years after the development of the human scalp electroencephalogram (EEG),[3] Loomis and colleagues[4] published the first attempt to classify different brain rhythms during sleep. They described 5 stages (A–E), with stages A and B approximately corresponding with the current stage N1, stage C corresponding with stage N2, and stages D and E corresponding with stage N3. They recognized such phenomena as the fragmentation and fallout of α rhythm, sleep spindles, and high-amplitude slow waves. Various modifications of this basic schema were suggested over the next 15 years[5,6] and, subsequently,[7,8] Gibbs and colleagues[6] described a stage with an EEG pattern similar to wakefulness that they called early morning sleep, probably an identification of the rapid eye movement (REM) state. However, it was the seminal discovery of periodic rapid eye movements by Eugene Aserinsky, a graduate student working in the laboratory of Nathaniel Kleitman at the University of Chicago, that laid

This article originally appeared in *Sleep Medicine Clinics* Volume 4, Issue 3.
Center for Sleep Medicine, Mayo Clinic, 200 1st Street Southwest, Rochester, MN 55905, USA
E-mail address: msilber@mayo.edu

Sleep Med Clin 7 (2012) 487–496
http://dx.doi.org/10.1016/j.jsmc.2012.06.009
1556-407X/12/$ – see front matter © 2012 Elsevier Inc. All rights reserved.

the groundwork for a more accurate classification of sleep stages.[9] In 1957, Dement and Kleitman[10] proposed the first classification based on an understanding that REM and non-REM (NREM) sleep alternate in successive cycles during the night. They suggested 4 stages (1–4), with stage 1 corresponding with stage N1 at the start of the night and stage R toward morning, stage 2 corresponding with stage N2, and stages 3 and 4 with stage N3. In the early 1960s, Williams and colleagues[11] developed a modified scoring system at the University of Florida based on 1-minute epochs and 3 EEG derivations.

In 1968, Rechtschaffen and Kales[12] led a team of sleep researchers in the production of the first sleep staging manual, based on expert consensus. The group made some fundamental, prescient decisions that have deeply influenced the course of sleep research and sleep medicine. They recommended the recording of at least 1 EEG derivation (C3 or C4 referenced to the opposite ear or mastoid), 2 electro-oculogram (EOG) derivations, and a channel recording submental electromyogram (EMG). They required that sleep be scored in arbitrary epochs of 20 to 30 seconds with a single stage being assigned to each epoch. They divided sleep into 5 stages: stages 1 to 4 of NREM sleep and stage REM sleep. Stage 1 consisted of low-voltage mixed frequency EEG activity with slow rolling eye movements. Stage 2 was defined by the appearance of K complexes, sleep spindles, or both. The presence of high-voltage (>75 μV) low-frequency (<2 Hz) EEG activity characterized stages 3 and 4 sleep: 20% to 50% of the epoch for stage 3 and greater than 50% of the epoch for stage 4. The EEG in stage REM showed low-voltage mixed frequency activity in association with rapid eye movements and low submental EMG activity.

Despite occasional suggestions for modifying the system,[13–18] the Rechtschaffen and Kales (R and K) manual remained the standard staging system for human sleep studies for almost 40 years. In 2004, the Board of Directors of the AASM commissioned the development of a new manual for the scoring of sleep, including not only sleep staging but also rules for the scoring of arousals, respiratory, cardiac, and movement events. This ambitious project was performed through 7 task forces overseen by a steering committee.[19] All proposals were peer reviewed and ultimately approved by the AASM Board of Directors. Published evidence was reviewed, followed by a rigorous consensus decision-making process. The Visual Task Force, consisting of 12 members, reviewed 128 relevant articles and voted on 71 questions before submitting its

recommendations in late 2005. Input was also received from the Geriatric Task Force, and the Pediatric Task Force produced separate recommendations for modifying the proposed rules in children. The Visual Task Force followed certain general principles: rules should be compatible with published evidence, they should be based on biologic principles, they should be applicable to both normal and abnormal sleep, and they should be easily used by clinicians, technologists, and scientists.[20] The *AASM Manual for the Scoring of Sleep and Associated Events* and 7 review articles, covering all aspects of sleep scoring, were published in 2007.[1] The AASM has mandated that AASM-accredited sleep centers and laboratories must follow the new scoring rules. The Manual Steering Committee continues to meet and publish answers to frequently asked questions and requests for clarification on the public portion of the AASM Web site (http://www.aasmnet.org/scoringmanualfaq.aspx).

DERIVATIONS AND MONTAGES

Based on the routine use of 8-channel electroencephalographs in the 1960s and the common practice of studying 2 subjects simultaneously with a single machine, the R and K manual recommended a single EEG derivation (C4-A1 or C3-A2).[12] With the availability of machines capable of recording 16 or more derivations, these limitations no longer apply. Studies have shown that K complexes and δ frequency slow waves are maximally represented frontally, with some K complexes not being evident using central electrodes alone.[21,22] Sleep spindles occur maximally centrally,[22,23] whereas α rhythm of wakefulness arises from the occipital regions. Three EEG derivations are therefore currently required, sampling the frontal, central, and occipital regions (**Box 1**). One of 2 sets of derivations is selected at the discretion of the laboratory, the recommended montage with active electrodes referenced to the opposite mastoid process (M1 or M2), or the alternative montage with a combination of 2 bipolar derivations, and a single referential derivation.[1]

Two EOG derivations are required (see **Box 1**).[1] As with the EEG montages, laboratories may select from 2 different sets of EOG derivations. The recommended montage, referring the active electrodes to M2, record all eye movements as phase reversing deflections, making differentiation from volume conducted EEG potentials or electrode artifacts simple. In contrast, the alternative montage (referring the active electrodes to a central forehead electrode [Fpz]) allows detection of eye movement direction by noting whether the deflections are in phase or out of phase, and is especially useful when such distinction is deemed important. A single EMG derivation (see **Box 1**) with electrodes applied above and below the chin records EMG activity from the submental muscles.

STAGE TERMINOLOGY AND SCORING PRINCIPLES

The AASM manual classifies wake and sleep into the following stages: stage W (wakefulness), stage N1 (NREM stage 1 sleep), stage N2 (NREM stage 2 sleep), stage N3 (NREM stage 3 sleep), and stage R (REM sleep).[1] The change in abbreviations was instituted to differentiate the scoring rules from those of the R and K manual and allow other investigators and clinicians to easily determine which staging system was used. Older classifications, including that of R and K, arbitrarily divided the deeper portion of NREM sleep into 2 stages, depending on the amount of recorded slow wave activity.[12] This distinction has been eliminated in the AASM classification, because there is no biologic basis for such a demarcation.

The basic principle of sleep staging is that the night is divided into 30-second sequential periods known as epochs. Each epoch is assigned a stage. If 2 or more stages can be identified during a single epoch, the stage comprising the greatest portion of the epoch is assigned. Although an assessment of the overall flow of sleep might be better obtained by relying on identifying the start and end of each stage irrespective of epochs, such a scoring method would be intensely cumbersome in the presence of highly fragmented sleep such as may be seen in patients with obstructive sleep apnea.

WAKEFULNESS
Criteria for Stage W

The state of wakefulness is defined by the presence of α rhythm on the EEG (**Fig. 1**).[1] α Rhythm is defined as sinusoidal activity of 8 to 13 Hz over the occipital head region with eye closure, attenuating with eye opening. Little or no α rhythm is generated by 10% to 20% of normal individuals.[24] When α rhythm is not clearly discernable by visual inspection of the EEG, wakefulness can still be scored if the EOG shows any 1 of 3 markers of alertness. First, eye blinks with the eyes open or closed indicate the wake state. Blinking results in conjugate vertical eye movements at a frequency of 0.5 to 2 Hz (Bell phenomenon), which are visible on the EOG, especially if the Fpz reference is used. Second, the presence of reading eye movements indicates that the subject is awake. These conjugate movements, easily identifiable with experience, consist of a slow phase followed by a rapid movement in the opposite direction. Third, the presence of irregular conjugate eye movements with normal or high chin muscle tone suggests that the subject is awake and looking at the environment.

The Problem of Sleep Onset

When does sleep commence? Two valid alternative constructs can be used in defining sleep onset. First, there is electrophysiologic and psychophysiologic evidence that the change from wakefulness to sleep is a slow continuum best described by a period of drowsiness interspersed between full wakefulness and unequivocal sleep. The earliest electrophysiologic sign of drowsiness is reduction in the blink rate with the eyes closed.[24] This reduction is followed by the development of slow eye movements, defined as conjugate, regular, sinusoidal eye movements with initial deflection usually lasting longer than 500 milliseconds.[1] These EOG changes usually precede loss of α rhythm. EEG changes also precede fallout of

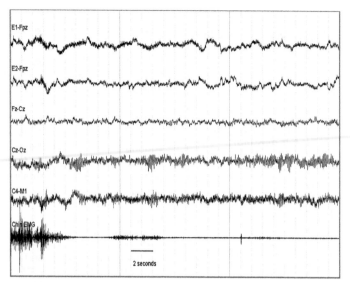

Fig. 1. Stage W. The Cz-Oz channel shows α rhythm, which defined the epoch as stage W, even though the EOG shows slow eye movements of drowsiness. See **Box 1** for electrode placements.

α: α amplitude either decreases or increases, frontocentral spread of α occurs, and θ or δ transients become interspersed within α activity.[24] The stage of wakefulness or sleep in which subjects fail to respond to auditory stimuli varies between individuals. Some stop responding in R and K stage wake, most during R and K stage 1, and a few only during R and K stage 2.[25]

In contrast, there is also a body of evidence suggesting that it is valid to define a single point on this continuum as the moment of sleep onset. In some psychophysiologic experiments, there is a 70% decrease in responses to auditory stimuli at the transition between R and K stage wake and stage 1 NREM sleep.[25] Many physiologic processes undergo changes, some abrupt, at the time α rhythm changes to slower θ frequencies. Minute ventilation,[26] phasic EMG activity in respiratory muscles,[27,28] and heart rate[29] decrease, whereas upper airway resistance increases.[30] Cerebral blood flow decreases in the frontal lobes and increases in the occipital lobes.[31,32]

Although the AASM manual recognizes that many signs of drowsiness are discernable before α rhythm is lost, it does specify a single time of sleep onset. This time is defined as the start of the first epoch scored as any stage other than stage W, recognizing that, in most subjects, this is stage N1[1] (discussed later).

NREM SLEEP
Stage N1 Sleep

Stage N1 sleep is defined by the presence of low-amplitude, mixed frequency (predominantly 4–7 Hz) activity (**Fig. 2**).[1] The EOG generally shows slow eye movements and the chin EMG is often lower in amplitude than in stage W. The EEG may show vertex sharp waves, which are sharply contoured waves maximal over the central region, distinguishable from the background EEG and lasting less than 0.5 seconds. None of these additional features are required for scoring stage N1, although their presence may be helpful in equivocal situations. In subjects who do not generate α rhythm and show low-amplitude mixed frequency activity with the eyes closed even in wakefulness, discerning sleep onset can be problematic. In these circumstances, stage N1 sleep should be scored when the first of the following phenomena is observed: slowing of background EEG frequencies by greater than or equal to 1 Hz, vertex sharp wave, or slow eye movements. The onset of slow eye movements antecedes the other changes in most subjects and thus is the criterion most likely to be applied. Because slow eye movements are usually seen while α rhythm is still present, the sleep latency is likely to be slightly shorter in subjects who do not generate α rhythm.

Stage N2 Sleep

Stage N2 sleep is defined by the presence of 1 or more K complexes without associated arousals or 1 or more trains of sleep spindles in the first half of the epoch or in the second half of the prior epoch (**Fig. 3**).[1] A K complex is a well-defined biphasic wave easily discernable from the background EEG with total duration greater than or equal to 0.5 seconds, usually maximal frontally. A sleep

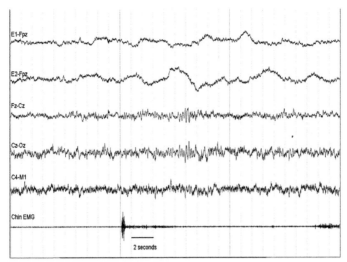

Fig. 2. Stage N1. The EEG shows low-amplitude, mixed frequency (predominantly 4–7 Hz) activity. Slow eye movements persist. See **Box 1** for electrode placements.

spindle is a train of waves with frequency 11 to 16 Hz, but usually 12 to 14 Hz, with duration greater than or equal to 0.5 seconds, usually maximal centrally. There are no defined amplitude criteria for a K complex or a sleep spindle. K complexes can be associated with arousals induced by environmental stimuli or by phenomena such as obstructive apneas. In some patients with obstructive sleep apnea, sleep can be fragmented by repeated apnea-induced arousals with frequent K complexes. K complexes with associated arousals do not represent a deeper level of sleep and so cannot be used to designate stage N2 sleep, unless a spontaneous K complex or sleep spindle is also present in the same epoch.

Because K complexes and sleep spindles are intermittent phenomena, they may not always be present in successive epochs. Their absence does not indicate that the sleep stage has reverted to stage N1 unless an arousal occurs or a major body movement (discussed later) followed by slow eye movements is present. Stage N2 sleep also terminates when there is a transition to stages W, N3, or R.

Stage N3 Sleep

Several lines of evidence indicate that slow wave sleep is sufficiently distinct from lighter stages of NREM sleep to warrant being defined as

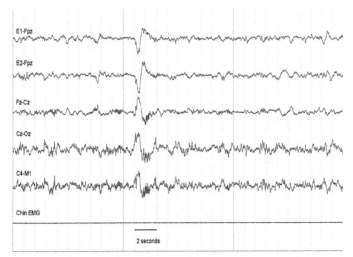

Fig. 3. Stage N2. The EEG shows sleep spindles and K complexes. Eye movements have ceased. See **Box 1** for electrode placements.

a separate stage. The neurophysiologic genesis of slow waves differs from that of K complexes.[33] Growth hormone is maximally released during slow wave sleep rather than stage N2.[34,35] Evening exercise and passive body heating increase slow wave sleep but not N2 sleep.[36,37] During the first recovery night after total sleep deprivation, there is rebound of slow wave sleep, but not N2 sleep.[38]

Stage N3 sleep is scored when greater than or equal to 20% of an epoch consists of slow wave activity, defined as waves of frequency 0.5 to 2 Hz with peak-to-peak amplitude greater than 75 μV recorded over the frontal regions (**Fig. 4**).[1] The frequency band is a subset of the classically defined δ frequency range (<4 Hz) and thus the term δ sleep should not be used. Sleep spindles may persist in stage N3 sleep, but are not required for scoring. The amplitude of slow waves decreases with age but similar age-related decreases in amplitude also occur in other sleep-related waves and frequency bands.[39] Although the choice of greater than 75 μV as the amplitude criterion for all ages of subjects is arbitrary, many experiments have shown that changes in slow wave percentage can be measured in subjects of any age in response to a wide range of interventions, including sleep deprivation,[40–42] sleep fragmentation,[42,43] and forced desynchronization.[44]

REM SLEEP

REM sleep is scored if an epoch includes low-amplitude, mixed frequency EEG, rapid eye movements, and low chin EMG tone (**Fig. 5**).[1] The EEG resembles that of stage N1, but some subjects have more prominent α frequencies, often at a frequency slower than that of their α rhythm while awake. Rapid eye movements are defined as conjugate, irregular, sharply peaked eye movements with the duration of the initial deflection usually less than 500 milliseconds. Low chin EMG tone implies that the chin EMG amplitude is no higher than in any other stage and is usually at the lowest level of the entire polysomnogram. Certain other phenomena, if present, may support scoring stage R but are not required. These include sawtooth waves (2–6 Hz sharply contoured or triangular, often serrated waves maximal over the central head regions and frequently preceding bursts of rapid eye movements) and transient muscle activity, previously known as phasic muscle twitches (burst of EMG activity lasting <0.25 seconds superimposed on low tone that may be present in the chin, anterior tibial, or EEG/EOG derivations).

Detailed rules have been established defining when a period of stage R sleep ends.[1] In broad outline, once stage R has been scored, subsequent epochs should continue to be scored as stage R until there has been a definite change to another stage, an arousal or major body movement is followed by slow eye movements, or K complexes or sleep spindles occur in the absence of rapid eye movements, even if chin EMG tone remains low. However, if an epoch contains rapid eye movements and the chin EMG tone is low, stage R should be scored even if K complexes or sleep spindles are present; this situation frequently occurs during the first REM period of the night when REM and NREM phenomena intermix. There are also rules concerning the scoring of transition epochs between epochs of definite stage N2 and

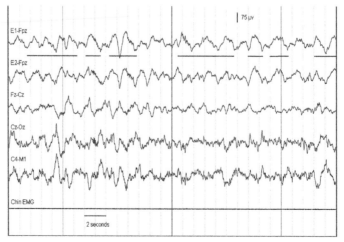

Fig. 4. Stage N3. The EEG shows slow waves with frequency less than 2 Hz and amplitude, measured frontally, greater than 75 μV (underlined) for more than 20% of the epoch. See **Box 1** for electrode placements.

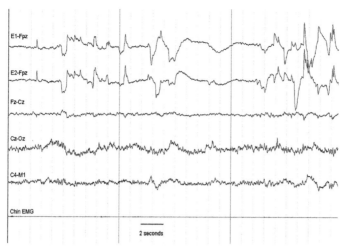

Fig. 5. Stage R. The EEG shows low-amplitude, mixed frequency activity. The EOG shows conjugate, irregular rapid eye movements. Chin EMG shows low tone. See **Box 1** for electrode placements.

definite REM sleep. In outline, stage R should be scored if chin EMG tone is low and K complexes or sleep spindles are absent, even if rapid eye movements have not yet commenced. However, if K complexes or sleep spindles are present in the transition epochs without rapid eye movements, these should be scored as stage N2, even if chin muscle tone is low.

MAJOR BODY MOVEMENTS

The term movement time was used in the R and K manual to classify epochs when more than 50% of the EEG was obscured by body movements and muscle artifact.[12] The AASM manual eliminated this term, replacing it with the concept of major body movements. Epochs with major body movements are scored as stage W if any α rhythm, even comprising less than half the epoch, is present, or if the preceding or following epoch is scored as stage W. Otherwise the epoch is given the same stage as the epoch following it.[1] The logic behind this rule is that major body movements generally result in an arousal or at least a change to a lighter stage of sleep.

PEDIATRIC CONSIDERATIONS

Maturational changes in the EEG with age make staging more challenging in children, especially in the first year of life. The AASM manual provides modifications for the staging of sleep in children from 2 months postterm onwards. For infants less than 2 months old, the 1971 Anders[2] manual for the scoring of states of sleep and wakefulness in newborn infants is recommended. Standard montages are used, but the distances between chin EMG electrodes and between EOG electrodes and the eyes may need to be reduced in infants and younger children.

Infant sleep should be scored using information derived from the EEG, eye movements, muscle tone, respiration, and behavior, including movements and vocalization. Three stages of sleep are recognized: (1) active sleep thought to be the precursor of REM sleep, (2) quiet sleep representing the precursor of NREM sleep, and (3) indeterminate sleep.[2] The EEG patterns of quiet sleep include high-voltage slow activity, trace alternant, and mixed rhythms. Trace alternant consists of bursts of moderate-voltage to high-voltage δ frequency activity lasting 3 to 8 seconds, alternating with 4-second to 8-second periods of lower amplitude, mixed frequency rhythms.

After 2 months of age, staging largely follows adult terminology. However, an undifferentiated stage N (NREM sleep) is used for appropriate epochs in records in which no K complexes/sleep spindles or no slow waves are present.[1] Sleep spindles usually develop at 2 to 3 months postterm and K complexes at 4 to 6 months.[45] Occipital α rhythm develops slowly with time, preceded by slower rhythms that attenuate with eye opening. Thus the term α rhythm is replaced by the concept of dominant posterior rhythm, which increases in frequency with age and can be as slow as 3.5 Hz in infants 3-months postterm. The patterns of drowsiness are also more varied in children. Stage N1 sleep can be characterized by hypnagogic hypersynchrony (paroxysmal bursts of high-amplitude sinusoidal waves of 3–4.5 Hz maximal frontocentrally, most common before age 5 years) or rhythmical anterior θ activity (runs of frontal activity of 5–7 Hz , most common in adolescents).[1,45]

EVALUATING THE AASM MANUAL

Since it was published in 2007, several studies have evaluated the staging methods of the AASM manual. The polysomnograms of 72 adult subjects (56 healthy, 5 with generalized anxiety disorder, 5 periodic limb movement disorder, and 6 Parkinson disease) were scored according to the R and K and AASM methods.[46] The duration and percentage of stages N1 (S1) and N3 (S3 and 4) sleep were significantly increased at the expense of less N2 (S2) sleep when studies were scored by AASM rules, and wake time after sleep onset was significantly longer. In subjects less than 60 years old, REM time was decreased. The increase in slow wave sleep was ascribed to the availability of a frontal derivation and the increase in N1 sleep to the rules no longer requiring an increase in muscle tone for an arousal to indicate the end of a period of N2 sleep. Interrater reliability of the AASM scoring rules was assessed using the same database.[47] Interrater agreement was higher using the AASM method for 10 of 13 variables, especially duration and percentage of N1 sleep. Epoch-by-epoch comparisons revealed substantial interrater agreement for both scoring methods, but higher for the AASM method. Agreement was least for stage N1. A study of 30 polysomnograms performed for suspected obstructive sleep apnea compared staging according to the AASM method with AASM staging modified by using only a single central EEG derivation.[48] Using 3 EEG derivations resulted in significantly less N1 and more N3 sleep being recorded, presumably because the frontal leads allowed better observation of K complexes and slow waves. However, there was no difference in interrater and intrarater reliability using the 2 methods.

FUTURE TRENDS

Although great care was taken to ensure that the new AASM staging system is compatible with published data and based on biologic principles, it is essentially a set of rules developed by expert consensus. It is encouraging that a study of interrater reliability[47] showed substantial agreement for predominantly normal subjects, but further studies of abnormal records of patients of different ages need to be performed. Validity studies may not be possible because there is no accepted gold standard for human sleep staging. The single study performed to date comparing the AASM and R and K methods showed differences

suggesting that the AASM method more reliably measures duration of sleep stages.[46]

The AASM rules may need modification for dealing with certain pathologic conditions, such as REM sleep behavior disorder, in which the atonia of REM sleep is lost.[49] In patients with advancing dementia, sleep architecture may deteriorate, resulting in an intermixture of wake rhythms and different states of sleep.[50] The phenomenon of α intrusion Into sleep[51] may also result in scoring difficulties, especially in the transition from wake to sleep. The AASM rules have been criticized for not addressing the microstructure of sleep.[52] Subpatterns of different stages, known as cyclic alternating patterns (CAP), have been described and an atlas with scoring rules published.[53] Although these concepts have resulted in insights into the nature of sleep and its disturbance by various disorders, the clinical benefit of scoring CAP is still uncertain.

The computerized scoring of sleep is beyond the scope of this article. Commercial systems based on digital algorithms largely using R and K rules are available and reliability data compared with human subjects have been published.[54,55] There is 1 report validating a computer-assisted scoring method using the AASM rules, but further studies using different software are needed. Further work is required to determine whether computerized scoring, with or without human revision, may reliably replace visual scoring in normal and abnormal sleep. At a research level, more sophisticated analyses, including quantitative EEG, spectral analysis, and period amplitude analysis, may provide novel insights into sleep and its disorders.[56] New hardware technology may also change the way physiologic signals are recorded, such as the use of direct current eye movement monitors to record changes of drowsiness.[57]

REFERENCES

1. Iber C, Ancoli-Israel S, Chessonn A, et al, American Academy of Sleep Medicine. The AASM manual for the scoring of sleep and associated events: rules, terminology and technical specifications. 1st edition. Westchester (IL): American Academy of Sleep Medicine; 2007.
2. Anders T, Emde R, Parmelee A. A manual of standardized terminology, techniques and criteria for scoring states of sleep and wakefulness in newborn infants. Los Angeles (CA): UCLA Brain Information Service, NINDS Neurological Information Network; 1971.
3. Berger H. Uber das elektroenkephalogramm des mensen. Arch Psychiatr Nervenkr 1929;87:527–70.

4. Loomis AL, Harvey EN, Hobart GA. Cerebral states during sleep, as studied by human brain potentials. J Exp Psychol 1937;1:24–38.

5. Blake H, Gerard R, Kleitman N. Factors including brain potentials during sleep. J Neurophysiol 1939; 2:48–60.

6. Gibbs E, Lorimer F, Gibbs F, editors. Atlas of encephalography, methodology and controls, vol. 1, 2nd edition. Reading (MA): Addison-Wesley; 1950.

7. Roth B. The clinical and theoretical importance of EEG rhythms corresponding to states of lowered vigilance. Electroencephalogr Clin Neurophysiol 1961;13:395–9.

8. Simon EW, Emmons WH. EEG, consciousness, and sleep. Science 1956;124:1066–9.

9. Aserinsky E, Kleitman N. Regularly occurring periods of eye motility and concomitant phenomena during sleep. Sleep 1953;118:273–4.

10. Dement W, Kleitman N. Cyclic variations in EEG during sleep and their relation to eye movements, body motility, and dreaming. Electroencephalogr Clin Neurophysiol 1957;9:673–90.

11. Williams RL, Karacan I, Hursch CJ. Electroencephalography (EEG) of human sleep: clinical applications. New York: John Wiley; 1974.

12. Rechtschaffen A, Kales A. A manual of standardized terminology, techniques, and scoring system for sleep stages of human subjects. Bethesda (MD): National Institute of Neurological Disease and Blindness; 1968.

13. Himanen SL, Hasan J. Limitations of Rechtschaffen and Kales. Sleep Med Rev 2000;4:149–67.

14. Hirshkowitz M. Standing on the shoulders of giants: the Standardized Sleep Manual after 30 years. Sleep Med Rev 2000;4:169–79.

15. McGregor P, Thorpy MJ, Schmidt-Nowara WW, et al. T-sleep: an improved method for scoring breathing-disordered sleep. Sleep 1992;15:359–63.

16. Shepard JW. Atlas of sleep medicine. Armonk (NY): Futura; 1991.

17. Van Sweden B, Kemp B, Kamphuisen HA, et al. Alternative electrode placement in (automatic) sleep scoring (Fpz-Cz/Pz-Oz versus C4-A1). Sleep 1990; 13:279–83.

18. Hori T, Sugita Y, Koga E, et al. Proposed supplements and amendments to "a manual of standardized terminology, techniques and scoring system for sleep stages of human subjects", the Rechtschaffen and Kales (1968) standard. Psychiatr Clin Neurosci 2001;55:305–10.

19. Iber C, Ancoli-Israel S, Chambers M, et al. The new sleep scoring manual-the evidence behind the rules. J Clin Sleep Med 2007;3:107.

20. Silber MH, Ancoli-Israel S, Bonnet MH. The visual scoring of sleep in adults. J Clin Sleep Med 2007; 3:121–31.

21. Happe S, Anderer P, Gruber G, et al. Scalp topography of the spontaneous K-complex and of delta-waves in human sleep. Brain Topogr 2002; 15:43–9.

22. McCormick L, Nielsen T, Nicolas A, et al. Topographical distribution of spindles and K-complexes in normal subjects. Sleep 1997;20:939–41.

23. De Gennaro L, Ferrara M, Bertini M. Topographical distribution of spindles: variations between and within NREM sleep cycles. Sleep Res Online 2000; 3:155–60.

24. Santamaria R, Chiappa KH. The EEG of drowsiness in normal adults. J Clin Neurophysiol 1987; 4:327–82.

25. Ogilvie RD, Wilkinson RT. Behavioral versus EEG-based monitoring of all night sleep/wake patterns. Sleep 1988;11:139–55.

26. Trinder J, Whitworth F, Kay A, et al. Respiratory instability during sleep onset. J Appl Physiol 1992;73: 2462–9.

27. Mezzanotte WS, Tangel DJ, White DP. Influence of sleep onset on upper-airway muscle activity in apnea patients versus normal controls. Am J Respir Crit Care Med 1996;153:1880–7.

28. Worsnop C, Kay A, Pierce R, et al. Activity of respiratory pump and upper airway muscles during sleep onset. J Appl Physiol 1998;85:908–20.

29. Burgess HJ, Kleiman J, Trinder J. Cardiac activity during sleep onset. Psychophysiology 1999;36: 298–306.

30. Fogel RB, White DP, Pierce RJ, et al. Control of upper airway muscle activity in younger versus older men during sleep onset. J Physiol 2003;553: 533–44.

31. Kjaer TW, Law I, Wiltschiotz G, et al. Regional cerebral blood flow during light sleep - a H15 O-PET study. J Sleep Res 2002;11:201–7.

32. Spielman AJ, Zhang G, Yang C, et al. Intracerebral hemodynamics probed by near infrared spectroscopy in the transition between wakefulness and sleep. Brain Res 2000;866:313–25.

33. Steriade M, Amzica F. Slow sleep oscillations, rhythmic K-complexes, and their paroxysmal developments. J Sleep Res 1998;7(Suppl 1):30–5.

34. Holl RW, Hartmann ML, Veldhuis JD, et al. Thirty-second sampling of plasma growth hormone in man: correlation with sleep stages. J Clin Endocrinol Metab 1991;72:854–61.

35. Van Cautier E, Plat L, Copinschi G. Interrelations between sleep and the somatotrophic axis. Sleep 1998;21:553–66.

36. Bunnell DE, Agnew JA, Horvath SM, et al. Passive body heating and sleep: influence of proximity to sleep. Sleep 1988;11:210–9.

37. Horne JA, Staff LH. Exercise and sleep: body-heating effects. Sleep 1983;6:36–46.

38. Aeschbach D, Cajochen C, Landolt H, et al. Homeostatic sleep regulation in habitual short sleepers and long sleepers. Am J Physiol 1996;270:R41–53.

39. Tan X, Campbell IG, Feinberg I. Inter-night reliability and benchmark values for computer analyses of non-rapid eye movement (NREM) and REM EGG in normal young adult and elderly subjects. Clin Neurophysiol 2001;112:1540–52.

40. Brendel DH, Reynolds CF, Jennings JR. Sleep stage physiology, mood, and vigilance responses to total sleep deprivation in healthy 80-year-olds and 20-year-olds. Psychophysiology 1990;27:667–85.

41. Carskadon MA, Dement WC. Sleep loss in elderly volunteers. Sleep 1985;8:207–21.

42. Reynolds CF, Kupfer DJ, Hoch CC, et al. Sleep deprivation in healthy elderly men and women: effects on mood and on sleep during recovery. Sleep 1986;9:492–501.

43. Reynolds CF, Kupfer DJ, Hoch CC, et al. Sleep deprivation as a probe in the elderly. Arch Gen Psychiatry 1987;44:982–90.

44. Dijk DJ, Duffy JF, Riel E, et al. Ageing and the circadian and homeostatic regulation of human sleep during forced desynchrony of rest, melatonin and temperature rhythms. J Physiol 1999;516:611–27.

45. Grigg-Damberger M, Gozal D, Marcus CL, et al. The visual scoring of sleep and arousal in infants and children. J Clin Sleep Med 2007;3:201–40.

46. Moser D, Anderer P, Gruber G, et al. Sleep classification according to AASM and Rechtschaffen & Kales: effects on sleep scoring parameters. Sleep 2009;32:139–49.

47. Danker-Hopfe H, Anderer P, Zeitlhofer J, et al. Inter-rater reliability for scoring according to the Rechtschaffen & Kales and the new AASM standard. J Sleep Res 2009;18:74–84.

48. Ruehland WR, O'Donoghue FJ, Pierce RJ, et al. The 2007 AASM recommendations for EEG electrode placement in polysomnography: impact on sleep and cortical arousal scoring. Sleep 2011;34:73–81.

49. Olson EJ, Boeve BF, Silber MH. Rapid eye movement sleep behavior disorder: demographic, clinical and laboratory findings in 93 cases. Brain 2000;123:331–9.

50. Mahowald MW, Schenck CH. Status dissociatus - a perspective on states of being. Sleep 1991;14:69–79.

51. Hauri P, Hawkins DR. Alpha-delta sleep. Encephalogr Clin Neurophysiol 1973;34:233–7.

52. Parrino L, Ferri R, Zucconi M, et al. Commentary from the Italian Association of Sleep Medicine on the AASM Manual for the Scoring of Sleep and Associated Events: for debate and discussion. Sleep Med 2009;10:799–808.

53. Terzano MG, Parrino L, Sherieri A, et al. Atlas, rules and recording techniques for the scoring of cyclic alternating pattern (CAP) in human sleep. Sleep Med 2001;2:537–53.

54. Anderer P, Gruber G, Parapatics S, et al. An E-health solution for automatic sleep classification according to Rechtschaffen and Kales: validation study of the Somnolyzer 24 x 7 utilizing the Siesta database. Neuropsychobiology 2005;51:115–33.

55. Prinz PN, Larsen LH, Moe KE, et al. C STAGE, automated sleep scoring: development and comparison with human sleep scoring for healthy older men and women. Sleep 1994;17:711–7.

56. Penzel T, Hirshkowitz M, Harsh J, et al. Digital analysis and technical specifications. J Clin Sleep Med 2007;3:109–20.

57. Atienza M, Cantero JL, Stickgold R, et al. Eyelid movements measured by Nightcap predict slow eye movements during quiet wakefulness in humans. J Sleep Res 2004;13:25–9.

Respiratory Physiology During Sleep

Vipin Malik, MD*, Daniel Smith, MD,
Teofilo Lee-Chiong Jr, MD

KEYWORDS

- Ventilatory regulation • Respiratory motoneurons • Hypoxemia • Hypercapnia
- Pneumotaxic center • Apneustic center • Chemoreceptors

KEY POINTS

- Ventilatory regulation is conceptually best understood as a 3-part system consisting of a central controller, sensors, and effectors.
- The effectors of respiration include the respiratory motoneurons and muscles, which are involved in inspiration and expiration.
- Positional changes during sleep (ie, nonupright position) affect the mechanics of breathing significantly.
- Both hypoxemia and hypercapnia can develop during sleep in patients with chronic obstructive pulmonary disease.
- Upper-airway narrowing and excess weight, if present, can increase the mechanical load on the respiratory system as well as breathing work.

The respiratory system provides continuous homeostasis of partial pressures of arterial oxygen (Pa_{O_2}), carbon dioxide (P_{CO_2}), and pH levels during constantly changing physiologic conditions. This elegant system responds promptly to subtle variations in metabolism occurring in both health and disease. During wakefulness, volitional influences can override this automatic control. Modifications occur in the regulation and control of respiration with the onset of sleep. Furthermore, these changes differ significantly with specific sleep stages. These alterations in respiratory control can result in the pathogenesis of sleep-related breathing disorders and limit the usual respiratory compensatory changes to specific disease states. This article reviews the normal physiology of respiration in both awake and sleep states, and discusses the effects of common disease processes and medications on the respiratory physiology of sleep.

CONTROL OF RESPIRATION

Ventilatory regulation is conceptually best understood as a 3-part system consisting of a central controller, sensors, and effectors. *Sensors* primarily include central and peripheral chemoreceptors, vagal pulmonary sensors, and chest-wall and respiratory muscle afferents. Data from these sensors regarding dynamic oxygen and CO_2 levels, lung volumes, and respiratory muscle activity are continuously transmitted to the central controller. Within the medulla, the *central controller* generates an automated rhythm of respiration that is constantly modified in response to an integrated input from the various receptors. The controller modulates motor output from the brainstem to influence the activity of the *effectors*, namely respiratory motoneurons and muscles. These effectors then alter minute ventilation and gas exchange accordingly (**Table 1**).

The medullary ventilatory center consists of neurons in the dorsal respiratory group (DRG)

A version of this article originally appeared in *Sleep Medicine Clinics Volume 5, Issue 2*.
Section of Sleep Medicine, National Jewish Medical and Research Center, Denver, CO, USA
* Corresponding author. Section of Sleep Medicine, Division of Critical Care and Hospital Medicine, National Jewish Health, 1400 Jackson Street, M323, Denver, CO 80206.
E-mail address: malikv@njhealth.org

Table 1
Control of respiration

Controllers/Effectors	Location	Afferents	Effects
Dorsal Respiratory group	Dorsomedial medulla, ventrolateral to the solitary tract	Upper airways, intra-arterial chemoreceptors, and lung afferents via the 5th, 9th and 10th cranial nerves, respectively	Increased frequency of a ramping pattern of firing during continued inspiration
Ventral Respiratory Group	Ventrolateral medulla	Response to the need for forced expiration occurring during exercise or with increased airways resistance	Respiratory effectors muscles are innervated from the VRG via phrenic, intercostal and abdominal motoneurons.
Pneumotaxic center	Rostral pons consists of the nucleus parabrachialis and the Kolliker-Fuse nucleus.	Pontine input serves to fine tune respiratory patterns and may additionally modulate responses to hypercapnia, hypoxia, and lung inflation	Duration of inspiration and provide tonic input to respiratory pattern generator
Apneustic center	Lower pons	Pneumotaxic center and vagal input	Provide signals that smoothly terminate inspiratory efforts
Central Chemoreceptors	Ventrolateral surface of medulla	Extracellular fluid [H+] concentration	Respond to changes in brain extracellular fluid [H+] concentration
Peripheral Chemoreceptors	Carotid bodies and the aortic bodies	Afferent input to the medulla through the 9th cranial nerve	Respond mainly to PaO_2, but also to changes in $PaCO_2$ and pH
Pulmonary Mechanoreceptors	1. PSRs are located in proximal airway smooth muscles. 2. J-receptors are located in the juxtacapillary area and appear to mediate dyspnea in the setting of pulmonary vascular congestion 3. Bronchial c-fibers		1. Respond to inflation, especially in the setting of hyperinflation 2. Mediate dyspnea in the setting of pulmonary vascular congestion 3. Affect bronchomotor tone and respond to pulmonary inflammation

and the ventral respiratory group (VRG) (**Fig. 1**).[1] Located in the dorsomedial medulla, ventrolateral to the solitary tract, the DRG was previously believed to be the site of rhythmic inspiratory drive. More recent research in animal models suggests that the respiratory rhythm is generated by a group of cells known as the pre-Bötzinger complex, a network of cells surrounding the Bötzinger complex in the ventrolateral medulla.[2]

The medullary centers respond to direct influences from the upper airways, intra-arterial chemoreceptors, and lung afferents via the fifth, ninth and tenth cranial nerves, respectively. The DRG appears to be active primarily during inspiration, with increased frequency of a ramping pattern of firing during continued inspiration. The VRG, located within the ventrolateral medulla, contains both inspiratory and expiratory neurons. VRG output increases in response to the need for forced expiration occurring during exercise or with increased airways resistance. Respiratory effectors muscles are innervated from the VRG via phrenic, intercostal, and abdominal motoneurons.

Poorly understood pontine influences further regulate and coordinate inspiratory and expiratory control. The pneumotaxic center in the rostral

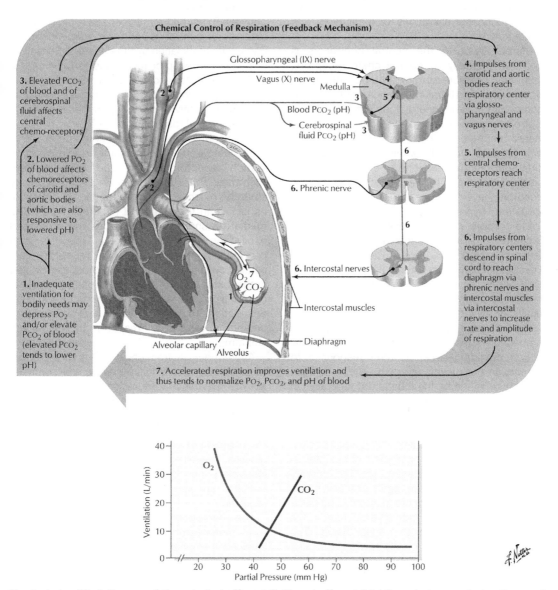

Fig. 1. A simplified diagram of the principal efferent (*left*) and afferent (*right*) respiratory control pathways. A section through the brain, brain stem, and spinal cord is shown (with pertinent respiratory areas indicated by *shading*), as are the central nervous system links with the respiratory apparatus. (Netter illustration from http://www.netterimages.com. © Elsevier Inc. All rights reserved.)

pons consists of the nucleus parabrachialis and the Kolliker-Fuse nucleus. This area appears to primarily influence the duration of inspiration and provide tonic input to respiratory pattern generators. Similarly, the apneustic center, located in the lower pons, functions to provide signals that smoothly terminate inspiratory efforts. The pontine input serves to fine-tune respiratory patterns and may additionally modulate responses to hypercapnia, hypoxia, and lung inflation.[3] The automatic central control of respiration may be influenced and temporarily overridden by volitional control from the cerebral cortex for a variety of activities, such as speech, singing, laughing, intentional and psychogenic alterations of respiration, and breath holding.

Afferent input to the central controllers is mediated primarily by central chemoreceptors, peripheral chemoreceptors, intrapulmonary receptors, and chest-wall/mechanoreceptors. Chemoreceptors provide a direct feedback to central controllers in response to the consequences of altered respiratory efforts. Central chemoreceptors, located primarily within the ventrolateral surface of medulla, respond to changes in brain extracellular fluid $[H^+]$ concentration. Other receptors have been recently identified in the brainstem, hypothalamus, and the cerebellum. These receptors are effectively CO_2 receptors, as central $[H^+]$ concentrations are directly dependent on central Pco_2 levels. Central $[H^+]$ may differ significantly from arterial $[H^+]$, as the blood brain barrier prevents polar solute diffusion into the cerebrospinal fluid (CSF). This isolation results in an indirect central response to most peripheral acid-base disturbances mediated through changes in partial pressure of arterial carbon dioxide ($Paco_2$). Central responses to changes in Pco_2 levels are also slightly delayed for a few minutes by the location of receptors in the brain only, rather than in peripheral vascular tissues.

Peripheral chemoreceptors include the carotid bodies and the aortic bodies. The carotid bodies, located bilaterally at the bifurcation of the internal and external carotid arteries, are the primary peripheral monitors. These highly vascular structures monitor the status of blood about to be delivered to the brain and provide afferent input to the medulla through the ninth cranial nerve. The carotid bodies respond mainly to Pao_2 but also to changes in $Paco_2$ and pH. Of importance, they do not respond to lowered oxygen content from anemia or carbon monoxide (CO) toxicity. Their mechanisms are integrated, and acute hypoxia induces an increased sensitivity to changes in $Paco_2$ and acidosis. Conversely, the response to low Pao_2 is markedly attenuated in the setting of low $Paco_2$.

Respiratory responses to increases in central $Paco_2$ levels above 28 mm Hg are linear with increases in respiratory rate, tidal volume, and minute ventilation.[4] Peripheral $Paco_2$-driven responses also vary with differences in levels of Pao_2. By contrast, the slope of the ventilatory response to Pao_2 varies based on sensitivity and threshold. The response to hypoxia is nonlinear and appears to be minimal above Pao_2 levels of 60 mm Hg.

Resultant interactions of chemoreceptor inputs regulate normal $Paco_2$ levels in humans to between 37 and 43 mm Hg at sea level. In effect, respiratory control is primarily dependent on $Paco_2$ with modulation by other factors. Sensitivity of peripheral receptor responses to hypercapnia and hypoxia also increases with a reduction in arterial pH. Whereas acute hypoxia stimulates increased sensitivity to $Paco_2$ peripherally, it might depress central respiratory drive.[5]

Additional feedback to the central controller is transmitted from the lung directly from pulmonary stretch receptors (PSRs) and other afferent pathways. PSRs are located in proximal airway smooth muscles, and respond to inflation, especially in the setting of hyperinflation. PSRs mediate a shortened inspiratory and prolonged expiratory duration. Additional input is also provided by rapidly adapting receptors that sense flow and irritation. J-receptors are located in the juxtacapillary area and appear to mediate dyspnea in the setting of pulmonary vascular congestion. Bronchial c-fibers also affect bronchomotor tone and respond to pulmonary inflammation.

Afferent activity from chest-wall and respiratory muscles additionally influences central controller activity. Feedback information regarding muscle stretch, loading, and fatigue may affect both regulatory and somatosensory responses. Upper-airway receptors promote airway patency by activation of local muscles including the genioglossus. These receptors may also inhibit thoracic inspiratory muscle activity. Thus, afferent activity enables an appropriate response by central regulation.

The effectors of respiration include the respiratory motoneurons and muscles, which are involved in inspiration and expiration. Descending motoneurons include two anatomically separate groups, the corticospinal tracts and the reticulospinal tracts. The phrenic nerve, arising from C3 to C5, innervates the diaphragm as the primary muscle of respiration. Accessory muscles that assist inspiration include the sternocleidomastoid, intercostal, scalene, and parasternal muscles. These muscles serve to collectively stabilize and expand the ribcage. Abdominal muscles are active in expiration and may also assist with inspiration during exercise, or in the setting of chronic obstructive pulmonary disease (COPD) or diaphragm weakness. Upper-airway muscles active in inspiration include the genioglossus, palatal muscles, pharyngeal constrictors, and muscles that pull the hyoid anteriorly. Collectively, these muscle groups and motoneurons effect responses generated from central control centers based on input from multiple receptors. This elegant system operates through the complex coordination and interaction of these subcomponents to continuously adapt to changing metabolic needs.

RESPIRATION DURING SLEEP

Regulation of respiration differs significantly between sleep and wakefulness. With sleep onset, important changes occur in the various processes that regulate respiratory control. Behavioral influences on respiration terminate with cessation of input from the waking state. Positional changes typically associated with sleep also result in significant alterations in respiratory mechanics. Sleep is a dynamic physiologic state with further varying effects on respiration seen in specific sleep stages, particularly in rapid eye movement (REM) in comparison with non–rapid eye movement (NREM) sleep.

Minute ventilation falls with the onset of sleep in response to decreased metabolism and decreased chemosensitivity to oxygen (O_2) and CO_2.[6,7] Ventilation during NREM sleep demonstrates an inherently more regular respiratory pattern than wakeful breathing, without significant reductions in mean frequencies. The nadir of minute ventilation in NREM sleep occurs during NREM stage 3 (N3) sleep (ie, slow-wave sleep), primarily as a result of reductions in tidal volume. As a result, end-tidal carbon dioxide ($ETCO_2$) during NREM sleep increases by 1 to 2 torr compared with the waking state.[8] During REM sleep, respiratory patterns and control vary more significantly. REM sleep respiration is typically characterized by an increased frequency and a reduced regularity. Tidal volume is reduced further in comparison with that of NREM sleep, resulting in the lowest level of normal minute ventilation. Accordingly, $ETCO_2$ increases of an additional 1 to 2 torr, often associated with a reduction in oxygen saturation, are seen with the onset of REM sleep. Metabolic reductions seen in sleep demonstrate sleep-stage variations with increased rates in REM compared to NREM sleep.

Ventilatory responses to CO_2 and O_2 differ in sleep in comparison with wakefulness, with important distinctions between REM and NREM sleep. The linear increases in ventilatory responses to $Paco_2$ persist during NREM sleep, albeit with a reduced slope compared to wakefulness. These changes appear more evident in males than in females, who demonstrate reduced CO_2 responses while awake with less apparent reductions during NREM sleep.[9] In addition, the threshold of the response to CO_2 is shifted upward, with a higher $ETCO_2$ required to drive respiration in sleep. Responses to increases in $ETCO_2$ are further reduced during REM sleep. Respiratory output in sleep, particularly NREM sleep, is significantly reduced in response to hypocapnia. Respiratory responses to hypoxia appear attenuated during NREM sleep as well, without significant gender-related differences; hypoxia-induced drive is reduced further in REM sleep.

Of importance, both hypoxia and hypercapnia may trigger arousals from sleep, resulting in a return to the more tightly regulated ventilatory control associated with wakefulness. Arousal thresholds for hypercapnia range between 56 and 65 torr, and vary among the different sleep stages. The threshold for arousal in response to hypoxia is more variable and seems less reliable. Severe oxygen desaturations in some individuals do not uniformly result in arousals.

In addition to the changes in controller responses during sleep, the effectors also demonstrate significant sleep-related functional variation. Of the various effectors of respiration, the upper-airway muscles appear to be the most dramatically affected by changes occurring with sleep. As described previously, these muscles function to maintain patency and prevent collapse of the upper airways during inspiration. These muscles primarily include the genioglossus, tensor palatini, and the sternohyoid, which are active during inspiration during wakefulness and are reduced activity during sleep. The genioglossus responds briskly to increases in $Paco_2$ during wakefulness; this response markedly diminishes during sleep. Indeed, the modest increase in $Paco_2$ seen with sleep onset does not appear to produce a significant increase in genioglossus activity. Human studies of upper-airway responses during REM sleep are limited, with most studies demonstrating that muscle activity is eliminated by generalized REM-sleep–associated skeletal muscle atonia; this effect is most prominent during phasic REM sleep. Upper-airway responses to hypoxia generally parallel the responses to hypercapnia. Studies consistently demonstrate more striking sleep-related reductions in muscle activity of the upper airways than of the diaphragm or accessory muscles of respiration.

Positional changes during sleep (ie, nonupright position) affect the mechanics of breathing significantly. Anatomic structures of the upper airways may be more predisposed to collapse, particularly with the concurrent reductions in upper-airway muscle tone. Redundant soft-tissue–related airway compromise and retroglossal narrowing of the upper airways may be significantly increased in the supine position. Subtle increases in vascular congestion of the airways in response to positional changes may also augment airways resistance. In the supine position, the contribution of chest-wall expansion does not exceed the effect of increased abdominal distention, and functional residual capacity is thus reduced. Intercostal muscle activity is significantly increased during NREM sleep compared with wakefulness, and results in proportional increases in the contribution of the chest wall to respiration. With REM-sleep–associated atonia, skeletal muscles associated with respiration are significantly impaired and ventilation is accomplished by the diaphragm alone. Chest-wall compliance is increased with this decreased intercostal tone, and paradoxic collapse of the chest during inspiration may occur. REM sleep is, therefore, associated with relative hypoventilation from both reduced respiratory mechanical capacities and decreased sensitivity of the respiratory drive to hypercapnia and hypoxia.

There are significant differences in the responses to increased airways resistance between sleep and wakefulness. During the waking state, increased ventilatory responses to both elastic loading and airways-resistance loading are present; this prompt compensation maintains appropriate ventilation and prevents development of hypercapnia. Load compensation is significantly reduced during sleep. During NREM sleep, moderate levels of elastic loading (18 cm H_2O/L) results in decreases in minute ventilation and increases in ETCO$_2$.[10] Ventilatory effort is then increased without normalization back to preload levels of ventilation. Lower levels of loading (12 cm H_2O/L) result in significant ventilatory changes over a few breaths resulting in full compensation without arousals.[11] Waking responses to resistance loads include an increase in the duration of respiration, an increase in tidal volume, and a decrease in respiratory rate. Minute ventilation is reduced. Responses to increased resistance during NREM sleep demonstrate a different pattern of reduced tidal volumes and increased respiratory rates, and no significant change in inspiratory time ratio. Reductions in minute ventilation in response

to resistance loading are more evident during NREM sleep than in waking states.

MEDICATIONS AND BREATHING DURING SLEEP

There are several drugs that can impair respiration during sleep, including alcohol, anesthetics, narcotics, and sedative hypnotics. Conversely, some agents, such as almitrine, acetazolamide, some antidepressants, nicotine, progesterone, theophylline, and thyroid hormones, can stimulate breathing during sleep.

Drugs that can Impair Respiration

Alcohol, when ingested while awake, can lead to reduction of both hypoxic and hypercapnic ventilatory responses. Irregular breathing with transient apneas can develop. When ingested close to bedtime, it depresses the upper-airway muscle tone and may precipitate obstructive sleep apnea, or aggravate a preexisting one; the latter is generally most evident during the first 1 to 3 hours of sleep when alcohol levels are at their highest. Hypercapnia and significant hypoxemia can occur with severe intoxication. The risk of sleep-disordered breathing remains elevated in some abstinent alcoholics following long-term habitual alcohol use, possibly caused by residual upper-airway muscle dysfunction or damage to the central nervous system.[12]

Anesthetics can impair the hypoxic ventilatory response, decrease lung volumes, and decrease upper-airway muscle tone, all of which can lead to significant deterioration of respiratory status in patients with an existing obstructive sleep apnea or advanced COPD.[13]

Narcotics are potent respiratory depressants which, when ingested at bedtime, can diminish upper-airway muscle tone, give rise to hypoxemia, and decrease the hypercapnic ventilatory response.[14]

Sedative hypnotics (eg, benzodiazepines or barbiturates) are mild respiratory depressants. Depression of breathing is be more pronounced during coingestion with other central nervous system depressants, such as alcohol, or in individuals with an underlying respiratory impairment (eg, severe COPD, neuromuscular weakness, or hypoventilation syndromes). Both agents can decrease upper-airway muscle activity and worsen sleep-disordered breathing; they have variable effects on central apneas. Whereas they may increase the frequency and prolong the duration of hypercapnic forms of central apneas (eg, neuromuscular disorders), sedative hypnotics may be beneficial for patients with certain types of nonhypercapnic form of central apnea, such as those that occur periodically at sleep onset.[15]

Drugs that can Stimulate Respiration

Almitrine is a respiratory stimulant that enhances peripheral chemoreceptor sensitivity. Although it can potentially improve nighttime oxygenation, this effect is generally mild and inconsistent.[16,17]

Acetazolamide administration induces metabolic acidosis from bicarbonate diuresis; this, in turn, can stimulate respiration.[18] Although it is beneficial for the treatment of high-altitude–related periodic breathing, its usefulness for patients with obstructive sleep apnea is limited, inconsistent, and unpredictable.

Certain *antidepressants*, such as protriptyline, a tricyclic antidepressant, and fluoxetine, a selective serotonin reuptake inhibitor, can decrease the frequency and duration of apneas-hypopneas by increasing upper-airway muscle tone and decreasing percentage of REM sleep, during which sleep-disordered breathing tends to be worse than during NREM sleep.[19]

Nicotine is a respiratory stimulant. Notwithstanding its effect of enhancing upper-airway muscle activity, it has no role in the treatment of obstructive sleep apnea.[20]

Progesterone can increase hypoxic and hypercapnic respiratory responses as well as minute ventilation; it can improve ventilation in patients with obesity-hypoventilation syndrome and decrease apnea-hypopneas in post-menopausal women.[21,22]

Theophylline can reverse the bronchospasm of nocturnal asthma, increase sleep-related oxygen saturation in patients with COPD, and improve Cheyne-Stokes crescendo-decrescendo periodic breathing.[23]

SLEEP PHYSIOLOGY AND RESPIRATORY DISORDERS
Nocturnal Asthma

Patients with nocturnal asthma often present with repetitive arousals and awakenings during the night accompanied by complaints of breathlessness, coughing, and wheezing secondary to bronchoconstriction.[24] A variety of factors may contribute to the worsening bronchial reactivity that occurs during sleep, including a relative increase in parasympathetic tone and decrease in nonadrenergic, noncholinergic discharge; comorbid gastroesophageal reflux or obstructive sleep apnea; circadian changes in levels of endogenous hormones (eg, catecholamines, cortisol, or histamine); or reduction of lung volumes and airway size. If severe, nocturnal asthma may give rise to significant hypoxemia.

Chronic Obstructive Pulmonary Disease

Both hypoxemia and hypercapnia can develop during sleep in patients with COPD. Respiratory impairment is more severe during REM sleep than during NREM sleep. Hypoxemia, the extent of which is related to the percentage of REM sleep in relation to total sleep time as well as daytime levels of Pa_{CO_2}, Pa_{O_2}, and oxygen saturation (Sa_{O_2}), can result from hypoventilation, ventilation/perfusion mismatching, and/or reduction of lung volume (eg, functional residual capacity). COPD can also occur concurrently with obstructive sleep apnea; referred to as the overlap syndrome; this is associated with worse hypoxemia and greater pulmonary artery pressures compared with patients with isolated COPD.[25,26]

Restrictive Lung Disease

Sleep of patients with *interstitial lung disease* is often accompanied by frequent arousals. Sleep disruption appears to be more pronounced in those with nocturnal oxygen desaturation, the extent of which is influenced by levels of awake Pa_{O_2}, lung compliance, and age of the patient.[27] The increase in respiratory drive that is present in patients with interstitial lung disease may reduce the prevalence of apneas-hypopneas.

Kyphoscoliosis, by blunting ventilatory drive due to a greater mechanical load of displacing the thoracic cage, can lead to a number of sleep-related breathing disorders, such as central and obstructive apnea-hypopneas, periodic breathing, hypercapnia and hypoxemia.

Obesity is associated with increased work of breathing and greater metabolic demands. Lower functional capacity, less efficient respiratory muscles, and increased mass loading of the thoracic cage (ie, decrease in compliance) can all give rise to hypoxemia, which is generally worse during sleep than during wakefulness because of the lower functional residual capacity of a supine position, relative hypoventilation, and the development of sleep-related apneas-hypopneas. If severe, obesity can lead to the development of the obesity hypoventilation syndrome with its associated reductions in hypoxic and hypercapnic ventilatory drives.

Pregnancy, like obesity, can reduce lung volumes (eg, functional residual capacity and residual volume), especially during the third trimester when weight gain and uterine displacement are maximal. Pregnancy may also be associated with an increase in the prevalence of snoring, owing to structural changes and increased compliance of the upper airways. However, apnea-hypopnea frequency and sleep-related hypoxemia tend to be less affected because of the augmented ventilatory drive produced by higher levels of progesterone.

Neuromuscular Disorders

Patients with *Duchene muscular dystrophy* can develop hypoventilation and oxygen desaturation during sleep. *Myotonic dystrophy* can involve the pharyngolaryngeal and diaphragm muscles; obstructive and central apneas-hypopneas, hypoventilation, and oxygen desaturation occurring during sleep has been described. *Poliomyelitis* is often associated with a defective central control of respiration and can give rise to apneas and hypopneas during sleep. *Diaphragm paralysis*, especially if bilateral, can lead to increases in $Paco_2$ and reductions in Pao_2; these derangements in arterial blood gases are generally worse during REM sleep in comparison with waking and NREM sleep, because of the REM-sleep–related inhibition of the intercostal and accessory respiratory muscles.

Obstructive Sleep Apnea

Upper-airway narrowing and excess weight, if present, can increase the mechanical load on the respiratory system as well as breathing work. Oxygen desaturation can result from repetitive episodes of apneas-hypopneas, the latter being more common during REM sleep than during NREM sleep. Episodes of oxygen desaturation, therefore, tend to more frequent and last longer during REM sleep. Hypoxemia and, to lesser extent, hypercapnia can also arise from the reduction in lung volume related to the supine sleep position and is made worse by comorbid obesity resulting in augmented respiratory muscle activity generated to compensate for the diminished or absent airflow secondary to upper-airway narrowing or collapse (ie, Müller maneuver).

REFERENCES

1. Ezure K. Synaptic connections between medullary respiratory neurons and considerations on the genesis of respiratory rhythm. Prog Neurobiol 1990;35:429–50.
2. Smith JC, Ellenberger HH, Ballanyi K, et al. Pre-Bötzinger complex: a brainstem region that may generate respiratory rhythm in mammals. Science 1991;254:726–9.
3. Mitchell RA, Berger AJ. Neural regulation of respiration. In: Horbein TF, editor. Regulation of breathing (part I). New York: Marcel Dekker; 1981. p. 541–620.
4. Nattie EE. Central chemosensitivity, sleep, and wakefulness. Respir Physiol 2001;129:257–68.
5. Bisgard GE, Neubauer JA. Peripheral and central effects of hypoxia. In: Demspey JA, Pack AI, editors. Regulation of breathing. 2nd edition. New York: Marcel Dekker; 1995. p. 617–68.
6. Douglas NJ, White DP, Weil JV, et al. Hypoxic ventilatory response decreases during sleep in normal men. Am Rev Respir Dis 1982;125(3):286–9.
7. Douglas NJ, White DP, Weil JV, et al. Hypercapneic ventilatory response in sleeping adults. Am Rev Respir Dis 1982;126(5):758–62.
8. Kreiger J. Respiratory physiology; breathing in normal subjects. In: Kryger M, Roth T, Dement WC, editors. Principles and practice of sleep medicine. Philadelphia: WB Saunders; 2000. p. 229–41.
9. Berthon-Jones M, Sullivan CE. Ventilation and arousal responses to hypercapnia in normal sleeping humans. J Appl Physiol 1984;57:59–67.
10. Wilson PA, Skatrud JB, Dempsey JA. Effects of slow wave sleep on ventilatory compensations to inspiratory loading. Respir Physiol 1984;55:103–20.
11. Badr MS, Skatrud JB, Dempsey JA, et al. Effect of mechanical loading on expiratory and inspiratory muscle activity during NREM sleep. J Appl Physiol 1990;68:1195–202.
12. Sisson JH. Alcohol and airways function in health and disease. Alcohol 2007;41:293–307.
13. Ho AM, Chen S, Karmakar MK. Central apnoea after balanced general anaesthesia that included dexmedetomidine. Br J Anaesth 2005;95:773–5.
14. Wang D, Teichtahl H, Drummer O, et al. Central sleep apnea in stable methadone maintenance treatment patients. Chest 2005;128(3):1348–56.
15. Nickol AH, Leverment J, Richards P, et al. Temazepam at high altitude reduces periodic breathing without impairing next-day performance: a randomized crossover double-blind study. J Sleep Res 2006;15:445–54.
16. Sans-Torres J, Domingo C, Morón A, et al. Long-term effects of almitrine bismesylate in COPD patients with chronic hypoxaemia. Respir Med 2003;97:599–605.
17. Daskalopoulou E, Patakas D, Tsara V, et al. Comparison of almitrine bismesylate and medroxyprogesterone acetate on oxygenation during wakefulness and sleep in patients with chronic obstructive lung disease. Thorax 1990;45:666–9.
18. Yasuma F, Murohara T, Hayano J. Long-term efficacy of acetazolamide on Cheyne-Stokes respiration in congestive heart failure. Am J Respir Crit Care Med 2006;174:479.
19. Qureshi A, Lee-Chiong TL. Medical treatment of obstructive sleep apnea. Semin Respir Crit Care Med 2005;26(1):96–108.
20. Morgenthaler TI, Kapen S, Lee-Chiong T, et al, Standards of Practice Committee, American Academy of Sleep Medicine. Practice parameters for the medical therapy of obstructive sleep apnea. Sleep 2006;29: 1031–5.

21. Javaheri S, Guerra LF. Effects of domperidone and medroxyprogesterone acetate on ventilation in man. Respir Physiol 1990;81:359–70.

22. Saaresranta T, Polo-Kantola P, Irjala K, et al. Respiratory insufficiency in postmenopausal women: sustained improvement of gas exchange with short-term medroxyprogesterone acetate. Chest 1999;115:1581–7.

23. Shigemitsu H, Afshar K. Nocturnal asthma. Curr Opin Pulm Med 2007;13:49–55.

24. McNicholas WT. Impact of sleep in COPD. Chest 2000;117:48S–53S.

25. Bhullar S, Phillips B. Sleep in COPD patients. COPD 2005;2:355–61.

26. Weitzenblum E, Chaouat A, Kessler R, et al. Overlap syndrome: obstructive sleep apnea in patients with chronic obstructive pulmonary disease. Proc Am Thorac Soc 2008;5(2):237–41.

27. Krachman SL, Criner GJ, Chatila W. Cor pulmonale and sleep-disordered breathing in patients with restrictive lung disease and neuromuscular disorders. Semin Respir Crit Care Med 2003;24:297–306.

Cardiac Activity and Sympathovagal Balance During Sleep

John Trinder, PhD

KEYWORDS

- Sleep • Sympathovagal balance • Heart rate • Blood pressure • Heart rate variability

KEY POINTS

- A variety of techniques have shown that non–rapid eye movement sleep is associated with reduced sympathovagal tone (vagal dominance).
- Because it has not been possible to isolate sympathetic effects on the heart during sleep, the central role of the sympathetic nervous system remains unproven.
- It remains unclear whether the change in sympathovagal balance reflects an influence of sleep mechanisms over the autonomic nervous system, or the reverse, although perhaps the most likely scenario is that there are reciprocal influences.
- Sleep deprivation seems to have only minor effects on sympathovagal balance. However, the effects of obstructive sleep apnea are substantial and are likely to mediate many of the pathophysiologic processes associated with the disorder.

INTRODUCTION

Two broad issues are considered in this article: the relationship between sleep and cardiac activity and sympathovagal balance in normal human sleepers, and in individuals with sleep disorders. The article is restricted to cardiac activity, reflecting the pervasive interest among sleep researchers in the relationship between obstructive sleep apnea (OSA) and heart disease.

Sympathovagal balance is a critical concept for understanding both the nature of sleep and the mechanisms by which disorders of sleep result in physiologic disorders. There is substantial evidence indicating that, during normal sleep, sympathovagal balance shifts toward parasympathetic dominance. This shift occurs particularly during non–rapid eye movement (NREM) sleep but, because NREM makes up 75% to 80% of a nights sleep, parasympathetic dominance characterizes the sleep period generally. However, the significance of the shift in sympathovagal balance during NREM sleep remains obscure. For example, it is unclear whether the normal sleep-related change is a functional consequence of sleep, endowing the sleeper with benefits that enhance waking activity, or is sleep promoting, facilitating the occurrence, quality, and maintenance of sleep.

There is evolving evidence that patients with various sleep disorders have relative sympathetic dominance of autonomic nervous system (ANS) activity during sleep compared with normal sleepers, an effect that can persist into wakefulness. The mechanisms that produce a shift to sympathetic nervous system (SNS) dominance are typically not well understood and likely differ between different sleep disorders. Nevertheless, there is a general view that increased SNS activity drives the shift in sympathovagal balance and plays a critical mediating role between sleep disorders and end organ damage.

A version of this article originally appeared in *Sleep Medicine Clinics Volume 2, Issue 2.*
Melbourne School of Psychological Sciences, University of Melbourne, Melbourne, Victoria 3010, Australia
E-mail address: johnat@unimelb.edu.au

Sleep Med Clin 7 (2012) 507–516
http://dx.doi.org/10.1016/j.jsmc.2012.06.012

Methodological considerations have compromised the assessment of sympathovagal balance during sleep, particularly in human studies. The difficulty is that the range of assessment techniques is limited by the requirement that the techniques do not excessively disturb sleep, because sleep quality and sympathovagal balance are closely related. The most commonly used method of assessing cardiac autonomic control, heart rate variability (HRV), is open to several methodological and interpretative caveats that have been widely ignored in the sleep literature. Because methodological considerations are critical in understanding the literature, this article begins with a brief review of these issues.

THE MEASUREMENT OF AUTONOMIC ACTIVITY DURING SLEEP: METHODOLOGICAL CONSIDERATIONS

Most studies that have assessed sympathovagal balance during sleep have measured heart rate (HR), blood pressure (BP), and baroreflex activity as measures of cardiac output, and HR variability (HRV) and BP variability (BPV) as measures of autonomic control. Although other methods, most notably muscle sympathetic nerve activity (MSNA) recordings and measures of catecholamine levels, have been applied, fewer studies have used these methods, in large part because they are intrusive, technically difficult, and, in the case of catecholamine levels, lack temporal sensitivity. Despite being widely used, HRV/BPV methods have often been inappropriately applied and misinterpreted, leading to some confusion in the literature.

Cardiac variability can be assessed in either the time domain or spectral domain. An example of a time domain measure is the standard deviation of all HR interbeat intervals (IBI) within a specified period. Although this measure provides an estimate of the total variability in the period analyzed, other time domain variables reflect different frequency components in the IBIs. An example of a spectral measure is the power within a specified frequency band (eg, 0.04 to 0.15 Hz) from a fast Fourier transform or autoregressive analysis of BP IBIs. Three broad concepts have been derived from variability analysis. The first, developed primarily from time domain methods, is that high HRV and low BPV are signs of cardiovascular health, because they indicate that HR is effectively varying to maintain BP within a narrow range. The second, seemingly contradictory, concept is that high HRV indicates sleep disturbance because disturbing events such as arousals from sleep and respiratory disturbances produce abrupt

alterations in HR. These 2 observations are not conceptually incompatible because they reflect different sources of variance. However, these contrasting perspectives raise an important point: HRV can only be interpreted when the source of the variability is known. The third concept is that variability within particular frequency ranges reflects particular physiologic processes, such as, for example, the identification of variation in BP IBI in the low-frequency (LF) range (0.04–0.15 Hz) with peripheral vasomotor tone. It is the third concept when applied to HR variability that has been widely used and widely misunderstood.

The spectral analysis of HR IBI shows several peaks in the resulting power-by-frequency distribution. Two of these have been intensively studied. One occurs at the respiratory frequency of approximately 0.25 Hz (range approximately 0.15–0.4 Hz). This high-frequency (HF) component is widely accepted as a measure of parasympathetic nervous system (PNS) activity, largely because the physiologic processes by which vagal activity is reflected in changes in IBI are well understood. Nevertheless, there are well-known measurement artifacts, such as variations in respiratory rate and intensity of respiratory drive, that distort the measure and that must be taken into account when interpreting data. The second peak occurs at approximately 0.1 Hz (range approximately 0.04–0.15 Hz) and is typically referred to as the LF component. The physiologic processes leading to variations in IBI over this frequency range are not well understood and there has been considerable debate as to what is measured by the LF component (see Refs.[1–3] for a range of views). The most widely held position is that it measures some combination of PNS and SNS activity. It has become common practice to neutralize the PNS contribution to the LF component by dividing the LF by the HF component (LF/HF ratio). The assumption of this strategy is that the PNS component in the numerator will be canceled. However, this is unlikely to be true, because the vagal components in the LF and HF ranges are derived from different physiologic processes,[1] and because there are significant nonlinear relationships between the various components.[2] As a consequence, the LF component reflects an indeterminate combination of SNS and PNS activity, whereas the LF/HF ratio reflects an approximate balance between sympathetic and vagal influences, although even this latter conclusion has been criticized.[3] Like any ratio, a change in LF/HF cannot be attributed to changes in a particular component and thus a change in the ratio is as likely to be caused entirely by a change in one or other of the PNS components as by a change in the sympathetic contribution to the LF component.

A further difficulty with the technique is shown by the observations that high HRV can indicate both cardiovascular health and disturbed sleep. This observation is seen because not all variability in IBIs is attributable to the PNS and SNS. For example, physical activity, body movements, and the apnea-hyperpnea cycle in patients with OSA all add power to a range of frequencies, resulting in variations in the total power (TP). If the intention of a study has been to identify ANS components, the generally adopted solution has been to express power within the frequency ranges of interest as a proportion of TP. For example, LF power is expressed as LF/TP. However, because TP is primarily made up of LF plus HF, the expressions LF/TP and HF/TP are highly correlated and both are highly correlated with the LF/HF ratio. In many articles, TP is defined as LF plus HF power, in which case the 3 quantities are perfectly correlated and all reflect the same ratio of PNS to SNS activity. In the light of these arguments, in this article normalized LF and HF power and the LF/HF ratio are interpreted as representing a single variable reflecting sympathovagal balance. There is an additional problem. A proportional representation assumes the additional power is evenly distributed over the 0.04 to 0.40 frequency range. If not, and there is no reason to think that variability associated with sleep disturbance would be evenly distributed, the various LF/HF ratios could be altered without any change in sympathovagal balance.

So what can be learned from HRV/BPV analyses? First, with appropriate care in the collection and analysis of the data, such that extraneous influences on TP are minimized, absolute HRV HF power reflects vagal influences on the heart moderately well. Further, the 0.04-Hz to 0.15-Hz component of BPV reflects sympathetically mediated vasomotor tone. In addition, with more sophisticated computational models, such as multivariate autoregressive analyses that allow the dynamic relationship between respiration, HR, and BP to be decomposed,[4] or autoregressive models with exogenous input that allow variations in the respiratory component to be partialled out,[5] it may be possible to identify more complex relationships from data collected during undisturbed sleep. However, the LF component of HRV only provides information on sympathovagal balance. Thus, there is no direct noninvasive measure of sympathetic influences on the heart that may be applied during sleep. This point is taken up again later.

AUTONOMIC CARDIOVASCULAR ACTIVITY DURING SLEEP IN HEALTHY INDIVIDUALS: SLEEP AS THE INDEPENDENT VARIABLE

Early studies of the relationship between sleep and cardiac activity implicitly conceptualized the association as one in which sleep altered cardiovascular function. The interest was in identifying the ways in which sleep mechanisms imposed regulatory controls over other physiologic process, reflecting some functionally significant role of sleep.[6] This article reflects this conceptual approach.

Cardiac activity shows a marked 24-hour activity cycle, with higher levels of activity during daytime wakefulness (eg, Refs.[7-10]). The 24-hour pattern reflects several processes in addition to sleep effects. These processes include direct effects of the circadian system, indirect effects via the relationship between heat production and HR and thermoregulatory influences on BP, and variations in physical activity and posture. Although it is clear that activity-inactivity, postural patterns, the circadian system, and sleep patterns are mutually dependent, laboratory studies that have isolated these effects have shown that there is a sleep-specific effect on both HR and BP[11-13] and a circadian influence on HR[14-17] that are independent of changes in posture and physical activity.[11,13]

The 24-hour variation in BP has been most successfully modeled by a square wave function with abrupt decreases in association with sleep onset and increases at morning wakefulness, and constant values during sustained wakefulness and sleep.[18] The decrease in BP during the sleep period has given rise to the expression, a dipping BP profile. The sleep-related decrease in BP occurs abruptly at sleep onset, such that the tonic NREM sleep level is reached soon after the attainment of stable NREM sleep, with systolic BP decreasing 15 mm Hg or more.[19] In laboratory studies in which posture is controlled, the sleep onset effect seems to consist of 2 components. The first consists of a decrease of ~7 mm Hg preceding electroencephalogram (EEG) indications of sleep.[20] This effect seems to be instigated by turning out the lights or perhaps the decision to go to sleep. The second is a decrease of equivalent magnitude that occurs once stable stage 2 sleep is attained.[20] During the sleep onset period, from the onset of stage 1 sleep until stable stage 2 sleep, when sleep-wake state is unstable with repetitive arousals, the sleep-related decrease in BP is suspended and BP may even increase slightly.[20] The dependence of the decrease in BP on the occurrence of sleep is further shown by the observation that the decrease is delayed if sleep onset is delayed.[11]

Although the increase in BP in the morning has been less intensely studied, it also occurs in close association with the transition to wakefulness. However, there seems to be little sleep-wake state influence, the BP surge being largely caused by postural and ambulatory changes.[21]

Within sleep, BP levels are sleep-stage dependent, being low during NREM sleep and approximating relaxed wakefulness during rapid eye movement (REM) sleep,[19] with transient increases in association with phasic REM events.[13,22] Within a particular sleep stage, BP is constant over time, although the average level increases because of the increasing proportion of REM sleep as the night progresses.[19]

Several studies have investigated the influence of the circadian system on BP using the constant routine procedure and have not shown circadian effects.[15,17] However, recent studies may contradict this conclusion. In a study using the constant routine technique, van Eekelen and colleagues[23] showed a circadian influence over several variables derived from HR. However, the effects were only observed when the protocol commenced early on day 1. If the protocol began in the evening of day 1, the circadian influence was lost, presumably obscured by sleep deprivation influences. This finding suggests that the constant routine technique may not be the most effective method for identifying circadian influences over cardiac activity. Consistent with this, in a recent study using a forced desynchrony protocol, we showed a strong circadian system influence over BP.[24]

In contrast with the equivocal results for BP, both constant routine and forced desynchrony studies consistently show a strong circadian influence over HR, reflecting the close relationship between HR and metabolic heat production.[14,15,17,24] However, the effect can be obscured under severe sleep deprivation conditions.[23] Nevertheless, under normal circumstances, the 24-hour variation in HR approximates a sine wave rather than the square wave of BP. The nadir of the oscillation occurs during the normal sleep period, with sleep onset occurring during the decreasing phase of HR. Thus sleep-specific effects can be difficult to isolate from the circadian oscillation. Nevertheless, several studies have identified a sleep onset–specific decrease in HR[11,14,19] that, as with BP, has 2 components, 1 related to preparation for sleep (lights out) and the other when stable sleep is attained.[20] During sleep, HR is higher during REM than during NREM at any particular sleep duration,[19] with transient tachycardia in

association with phasic REM events.[13,22] However, because HR decreases under circadian influence in both sleep states and because REM sleep is concentrated in the second half of the night, whole-night averages do not always show REM-NREM differences.

In summary, in normal healthy individuals, cardiac activity is markedly reduced in NREM sleep. This effect is the result of several physiologic processes including direct influences from sleep and circadian mechanisms. However, the relative importance of circadian versus sleep mechanisms differs between BP and HR. Because NREM sleep constitutes 75% to 80% of the sleep period, sleep is a period of cardiovascular quiescence, a state that has been referred to as a cardiovascular holiday.

Changes in cardiac activity during sleep are typically attributed to changes in autonomic control. Several studies have indicated that sleep is associated with an increase in baroreflex sensitivity (BRS),[10,25,26] an effect that may be initiated during the sleep onset period.[20] An increase in BRS suggests that the capacity to defend BP is retained during sleep and, as a consequence, the simultaneous decreases in HR and BP over sleep onset strongly suggests a downward resetting of the reflex. Further, baroreflex resetting is indicated by pharmacologic studies.[27] Sleep onset is also associated with rapid and substantial peripheral vasodilatation, reflecting peripheral sympathetic withdrawal. The time course of the changes in these variables suggests that peripheral vasodilatation results in a decrease in BP, unloading the system and producing peripheral resetting of the baroreflex. However, central resetting has not been ruled out.

Time domain analyses of HRV indicate that sleep, compared with wakefulness, is associated with greater activity in the higher frequency components and slightly less activity in LF components with greater overall variability.[28] Both 24-hour variability and the sleep-related increase in higher frequency activity decrease with increasing age,[28] effects attributed to an age-related decrease in parasympathetic activity. A range of disorders that are associated with cardiovascular dysfunction have also been shown to be associated with reduced HRV.[29]

PNS activity, as reflected in both time and frequency domain measures, has been shown to increase during NREM sleep. In the case of frequency domain measures, several studies have identified increases in absolute power in the respiratory frequency range (respiratory sinus arrhythmia) that could not be attributed to changes in total spectral power.[10,19,22,30] There is evidence that, in humans, HRV in the HF range can be eliminated by pharmacologic blockade of the PNS by atropine,[31] and that atropine eliminates the sleep-related increase in HRV.[22]

There is also strong evidence of a decrease in sympathetic vascular tone during NREM sleep. Thus, sleep is associated with peripheral vasodilation[32,33]; the 0.4-Hz to 0.15-Hz component of BPV, which is thought to reflect sympathetic vascular tone, is reduced during NREM sleep[34]; and MSNA is reduced.[35,36] Both increased PNS activity and decreased vascular tone are reversed in REM sleep.[10,22,30,36]

Thus, in young healthy individuals, the assessment of sympathovagal balance in sleep and its different stages has indicated that cardiovascular activity is reduced during NREM sleep through baroreflex resetting, reduced sympathetic vascular tone, and increased PNS activity. As noted earlier, the implicit conceptual understanding in this literature is that changes in sympathovagal balance during sleep reflect an influence of sleep on cardiovascular control. Further, these changes are thought to be beneficial for cardiovascular health, providing what has been referred to as a cardiovascular holiday. Consistent with this, failure to achieve parasympathetic dominance during sleep has been linked to cardiovascular morbidity (discussed later).

As an additional point, there is no direct evidence of a change in SNS input to the heart during NREM sleep, because neither absolute measures of LF activity nor the various ratios of LF to HF activity uniquely reflect SNS activity. The commonly held view that sympathetic cardiac influences on the heart are reduced during NREM sleep depends on the application of 2 basic principles of autonomic control. The first is that activation of the SNS is a diffuse, generalized process such that it is valid to infer central sympathetic withdrawal from peripheral sympathetic withdrawal. The second is that the PNS and SNS branches are considered to have a reciprocal relationship, allowing the inference that SNS activity has changed when the LF/HF ratio has changed. Whether these general characteristics of ANS control hold during the subtle changes that occur during sleep is not known, although it is known that there are frequent exceptions to both principles. Thus, the contribution of the withdrawal of sympathetic influences on the heart during NREM sleep remains uncertain.

AUTONOMIC CARDIOVASCULAR ACTIVITY DURING SLEEP IN HEALTHY INDIVIDUALS: SLEEP AS THE DEPENDENT VARIABLE

There is an alternative approach to the relationship between sleep and sympathovagal balance.

Otzenberger and colleagues[37] proposed a coupling between cortical synchronization, as reflected in EEG δ activity, and parasympathetic dominance. The experimental strategy used in this approach has been to correlate changes in EEG δ activity with measures of sympathovagal balance over time within sleep. Thus, in their initial study, using the Poincare plot method to assess sympathovagal activity, the development of cortical synchronization was associated with an increase in HF activity. (Poincare plots compare the relationship between successive RR intervals. The correlation of $RR_n - RR_{n+1}$ intervals is thought to reflect HF activity, because rapid changes in RR interval reduce the correlation.) Subsequent studies from this and other groups using the LF/HF ratio (or normalized power in LF and HF bands) have also reported a relationship between lower sympathovagal balance (parasympathetic dominance) and cortical synchronization.[38–40] Two studies reported that sympathovagal balance anticipates the development of δ EEG activity, suggesting that the ANS change precedes the cortical synchronization.[41,42] However, EEG events reflecting synchronization, such as tone-elicited K complexes, are also increased in anticipation of EEG δ.[43] Thus, rather than autonomic activity preceding cortical activity, it may simply be that traditional sleep measures fail to reflect the dynamic nature of the state.

Other studies using this approach have observed significant correlations between EEG δ activity and both absolute LF activity and the LF/HF ratio, in the absence of a correlation between δ activity and absolute HF activity.[44–46] This pattern of activity suggests that LF activity may be the critical component. However, these studies do not resolve the interpretive dilemma from a sympathovagal perspective, because the data do not distinguish between the sympathetic and vagal components of LF activity.

In addition to the relationship between sympathovagal balance and EEG δ activity observed within a night's sleep, there is accumulating evidence that the relationship holds between individuals. For example, aging is associated with a reduction in δ activity and an increase in the LF/HF ratio during NREM sleep.[42,47] Jurysta and colleagues[42] reported that, although δ activity and sympathovagal balance altered with age, the coherence between the 2 measures within a night did not alter. Several disorders have been identified that are characterized by low levels of δ activity and high sympathovagal balance, including insomnia,[48] fibromyalgia,[49] and alcohol dependence.[50] In addition, acute stress imposed before sleep has been shown to reduce the amount of δ activity and increase sympathovagal balance during sleep.[51]

In summary, there is good evidence for an association between the vagal dominance normally observed during NREM sleep and EEG δ power. However, although this literature has implicitly assumed that sleep is the dependent variable, it has not been determined that the relationship is causal. It is also unclear whether the change in sympathovagal balance primarily reflects changes in SNS or PNS activity. Nevertheless, the speculation that vagal activity during NREM sleep is necessary for the full development of EEG synchronization and that a shift to sympathetic dominance caused by stress, or a sleep or medical disorder, will disrupt the development of EEG δ activity, is an intriguing hypothesis.

SLEEP DEPRIVATION

The relationship between sleep deprivation and sympathovagal balance has been of interest for several reasons. First, as noted earlier, the sleep-related reduction in cardiac activity and shift to vagal dominance can be viewed as a consequence of sleep and as reflecting a restorative physiologic process.[52] According to this view, sleep deprivation should be associated with an exaggeration of these changes during recovery sleep. However, Rosanky and colleagues[52] did not observe such an effect.

Second, disturbed sleep, such as frequently occurs in shift workers or in sleep disorders such as OSA, is known to be associated with cardiovascular morbidity. Although the mechanisms remain unclear, heightened sympathetic activity has been considered a strong possibility. Thus, there has been interest in the extent to which laboratory manipulations of sleep, particularly total sleep deprivation, affect cardiac activity and sympathovagal balance during sleep-deprived wakefulness. However, the data have been equivocal on this issue.

Several studies have reported an increase in BP as a consequence of total[53,54] or partial[55,56] sleep deprivation, although the finding is not universal.[57] The results for HR have been particularly inconsistent, with both positive[55,56,58] and negative outcomes.[53,54,58,59] Two studies measured MSNA following a night's sleep deprivation and both reported a decrease in activity.[53,54] In addition, discrepant results have been reported for catecholamine levels, with some studies reporting increased levels following sleep deprivation,[55,56,58] whereas other have reported no effect.[53,59]

HRV analyses suggest a shift to greater sympathetic dominance following sleep disruption.

Spiegel and colleagues[60] reported decreased RRn/RRn+1 correlations following 6 nights of sleep restriction, whereas other studies have reported an increase in the LF/HF ratio following partial[56] or total[57] sleep deprivation. However, none of the studies reported absolute power in the frequency bands and, as a consequence, the data are difficult to interpret.

As Kato and colleagues[53] have concluded, although BP is likely to be increased following sleep deprivation, the effect does not seem to be caused by peripheral sympathetically mediated vasoconstriction, or by increased HR. These investigators suggested 2 alternative mechanisms: local endothelial changes or modification of the baroreflex. Consistent with the latter suggestion, Ogawa and colleagues[54] subsequently reported that the baroreflex is reset to a higher BP following sleep deprivation.

AUTONOMIC CARDIOVASCULAR ACTIVITY IN OSA

In patients with OSA during sleep, cardiovascular activity varies in synchrony with the apnea-hyperpnea respiratory cycle, with bradycardia and hypotension during apneas and tachycardia and hypertension following apnea termination.[61] Average HR and BP levels are often higher in patients with OSA over the sleep period compared with control subjects. This effect is sufficiently strong in some patients to eliminate the normal sleep-related decrease in BP, producing what has been referred to as a nondipping profile.[62] In addition, an increase of waking BP is common in patients with OSA.[61]

The elimination of the sleep-related decrease in BP and waking hypertension seem to be caused by the accumulated effect of 3 factors: an exacerbation of negative intrathoracic pressure in response to inspiratory effort during obstructions; hypoxia; and arousal from sleep. The mechanisms by which these pathophysiologic processes result in abnormal cardiovascular patterns are complex and beyond the scope of this article. Nevertheless, there seem to be common final pathways. In particular, all 3 processes lead to alterations in baroreflex and sympathetic vasomotor control.[61]

In view of the marked effect of the apnea-hyperpnea cycle on cardiac activity, the finding that time domain measures of variability indicate increased HR and BP variability is not surprising. Increased HRV has been suggested as a screening tool for OSA,[63] although other investigators have suggested that high HRV indicates sleep fragmentation in general, rather than being a specific marker of OSA.[64] In contrast with measures during sleep, time domain measures of HR and BP variability in patients with OSA during relaxed wakefulness in the supine position (without apneas) indicate reduced HR and increased BP variability.[65] These results suggest impaired baroreflex function in patients with OSA.

Consistent with impaired baroreflex activity, there is evidence from some studies,[66,67] but not all,[68] that BRS is reduced in patients with OSA. Several studies have shown increases in BRS with acute application of continuous positive airway pressure (CPAP). For example, Tkacova and colleagues[69] identified an increase in BRS in patients with OSA with congestive heart failure after acute treatment with CPAP. They also reported indirect evidence of resetting of the baroreflex to a lower BP level. The data were interpreted as indicating that the OSA before treatment was associated with an increased set point and reduced BRS. A small increase in BRS has also been observed in patients with severe OSA during acute CPAP treatment.[70] In addition to impaired control of BP, these effects would contribute to sympathetic activation of vasomotor tone. However, a reciprocal effect is also likely, in which increased vasomotor tone, if maintained, would upwardly reset the baroreflex.

The literature is consistent in showing an increase in sympathetic vasomotor tone in patients with OSA. Thus, patients with OSA have greater MSNA,[71–73] although CPAP treatment reduces MSNA.[74–76] Imadojemu and colleagues[77] showed that higher MSNA in patients with OSA at apnea termination results in greater peripheral vasoconstriction. Thus, the surge in BP following an apnea is caused by peripheral sympathetic activity rather than greater cardiac output. The higher MSNA seems to be largely mediated by hypoxia,[78,79] with consequent endothelial dysfunction.[80]

Catecholamine levels have been consistently shown to be higher in patients with OSA during both sleep and wakefulness, indicating increased sympathetic arousal.[81] However, the effect may relate to the occurrence of movement arousals during sleep,[82] although the organs involved in the increased sympathetic activity remain unknown from the catecholamine measures themselves. Further, norepinephrine levels are reduced by acute CPAP treatment.[83,84]

Spectral measures of HRV have been of limited value in evaluating autonomic control in patients with OSA during sleep because the repetitive apnea-hyperpnea cycles, although primarily adding variance to the very-low-frequency range, also contribute to the LF and HF components,[85] which has the effect of masking the direct respiratory-cardiac neural coupling.[5]

Several groups have introduced more sophisticated mathematical models to analyze HRV and applied these techniques to patients with OSA. Khoo and colleagues[5,86] introduced a technique in which perturbations are introduced to the respiratory system via random presentations of positive airway pressure. Respiratory, cardiac, and hemodynamic responses are then analyzed by computational models that decompose the components of HRV in different ways. As described earlier, these models include the ability to characterize the dynamic relationships between respiration, HR, and BP, including feed-forward and feedback influences (closed loop analyses[87]), and the separation of respiratory contributions into direct respiratory-cardiac neural coupling from the effect of feedback from pulmonary stretch receptors.[88] In general, these studies have shown impaired parasympathetic control in OSA, as indicated by reduced baroreflex gain and reduced respiratory-cardiac neural coupling in patients,[88] with the effect of OSA on baroreflex gain being greater during sleep than during wakefulness.[89] These effects have been shown to be ameliorated by CPAP treatment.[86,87]

SUMMARY

A variety of techniques have shown that NREM sleep is associated with reduced sympathovagal tone (vagal dominance). The effect is characterized by sympathetic vasomotor tone, downward resetting of the baroreflex, marginally increased BRS, and increased parasympathetic activity. However, because it has not been possible to isolate sympathetic effects on the heart during sleep, the central role of the SNS remains unproven. It also remains unclear whether the change in sympathovagal balance reflects an influence of sleep mechanisms over the ANS, or the reverse, although perhaps the most likely scenario is that there are reciprocal influences. Sleep deprivation seems to have only minor effects on sympathovagal balance. However, the effects of OSA are substantial and are likely to mediate many of the pathophysiologic processes associated with the disorder.

REFERENCES

1. Berntson GG, Bigger JT Jr, Eckberg DL, et al. Heart rate variability: origins, methods, and interpretive caveats. Psychophysiology 1997;34:623–48.
2. Zhong Y, Wang H, Ju KH, et al. Nonlinear analysis of the separate contributions of autonomic nervous systems to heart rate variability using principal dynamic modes. IEEE Trans Biomed Eng 2004;51: 255–62.

3. Eckberg DL. Sympathovagal balance: a critical appraisal. Circulation 1997;96:3224–32.

4. Barbieri R, Parati G, Saul JP. Closed- versus open-loop assessment of heart rate baroreflex. IEEE Eng Med Biol Mag 2001;20:33–42.

5. Khoo MC, Kim TS, Berry RB. Spectral indices of cardiac autonomic function in obstructive sleep apnea. Sleep 1999;22:443–51.

6. Trinder J. Respiratory and cardiac activity during sleep onset. In: Bradley TD, Floras JS, editors. Sleep disorders and cardiovascular and cerebrovascular disease. New York: Marcel Dekker; 2000. p. 337–54.

7. Bevan AT, Honour AJ, Stott FH. Direct arterial pressure recording in unrestricted man. Clin Sci 1969; 36:329–44.

8. Furlan R, Guzzetti S, Crivellaro W, et al. Continuous 24-hour assessment of the neural regulation of systemic arterial pressure and RR variabilities in ambulant subjects. Circulation 1990;81:537–47.

9. Mancia G, Ferrari A, Gregorini L, et al. Blood pressure and heart rate variabilities in normotensive and hypertensive human beings. Circ Res 1983;53: 96–104.

10. Parati G, Castiglioni P, Di Rienzo M, et al. Sequential spectral analysis of 24-hour blood pressure and pulse interval in humans. Hypertension 1990;16: 414–21.

11. Carrington M, Walsh M, Stambas T, et al. The influence of sleep onset on the diurnal variation in cardiac activity and cardiac control. J Sleep Res 2003;12:213–21.

12. Snyder F, Hobson JA, Morrison DF, et al. Changes in respiration, heart rate, and systolic blood pressure in human sleep. J Appl Physiol 1964;19:417–22.

13. Van de Borne P, Nguyen H, Biston P, et al. Effects of wake and sleep stages on the 24-h autonomic control of blood pressure and heart rate in recumbent men. Am J Physiol 1994;266:H548–54.

14. Burgess HJ, Trinder J, Kim Y, et al. Sleep and circadian influences on cardiac autonomic nervous system activity. Am J Physiol 1997;273:H1761–8.

15. Kerkhof GA, Van Dongen HP, Bobbert AC. Absence of endogenous circadian rhythmicity in blood pressure? Am J Hypertens 1998;11:373–7.

16. Krauchi K, Wirz-Justice A. Circadian rhythm of heat production, heart rate and skin and core temperature under unmasking conditions in men. Am J Physiol 1994;267:R819–29.

17. Van Dongen HP, Maislin G, Kerkhof GA. Repeated assessment of the endogenous 24-hour profile of blood pressure under constant routine. Chronobiol Int 2001;18:85–98.

18. Idema RN, Gelsema ES, Wenting GJ, et al. A new model for diurnal blood pressure profiling. Square wave fit compared with conventional methods. Hypertension 1992;19:595–605.

19. Trinder J, Kleiman J, Carrington M, et al. Autonomic activity during human sleep as a function of time and sleep stage. J Sleep Res 2001;10:253–64.

20. Carrington MJ, Barbieri R, Colrain IM, et al. Changes in cardiovascular function during the sleep onset period in young adults. J Appl Physiol 2005;98:468–76.

21. Khoury GA, Sunderajan P, Kaplan NM. The early morning rise in blood pressure is related mainly to ambulation. Am J Hypertens 1992;5:373–7.

22. Zemaityte D, Varoneckas G, Sokolov E. Heart rhythm control during sleep. Psychophysiology 1984;21: 279–89.

23. van Eekelen APJ, Houtveen JH, Kerkhof GA. Circadian variation in base rate measures of cardiac autonomic activity. Eur J Appl Physiol 2004;93:39–46.

24. Trinder J. Circadian versus sleep influences on cardiovascular activity. J Sleep Res 2006;15(Suppl 1):12.

25. Parati G, Di Rienzo M, Bertinieri G, et al. Evaluation of the baroreceptor-heart rate reflex by 24-hour intra-arterial blood pressure monitoring in humans. Hypertension 1988;12:214–22.

26. Smyth HS, Sleight P, Pickering GW. Reflex regulation of arterial pressure during sleep in man. A quantitative method of assessing baroreflex sensitivity. Circ Res 1969;24:109–21.

27. Bristow JD, Honour AJ, Pickering TG, et al. Cardiovascular and respiratory changes during sleep in normal and hypertensive subjects. Cardiovasc Res 1969;3:476–85.

28. Bonnemeier H, Wiegand UK, Brandes A, et al. Circadian profile of cardiac autonomic nervous modulation in healthy subjects. J Cardiovasc Electrophysiol 2003;14:791–9.

29. Task Force of the European Society of Cardiology and the North American Society of Pacing and Electrophysiology. Heart rate variability: standards of measurement, physiological interpretation and clinical use. Circulation 1996;93:1043–65.

30. Berlad II, Shlitner A, Ben-Haim S, et al. Power spectrum analysis and heart rate variability in Stage 4 and REM sleep: evidence for state-specific changes in autonomic dominance. J Sleep Res 1993;2:88–90.

31. Medigue C, Girard A, Laude D, et al. Relationship between pulse interval and respiratory sinus arrhythmia: a time- and frequency-domain analysis of the effects of atropine. Pflugers Arch 2001;441:650–5.

32. Krauchi K, Cajochen C, Werth E, et al. Functional link between distal vasodilation and sleep-onset latency? Am J Physiol Regul Integr Comp Physiol 2000;278:R741–8.

33. van Someren EJ. Mechanisms and functions of coupling between sleep and temperature rhythms. Prog Brain Res 2006;153:309–24.

34. Lombardi F, Parati G. An update on: cardiovascular and respiratory changes during sleep in normal and hypertensive subjects. Cardiovasc Res 2000;45: 200–11.

35. Hornyak M, Cejnar M, Elam M, et al. Sympathetic muscle nerve activity during sleep in man. Brain 1991;114:1281–95.

36. Somers VK, Dyken ME, Mark AL, et al. Sympathetic-nerve activity during sleep in normal subjects. N Engl J Med 1993;328:303–7.

37. Otzenberger H, Simon C, Gronfier C, et al. Temporal relationship between dynamic heart rate variability and electroencephalographic activity during sleep in man. Neurosci Lett 1997;229:173–6.

38. Brandenberger G, Ehrhart J, Piquard F, et al. Inverse coupling between ultradian oscillations in delta wave activity and heart rate variability during sleep. Clin Neurophysiol 2001;112:992–6.

39. Gronfier C, Simon C, Piquard F, et al. Neuroendocrine processes underlying ultradian sleep regulation in man. J Clin Endocrinol Metab 1999;84:2686–90.

40. Jurysta F, van de Borne P, Migeotte PF, et al. A study of the dynamic interactions between sleep EEG and heart rate variability in healthy young men. Clin Neurophysiol 2003;114:2146–55.

41. Branderberger G, Ehrhart J, Buchheit M. Sleep stage 2: an electroencephalographic, autonomic, and hormonal duality. Sleep 2005;28:1535–40.

42. Jurysta F, van de Borne P, Lanquart JP, et al. Progressive aging does not alter the interaction between autonomic cardiac activity and delta EEG power. Clin Neurophysiol 2005;116:871–7.

43. Nicholas CL, Trinder J, Crowley KE, et al. The impact of slow wave sleep proximity on evoked K-complex generation. Neurosci Lett 2006;404:127–31.

44. Yang CC, Lai CW, Lai HY, et al. Relationship between electroencephalogram slow-wave magnitude and heart rate variability during sleep in humans. Neurosci Lett 2002;329:213–6.

45. Miyashita T, Ogawa K, Itoh H, et al. Spectral analyses of electroencephalography and heart rate variability during sleep in normal subjects. Auton Neurosci 2003;103:114–20.

46. Ako M, Kawara T, Uchida S, et al. Correlation between elctroencephalography and heart rate variability during sleep. Psychiatry Clin Neurosci 2003; 57:59–65.

47. Brandenberger G, Viola AU, Ehrhart J, et al. Age-related changes in autonomic control during sleep. J Sleep Res 2003;12:173–80.

48. Bonnet MH, Arand DL. Heart rate variability in insomniacs and matched normal sleepers. Psychosom Med 1998;60:610–5.

49. Martinez-Lavin M, Hermosillo AG, Rosas M, et al. Circadian studies of autonomic nervous balance in patients with fibromyalgia. Arthritis Rheum 1998;41: 1966–71.

50. Irwin MR, Valladares EM, Motivala S, et al. Association between nocturnal vagal tone and sleep depth, sleep quality, and fatigue in alcohol dependence. Psychosom Med 2006;68:159–66.

51. Hall M, Vasko R, Buysse D, et al. Acute stress affects heart rate variability during sleep. Psychosom Med 2004;66:56–62.

52. Rosansky SJ, Menachery SJ, Whittman D, et al. The relationship between sleep deprivation and the nocturnal decline of blood pressure. Am J Hypertens 1996;9:1136–8.

53. Kato M, Phillips BG, Sigurdsson G, et al. Effects of sleep deprivation on neural circulatory control. Hypertension 2000;35:1173–5.

54. Ogawa Y, Kanbayashi T, Saito Y, et al. Total sleep deprivation elevates blood pressure through arterial baroreflex resetting: a study with microneurographic technique. Sleep 2003;26:986–9.

55. Lusardi P, Mugellini A, Preti P, et al. Effects of a restricted sleep regimen on ambulatory blood pressure monitoring in normotensive subjects. Am J Hypertens 1996;9:503–5.

56. Tochikubo O, Ikeda A, Miyajima E, et al. Effects of insufficient sleep on blood pressure monitored by a new multibiomedical recorder. Hypertension 1996;27:1318–24.

57. Zhong X, Hilton J, Gates GJ, et al. Increased sympathetic and decreased parasympathetic cardiovascular modulation in normal humans with acute sleep deprivation. J Appl Physiol 2005;98:2024–32.

58. Froberg JE, Karlsson CG, Levi L, et al. Circadian variations in performance, psychological ratings, catecholamine excretion, and diuresis during prolonged sleep deprivation. Int J Psychobiol 1972;2: 23–36.

59. Fiorica V, Higgins EA, Iampietro PF, et al. Physiological responses of men during sleep deprivation. J Appl Physiol 1968;24:167–76.

60. Speigel K, Leprouit R, Van Cauter E. Impact of sleep debt on metabolic and endocrine function. Lancet 1999;354:1435–9.

61. Leung RS, Bradley TD. Sleep apnea and cardiovascular disease. Am J Respir Crit Care Med 2001;164: 2147–65.

62. O'Brien E, Sheridan J, O'Malley K. Dippers and non-dippers. Lancet 1988;2(8607):397.

63. Roche F, Gaspoz JM, Court-Fortune I, et al. Screening of obstructive sleep apnea syndrome by heart rate variability analysis. Circulation 1999;100: 1411–5.

64. Sforza E, Pichot V, Cervena K, et al. Cardiac variability and heart rate increment as a marker of sleep fragmentation in patients with a sleep disorder: a preliminary study. Sleep 2007;30:43–51.

65. Narkiewicz K, Montano N, Cogliati C, et al. Altered cardiovascular variability in obstructive sleep apnea. Circulation 1998;98:1071–7.

66. Carlson JT, Hedner JA, Sellgren J, et al. Depressed baroreflex sensitivity in patients with obstructive sleep apnea. Am J Respir Crit Care Med 1996; 154:1490–6.

67. Parati G, Di Rienzo M, Bonsignore MR, et al. Autonomic cardiac regulation in obstructive sleep apnea syndrome: evidence from spontaneous baroreflex analysis during sleep. J Hypertens 1997;15:1621–6.

68. Ziegler MG, Nelesen RA, Mills PJ, et al. The effect of hypoxia on baroreflexes and pressor sensitivity in sleep apnea and hypertension. Sleep 1995;18:859–65.

69. Tkacova R, Dajani HR, Rankin F, et al. Continuous positive airway pressure improves nocturnal baroreflex sensitivity of patients with heart failure and obstructive sleep apnea. J Hypertens 2000;18:1257–62.

70. Bonsignore MR, Parati G, Insalaco G, et al. Baroreflex control of heart rate during sleep in severe obstructive sleep apnoea: effects of acute CPAP. Eur Respir J 2006;27:128–35.

71. Carlson JT, Hedner J, Elam M, et al. Augmented resting sympathetic activity in awake patients with obstructive sleep apnea. Chest 1993;103:1763–8.

72. Hedner J, Ejnell H, Sellgren J, et al. Is high and fluctuating muscle nerve sympathetic activity in the sleep apnoea syndrome of pathogenetic importance for the development of hypertension? J Hypertens Suppl 1988;6:S529–31.

73. Somers VK, Dyken ME, Clary MP, et al. Sympathetic neural mechanisms in obstructive sleep apnea. J Clin Invest 1995;96:1897–904.

74. Hedner J, Darpo B, Ejnell H, et al. Reduction in sympathetic activity after long-term CPAP treatment in sleep apnoea: cardiovascular implications. Eur Respir J 1995;8:222–9.

75. Narkiewicz K, Kato M, Phillips B, et al. Nocturnal continuous positive airway pressure decreases daytime sympathetic traffic in obstructive sleep apnea. Circulation 1999;100:2332–5.

76. Waradekar NV, Sinoway LI, Zwillich CW, et al. Influence of treatment on muscle sympathetic nerve activity in sleep apnea. Am J Respir Crit Care Med 1996;153:1333–8.

77. Imadojemu VA, Gleeson K, Gray KS, et al. Obstructive apnea during sleep is associated with peripheral vasoconstriction. Am J Respir Crit Care Med 2002;165:61–6.

78. Xie A, Skatrud JB, Crabtree DC, et al. Neurocirculatory consequences of intermittent asphyxia in humans. J Appl Physiol 2000;89:1333–9.

79. Xie A, Skatrud JB, Puleo DS, et al. Exposure to hypoxia produces long-lasting sympathetic activation in humans. J Appl Physiol 2001;91:1555–62.

80. Lavie L. Sleep apnea syndrome, endothelial dysfunction and cardiovascular morbidity. Sleep 2004;27:1053–5.

81. Coy TV, Dimsdale JE, Ancoli-Israel S, et al. Sleep apnoea and sympathetic nervous system activity: a review. J Sleep Res 1996;5:42–50.

82. Loredo JS, Ziegler MG, Ancoli-Israel S, et al. Relationship of arousals from sleep to sympathetic nervous system activity and BP in obstructive sleep apnea. Chest 1999;116:655–9.

83. Sukegawa M, Noda A, Sugiura T, et al. Assessment of continuous positive airway pressure treatment in obstructive sleep apnea syndrome using 24-hour urinary catecholamines. Clin Cardiol 2005;28:519–22.

84. Ziegler MG, Mills PJ, Loredo JS, et al. Effect of continuous positive airway pressure and placebo treatment on sympathetic nervous activity in patients with obstructive sleep apnea. Chest 2001;120:887–93.

85. Keyl C, Lemberger P, Dambacher M, et al. Heart rate variability in patients with obstructive sleep apnea. Clin Sci 1996;91(Suppl):56–7.

86. Khoo MC, Belozeroff V, Berry RB, et al. Cardiac autonomic control in obstructive sleep apnea: effects of long-term CPAP therapy. Am J Respir Crit Care Med 2001;164:807–12.

87. Belozeroff V, Berry RB, Sassoon CS, et al. Effects of CPAP therapy on cardiovascular variability in obstructive sleep apnea: a closed loop analysis. Am J Physiol 2002;282:H110–21.

88. Jo JA, Blasi A, Valladares E, et al. Determinants of heart rate variability in obstructive sleep apnea syndrome during wakefulness and sleep. Am J Physiol Heart Circ Physiol 2005;288:H1103–12.

89. Jo JA, Blasi A, Valladares E, et al. Model-based assessment of autonomic control in obstructive sleep apnea syndrome during sleep. Am J Respir Crit Care Med 2003;167:128–36.

Sleep and Cytokines

Christopher J. Davis, PhD, James M. Krueger, PhD*

KEYWORDS

- Tumor necrosis factor • Interleukin1 • Sleep function • Adenosine triphosphate
- Humoral regulation • Sleep homeostasis

KEY POINTS

- Interleukin 1 (IL-1) and tumor necrosis factor (TNF) are well-characterized sleep regulatory substances that form part of the sleep homeostat.
- A large literature showing of cytokine involvement in the brain organization of sleep corroborates the view that sleep is an emergent property of neural networks such as cortical columns.
- Cortical columns oscillate between functional states; the sleeplike state of cortical columns is promoted by cytokines. Further, cytokines are involved in synaptic scaling mechanisms and are therefore capable of modulating network activity.
- The function(s) of sleep is still debated; however cytokine-mediated sleep mechanisms support the hypothesis that sleep serves a synaptic-connectivity function.
- How the brain tracks activity and mediates sleep homeostasis is posited in our ATP-cytokine-adenosine hypothesis, wherein IL-1 and TNF release from glia is enhanced by neuronal activity via adenosine triphosphate and, in turn, IL-1 and TNF activate nuclear factor κ B, adenosine, and other downstream effectors to locally influence state.

INTRODUCTION

Physiologic processes including sleep are regulated in part by humoral substances. Cytokines as pleiotropic signaling molecules are involved in the regulation of many such processes. The study of the humoral regulation of sleep began almost 100 years ago with the publication of Ishimori's[1] and Legendre and Pieron's[2] work showing that the transfer of cerebrospinal fluid from sleep-deprived dogs into normal dogs enhanced sleep in the recipients. These findings led to several searches dedicated to the identification of the responsible substances. These searches were conceptually based on the hypotheses that; (1) sleep is regulated, in part, by humoral agents

within the nervous system, and (2) those agents undergo concentration or conformational changes that track, and thereby potentially provide an index of, cumulative sleep/wake history. Although many have replicated those original findings in similar experiments (eg, Ref.[3] and reviewed in Ref.[4]), this search continues. Many substances are implicated in sleep regulation. These sleep regulatory substances (SRSs) range from low-molecular-weight substances with short half-lives (eg, adenosine, nitric oxide [NO]), to longer-lived peptides, such as growth hormone-releasing hormone and orexin, and proteins including the cytokines. Until recently, the brain mechanisms that index sleep/wake history to SRS activity were unknown. Two cytokines, interleukin 1 β (IL-1) and tumor necrosis

This article originally appeared in *Sleep Medicine Clinics Volume 2, Issue 2*.
This work was supported by the National Institutes of Health grant numbers NS031453, NS025378 and HD036520.
Sleep and Performance Research Center, WWAMI Medical Education and Program in Neuroscience, Washington State University, 412 E Spokane Falls Boulevard, Spokane, WA 99210-1495, USA
* Corresponding author.

E-mail address: Krueger@vetmed.wsu.edu

factor α (TNF), are well characterized for their roles in sleep regulation and are used to show these newer ideas in this review.

Many experimental approaches have been used to discover and characterize SRSs (reviewed in Refs.[4–6]). All of these approaches, including methods such as the use of transgenic animals, epigenetic and posttranslational modifications, and proteomic and genome-wide searches, are limited because sleep cannot be isolated as an independent variable. Virtually every physiologic parameter (eg, body temperature, hormonal levels, respiration rate, urinary output, brain metabolism, feeding and reproductive behaviors) changes with sleep. As a consequence, it is not possible to definitively know, for example, whether the change in expression of a particular molecule that correlates with sleep or sleep loss does so as a direct consequence of sleep or of some other concurrent physiologic process. Sleep researchers have developed lists of criteria that candidate SRSs need to meet before they can be reasonably proposed as being involved in sleep regulation (**Box 1**).[6–9] The usefulness of a multiple criteria approach to identify SRSs is that it limits false detection. Adherence to these criteria is especially important because many substances are capable of altering sleep (eg, alcohol). To date, only a few substances have met all of these criteria; IL-1 and TNF are among them.

Our knowledge of SRS involvement in processes believed to be unrelated to sleep has led to unexpected developments in our understanding of sleep mechanisms and how the brain organizes sleep. For example, our view of what exactly it is that sleeps has shifted from whole organisms to neural networks such as cortical columns (also called neuronal assemblies or neuronal groups).

Our departure from the canonical view that sleep is a global process distributed across the brain was deduced from the fact that all SRSs identified play a role in activity-dependent neural plasticity. This finding suggests that 1 important function of sleep is to facilitate neural connectivity. The roles that cytokines play in these developments are discussed later.

TNF AND IL-1 MEET ALL THE CRITERIA FOR SRSs

Systemic or central injection of either TNF or IL-1 enhances duration of NREMS and EEG δ wave power during NREMS in every species thus far tested including, mice, rats, rabbits, cats, sheep, monkeys, and humans (criterion 1; see **Box 1**) (reviewed in Refs.[4,10,11]). After intracerebroventricular (ICV) or intraperitoneal (IP) injections of either IL-1 or TNF, increases in NREMS manifest within the first hour and, depending on dose, last up to 8 to 12 hours. The effects on NREMS can be large (eg, after 3 μg of TNF IP, mice spent an extra 90 minutes of NREMS over the first 9 postinjection hours[12] and after 600 fmol ICV IL-1 rabbits spent an extra 2 hours in NREMS over the first 12 postinjection hours).[10] The effects on rapid eye movement sleep (REMS) are dependent on route of administration, time of day, and dose. For instance, low somnogenic doses usually do not alter duration of REMS, whereas high somnogenic doses inhibit REMS. High doses of either IL-1 or TNF inhibit sleep; the sleep responses after these high doses resemble the sleep that occurs during severe infectious disease (eg, sleep episode duration is shortened). Somnogenic doses of IL-1 or TNF also increase δ wave power during NREMS,[12,13] a measure of sleep intensity.

The brain is susceptible to sleep disruptions, often over periods of days or more. Prolonged bouts of wakefulness are followed by sleep rebound, sometimes over multiple subsequent sleep periods. Sleep rebound is characterized by increased time spent in sleep and increased sleep intensity as defined by larger amplitude of EEG δ waves. Sleep homeostasis is a defining characteristic of sleep and its mechanisms likely involve the production and release of SRSs, including IL-1 and TNF. Thus, injection of exogenous IL-1 or TNF induces an NREMS that resembles sleep after sleep loss in that its duration and intensity are greater. Further, if either IL-1 or TNF is inhibited during sleep loss, the expected subsequent sleep rebound is greatly attenuated (reviewed in Ref.[14]). These latter findings coupled with the evidence presented in the previous paragraph strongly implicate IL-1 and TNF in sleep homeostasis.

Box 1
Criteria for SRSs

1. The SRS should enhance a sleep phenotype (eg, duration of non–rapid eye movement sleep (NREMS) or electroencephalographic (EEG) δ wave power).

2. Inhibition of the SRS should reduce spontaneous sleep.

3. The SRS levels in the brain should correlate with sleep propensity.

4. The SRS should act on putative sleep regulatory circuits

5. The SRS levels in disease should correlate with sleepiness.

Derived from Refs.[6–9]

Inhibition of either IL-1 or TNF using several different approaches reduces spontaneous NREMS (criterion 2; see **Box 1**). For example, the IL-1 receptor antagonist (an endogenous gene product), IL-1 and TNF soluble receptors (also endogenous substances), and anti-IL-1 or anti-TNF antibodies inhibit NREMS if given to experimental animals [reviewed in Ref.[4]). In humans, the TNF soluble receptor is a normal constituent of cerebrospinal fluid and inhibits sleep[15] and fatigue.[16] Substances that inhibit the production, release, or actions of IL-1 or TNF also inhibit duration of NREMS. For example, glucocorticoids, IL-4, IL-10, and IL-13, and corticotrophin-releasing hormone all inhibit IL-1 and TNF and reduce spontaneous NREMS (reviewed in Ref.[4]).

Another approach to inhibit SRSs is to remove 1 or more of the genes in its signaling pathway. Knockout mice that lack either the IL-1 type I receptor (IL1R1),[13] the brain-specific IL1R1 accessory protein,[17] the TNF 55-kD receptor[12] or both IL1R1 and TNF receptor (TNFR)[18] have less spontaneous sleep than control strains of mice. The NREMS deficits in the TNF 55-kD receptor knockout mice occur mostly during the first hours of daylight, whereas the NREMS deficits in the IL1R1 and double TNF/IL-1 receptor knockout mice occur mostly during the nighttime. The results from those studies suggest some independence of the somnogenic actions of IL-1 and TNF, although these cytokines induce each other in brain in vivo.[13] Further, the TNF receptor knockout mice show NREMS responses if given IL-1[13] and the IL-1 receptor knockout mice do likewise if given TNF.[12]

Brain levels of either IL-1 or TNF or their respective mRNAs vary with sleep propensity (criterion 3; see **Box 1**). For example, IL-1 cerebrospinal fluid levels in cats vary with the sleep/wake cycle.[19] Spontaneous brain levels of IL-1 mRNA and TNF mRNA vary with sleep propensity in rats, with highest levels occurring at the onset of daylight hours (reviewed in Ref.[4]). Rat hypothalamic (an NREMS regulatory network) levels of both IL-1[20] and TNF[21] are highest at the time when spontaneous NREMS duration is greatest. Cerebral cortical levels of IL-1 and TNF also vary with the time of day. If sleep propensity is enhanced by sleep deprivation, both IL-1 mRNA and TNF mRNA levels increase in brain (reviewed in Ref.[4]). Further, if rats are fed a cafeteria diet their NREMS is enhanced, as are their hypothalamic IL-1 mRNA levels.[22] During infectious disease states when sleep in enhanced, brain levels of IL-1 and TNF mRNAs are enhanced (eg, during influenza virus infections in mice).[23]

If either IL-1 or TNF is microinjected into sleep regulatory circuits, NREMS is enhanced (criterion 4; see **Box 1**). Thus, microinjection of TNF into the anterior hypothalamus is associated with dose-dependent increases in NREMS.[24] In contrast, injection of the TNF soluble receptor into the anterior hypothalamus inhibits spontaneous NREMS. Similarly, an extensive study of IL-1-responsive sites indicated that sites near the ventricles and subarachnoid sites near the hypothalamus are associated with enhanced NREMS.[25] Further, IL-1 receptive hypothalamic neurons also are receptive to growth hormone-releasing hormone, another well-characterized SRS (reviewed in Ref.[4]), and those neurons are γ-aminobutyric acid-releasing (GABA)-ergic.[26] If growth-hormone-releasing hormone (GHRH) is microinjected into the hypothalamus, it induces sleep responses and activity in sleep-active neurons.[27,28] Sleep-active hypothalamic neuron firing rates are enhanced by IL-1, whereas wake-active hypothalamic neurons are inhibited.[29] Classic brain stem sleep/wake circuits are also modulated by SRSs. For example, microinjection of either IL-1 or TNF into the locus coeruleus[30] or IL-1 into the dorsal raphe[31] enhances NREMS. IL-1 suppresses wake-active serotonergic neurons in the dorsal raphe[32] by affecting GABA[33] and possibly its receptor availability.[34] Collectively, these data indicate that IL-1 and TNF act on sleep regulatory circuits to enhance NREMS. Both cytokines also have the capacity to act directly on the cerebral cortex to enhance sleep intensity regionally, and that suggests that these substances can act throughout the neuraxis to alter state within neuronal assemblies. This view of brain organization of sleep is discussed later.

Many diseases with associated changes in sleep propensity also alter cytokines (criterion 5; see **Box 1**). The changes in hypothalamic cytokines associated with influenza virus in mice have already been mentioned. Human studies have greatly enriched the literature relating circulating cytokines to disease-associated sleepiness. TNF plasma levels are increased in multiple diseases associated with enhanced sleepiness, including patients with AIDS, chronic fatigue, insomnia, myocardial infarct, excessive daytime sleepiness, postdialysis fatigue, preeclampsia, alcoholism, obesity, sleep apnea (reviewed in Ref.[4]), and Alzheimer disease.[35] The TNF polymorphic variant, G-308A, is linked to metabolic syndrome[36] insulin resistance,[37] sleep apnea,[38] and heart disease.[39] Systemic endotoxin, a gram-negative bacterial cell wall product, enhances sleep and plasma TNF levels in humans.[40] Clinically approved inhibitors of TNF (eg, etanercept) reverse the sleepiness and fatigue associated with sleep apnea,[15] rheumatoid arthritis,[16] ankylosing spondylitis,[41] and alcoholism.[42] Surgical treatment of, or CPAP treatment of, obstructive sleep apnea reduces TNF/TNFR plasma levels.[43–45]

Blood levels of IL-1 in humans may also vary with sleep propensity, but this literature is not as clear as that for TNF. IL-1 plasma levels peak at the onset of sleep[46] and are enhanced during sleep deprivation.[47,48] Circulating levels of either TNF or IL-1 affect sleep via the vagus nerve because vagotomy blocks IP TNF-enhanced[49] or IL-1-enhanced[50] NREMS. Systemic injections of either IL-1 or TNF enhance brain levels of IL-1 and TNF mRNAs.[51] Vagotomy also blocks the IP IL-1-enhanced hypothalamic IL-1 mRNA.[52] Collectively, it seems that the sleep disturbances associated with disease are mediated in part via IL-1 and TNF (reviewed in Ref.[53]). Given the strong relationship of IL-1 and TNF with sleep in both health and disease states, their importance in sleep medicine will continue to grow.

ASSOCIATED MECHANISMS OF IL-1-ENHANCED AND TNF-ENHANCED SLEEP

The regulation of the brain cytokine network is not fully understood. Regardless, a variety of cytokines and cytokine-associated substances have been shown to alter sleep. Several of these such as the IL-1 and TNF soluble receptors have already been mentioned. Cytokine-associated substances such as the IL-1 receptor antagonist and several antisomnogenic substances, such as IL4, IL-10, IL-13, and transforming growth factor β, inhibit spontaneous NREMS. In contrast, other cytokines such as IL-6, IL-18, acidic fibroblast growth factor, interferon γ, nerve growth factor, brain-derived neurotrophic factor, and glia-derived neurotrophic factor, promote NREMS (reviewed in Ref.[4]). There are some cytokines that apparently do not affect sleep, at least under the conditions tested; these include interferon β[54] and basic fibroblast growth factor.[55] Nevertheless, IL-1 and TNF affect many other molecules that in turn affect sleep. Nuclear factor κ B (NFκB) and c-Fos (AP-1) are transcription factors that are activated by IL-1 and TNF (reviewed in Refs.[4,53]). These transcription factors promote production of IL-1 and TNF and many other substances implicated in sleep regulation including multiple cytokines, the purine type 1 receptor adenosine A1 receptor (A1AR), cyclooxygenase 2, and GHRH receptor. NFκB is activated within the hypothalamus and cortex by sleep deprivation.[56,57] Adenosine also elicits NFκB nuclear translocation in basal forebrain slices via the A1AR.[58] An inhibitor of NFκB inhibits NREMS.[59] IL-1 and TNF also affect many small molecules with short half-lives that are involved in sleep regulation. including NO, adenosine and prostaglandins (reviewed in Ref.,[4] eg, Ref.[60]). For example, inhibition of NO synthase blocks IL-1-induced increased NREMS responses.[61] Cytokines also interact with multiple neurotransmitters involved in sleep regulation including GABA, norepinephrine, serotonin, and acetylcholine (reviewed in Ref.[4]). The cytokine network is characterized by redundancy, positive feedback loops, extensive cross-talk, autoregulation, and many other complexities; most of it remains to be studied within the context of sleep. The exact somnogenic biochemical pathways affected by cytokines likely depend on circumstances such as time of day, waking activity, and disease, although it seems clear that known SRSs work in concert with each other to affect sleep.

BRAIN ORGANIZATION OF SLEEP: CYTOKINE INVOLVEMENT IN CORTICAL COLUMN STATE

Sleep researchers have yet to reach consensus as to exactly what it is that sleeps. This problem has the potential to confuse discussions of sleep regulation. For instance, traditionally sleep was considered a whole-animal phenomenon: either the subject was asleep or awake. However, it is now clear that some marine mammals show unihemispheric sleep (reviewed in Ref.[62]). Further, some characteristics of sleep such as EEG δ wave activity, metabolism, and blood flow manifest regionally depending on previous waking activity in those regions. In addition, a fundamental metafinding within sleep research is that regardless of where a lesion in the brain may occur, if the subjects survive, they sleep. This finding strongly indicates that sleep is an intrinsic property of any viable neuronal network and, contrary to the prevailing sleep regulatory paradigm, that sleep regulatory circuits do not impose sleep on the brain, because if they are lesioned, the animal sleeps (reviewed in Ref.[63]).

These considerations led us and others to propose that sleep is a fundamental property of neural networks.[64–67] It is possible that individual cells may sleep, but if one entertains this hypothesis, definitional problems are confronted (eg, is a silent neuron, or a bursting neuron, asleep? Most likely not, because such firing patterns can be found in conditions not associated with sleep). There also seems to be little chance of causally connecting activity of a single neuron to a state beyond correlation of firing rates. The positing of a brain organization level at which sleep emerges allows falsifiable hypotheses to be made at the appropriate level of organization. By way of analogy, to study the heat capacity, osmotic properties, vapor pressure, or taste of water, one does not study H or O; these emergent properties are the result of combining H and O and are fundamentally not predictable from our current knowledge of H or O. To relate our hypothesis to our past work with cytokines, we framed it within a biochemical mechanistic causal proposal (**Box 2**). There is now considerable evidence for the hypothesis and it is discussed in this section.

There is cell activity-dependent expression of cytokines in brain (step 1; see **Box 2**). This is well known for cytokines such as nerve growth factor (NGF) and brain-derived neurotrophic factor (BDNF) (reviewed in Ref.[68]), but is less studied for IL-1 and TNF. Conditions such as kindling, sleep deprivation, or extracellular glutamate enhance brain IL-1 or TNF, suggesting that excessive activity or excitatory stimuli are responsible.[69–72] Data from our laboratory indicate that within cerebral cortical neurons or glia, TNF and IL-1 are enhanced if afferent neuronal activity into the specific column is enhanced.[73,74] Collectively, such data strongly suggest that cytokine expression in neurons/glia is activity dependent.

The activity-dependent cytokines act on neurons to change their electrical and responsive properties (step 2; see **Box 2**). For some cytokines such as NGF and BDNF, this process is well established. For IL-1 and TNF, it has also been studied, but within the context of the fever literature (reviewed in Ref.[75]). For instance, IL-1 or TNF alter hypothalamic neuron sensitivity to temperature. TNF upregulates, whereas IL-1 downregulates glutamatergic α-amino-3-hydroxy-5-methyl-4-isoxazolepropionic acid

(AMPA) receptor expression in neurons (see later discussion), and changed populations of AMPA receptors alter neuronal response patterns. IL-1 receptors on hypothalamic neurons colocalize with GHRH receptors on GABAergic cells.[26] IL-1 enhances presynaptic release of GABA in hypothalamic cells.[76] IL-1 enhances hypothalamic sleep-active neurons and inhibits wake-active neurons.[29] There is thus ample evidence indicating that cytokines act on neurons to change their electrical properties.

These cytokine-induced altered neuronal properties affect sleep phenotype. Thus if either IL-1[77] or TNF[78] is applied to the surface of the cortex unilaterally, there is a dose-dependent and state-dependent increase in EEG δ power on the side receiving the cytokine. The increases occur during NREMS but not during REMS or waking and are confined to the 0.5-Hz to 4-Hz frequency band. Further, if TNF expression is unilaterally inhibited using a small-interfering RNA (siRNA) within the cortex, there is a reduction of EEG δ power unilaterally.[79] If rats are deprived of sleep and pretreated with a TNF soluble receptor or an IL-1 soluble receptor, the enhanced EEG δ wave power that occurs during subsequent NREMS is attenuated.[77,78] Together, these data suggest that TNF and IL-1 are produced in response to activity and act locally on networks to change input-output properties, resulting in a regionally more intense sleep or if inhibited a regionally less intense NREMS.

There is direct evidence that neuronal assemblies oscillate between 2 or more functional states and one of these states is induced by TNF and is sleeplike in character (step 3; see **Box 2**). If cortical columns are probed with afferent stimulation and subsequent amplitudes of evoked potentials are measured, different functional states can be determined.[80] One of those states correlates with whole-animal sleep and the probability of entering that state is dependent on previous afferent input to the column and past state status. Excessive afferent input to a cortical column increases the likelihood that the column enters the sleeplike state. Similarly, the longer the column is in a wakelike state, the higher the probability that later it enters the sleeplike state. These properties of cortical column sleeplike states are also properties of whole-animal sleep. Further, cortical column state affects behavior. If rats are trained to lick in response to stimulation of a whisker, the error rate is higher if the cortical column of the stimulated whisker is in the sleeplike state than if it is in the wakelike state.[81,82] Localized injection of TNF onto cortical columns induces the sleeplike state in the affected columns.[78] These data

---

Box 2
Sleep mechanisms

1. There is activity-dependent production of SRSs.

2. Activity-dependent SRSs act locally on nearby neurons/glia to change their electrical/receptive properties and thereby alter the input-output relationships of the networks within which they are found.

3. Altered input-output relationships within neuronal assemblies indicate functional state changes of the assemblies.

4. Synchrony of state between semiautonomous neural assemblies occurs because they are loosely connected via neurons and humoral substances.

5. Sleep regulatory circuits coordinate neuronal assembly functional state changes into organism sleep.

suggest that sleep is a fundamental property of neuronal assemblies.

During organism sleep and wake, most of the columns are in their respective sleeplike and wakelike states, suggesting synchrony of state between columns (step 4; see **Box 2**). Columns are topographically organized, and in general, the closer a column is to another, the more tightly the 2 are linked by neural and humoral connections. Because they are linked, it is likely from a theoretic view that they functionally synchronize with each other.[83,84]

Cortical columns are also connected to subcortical sleep regulatory circuits (step 5; see **Box 2**). Unilateral injection of either TNF or IL-1 onto the cerebral cortex activates reticular thalamic neurons as determined by fos expression.[85,86] Further, prefrontal cortical neurons, ventral lateral preoptic neurons, and medial preoptic neurons are also activated by IL-1.[86] These data suggest that the status of cortical column state could be relayed to these NREMS regulatory networks. It is also possible that these regulatory networks are thus involved in coordinating whole-animal sleep using cortical column state status information. Thus in this view sleep is (1) dependent on previous cellular activity, (2) initiated at the cortical column level, (3) a self-organized state being coordinated between columns and being a statistical property of the number of columns is the sleeplike state, and (4) it is refined and timed into whole-animal sleep by sleep regulatory networks. Each of these is a falsifiable hypothesis.

A NEUROCONNECTIVITY FUNCTION FOR SLEEP: CYTOKINE INVOLVEMENT

Sleep as a subject of neurobiology is unusual because its function has not been experimentally defined. Its importance is shown by the facts that during sleep one does not reproduce, eat, drink, or socialize and one is subject to predation. These are high evolutionary costs to overcome by whatever the beneficial effects of sleep are. So what could be so important to the brain to allow such a disadvantaged state to persist? There are many theories of sleep function positing that the answer is neural connectivity.[66,87–91] In this review, we focus on just 2 (our own[89] and that of Kavanau[66]) because the logic of the 2 is similar and both are derived in part from the earlier proposal of Roffwarg.[92] The central idea of both theories was the recognition that use-dependent changes in synaptic efficacy and connectivity would lead to dysfunction unless there were processes to stabilize synaptic networks that are constantly being modified by activity. This process is now termed synaptic scaling. Synaptic scaling serves to regulate Hebbian plasticity; thus, an increase in network activity causes a slow compensatory decrease in excitatory synaptic efficacy, whereas a decrease in network activity enhances excitatory synaptic strength.[93] The stabilization mechanism proposed by us was SRS-induced changes in local electrical properties, whereas the mechanism proposed by Kavanau was intrinsic spontaneous electrical activity. These mechanisms are not mutually exclusive and both are scaling mechanisms. More recent sleep-connectivity theories have also invoked synaptic scaling (reviewed in Refs.[94,95]).

Of importance to this review is that TNF is involved in synaptic scaling. Thus, TNF promotes AMPA receptor expression and enhances cytosolic Ca^{++} levels.[96] This TNF action is physiologic because an inhibitor of TNF inhibits AMPA-induced postsynaptic potentials[97] and AMPA-induced changes in cytosolic Ca^{++}.[96] A TNF siRNA applied to the cortex inhibits gluR1 mRNA levels[79]; gluR1 is a subunit of the AMPA receptor. AMPA receptors are involved in EEG synchronization[98] and synaptic plasticity.[99] Direct evidence for the involvement of TNF in synaptic scaling has been described.[100] IL-1 may also affect AMPA receptor expression.[101] AMPA receptors in layer V are involved in downscaling during NREMS.[102] Overall, these data suggest a cytokine-dependent mechanism for the reconfiguration of synaptic weights during NREMS.

CONNECTING ACTIVITY TO CYTOKINES: THE ADENOSINE TRIPHOSPHATE-CYTOKINE-ADENOSINE HYPOTHESIS

A major tenant of the neuroconnectivity theories is their dependence on activity. Indeed, within the brain, a major stimulus for IL-1 and TNF production and release is neuronal activity. Adenosine triphosphate (ATP) is coreleased with neurotransmitters.[103] ATP in turn induces IL-1[104] and TNF[105] release from glia via P2X receptors (reviewed in Refs.[106,107]). ATP is present in neuronal synaptic vesicles. The concentration of ATP in the vesicles is 10 to 50 times higher than in the cytosol. In the brain, ATP is coreleased in GABAergic, cholinergic, noradrenergic, and glutamatergic synapses. ATP is also considered a gliotransmitter. Once released, some extracellular ATP is converted to adenosine. In turn, adenosine binds to the other major purine receptor types, P1 receptors (**Fig. 1**). The action of adenosine is fast, occurring within milliseconds to seconds, and it results in increased K+ permeability and hyperpolarization.

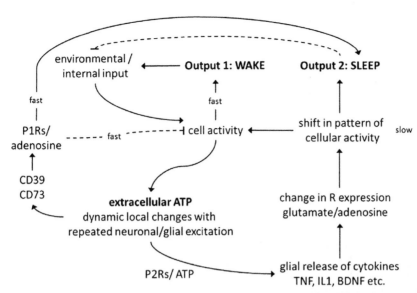

Fig. 1. The sleep homeostat. Molecular networks operating on different timescales (fast vs slow) comprise the sleep homeostat. Cellular activity is induced and sustained by environmental stimuli. Cellular activity increases arousal (*output 1*) and causes ATP to be coreleased with glutamate and other neurotransmitters. This extracellular ATP provides a way for the brain to track previous activity; some ATP is enzymatically converted to adenosine (fast) and some binds with glial P2 receptors to facilitate SRS secretion. SRSs induce fast-acting labile substances like adenosine and NO. Alternatively, SRSs and their effectors can lead to alterations (slow) in receptor content and receptor-mediated ion gating, causing a shift in overall cellular activity. Resulting changes in receptor populations predispose affected networks (within the diffusible range of extracellular ATP) to sleep (*output 2*).

Some of the released extracellular ATP acts on glial P2Rs and causes the release of IL-1, TNF, and BDNF as well as additional ATP (see **Fig. 1**). IL-1 precursor is processed by caspase 1, which is triggered via ATP activation of P2X7 receptors.[108,109] TNF and IL-1 released from glia act more slowly (minutes to hours) on adjacent neurons, leading to the activation of NFκB. NFκB promotes transcription of receptor mRNAs such as the adenosine A1R and the glutamate AMPA receptor-gluR1 mRNAs. Translation of those mRNAs into their respective proteins and their subsequent expression on the cell membrane would change sensitivity of the postsynaptic neuron over longer periods. This is a prototypical scaling effect, because the expression of postsynaptic receptors is modulated by the activity of the presynaptic neuron (ie, the amount of released ATP). Thus, the sensitivity of the postsynaptic neuron is scaled to the previous use of the synapse. As mentioned, TNF and BDNF are the 2 molecules most firmly linked to synaptic scaling. Thus, ATP levels are affected by metabolism and neural activity and in turn affect extracellular levels of adenosine and cytokines, thereby providing direct links between neural activity, metabolism, and sleep regulation. This idea fostered our ATP-adenosine-cytokine hypothesis.[89] Mechanistically, our hypothesis is summarized as follows:

(1) neuronal activity is associated with gliotransmission and neurotransmission corelease of ATP; (2) the consequent increase in extracellular ATP thus provides an index of previous local neuronal activity; (3) the ATP is detected by nearby purine type 2 receptors, causing the release of sleep regulatory cytokines such as TNF, IL-1, and BDNF, and this provides for the translation of previous neuronal activity into local levels of SRSs; (4a) these substances in turn, by a slow process (gene transcription/translation), alter electrical properties of nearby neurons by altering their own production and that of receptor populations, such as glutamate and adenosine receptors; (4b) the SRSs also, by a fast process (diffusion for short distances), directly interact with their receptors on neurons and alter electrical properties; (4c) further, ATP itself breaks down, releasing extracellular adenosine, which in turn acts on adenosine receptors, again altering electrical potentials on the nearby neurons. These events are happening locally and the collective electrical changes result in a shift in input-output relationships within the local neuronal assemblies that originally showed the increase in activity (ie, a state shift). In a mathematical model, the local states of neuronal assemblies rapidly synchronize, or phase lock, with each other because they are loosely connected to each other via neurons and humoral

substances.[84] Well-characterized sleep regulatory circuits and associated activation networks play a critical role in both sleep and waking by ensuring the synchronization of neuronal assembly state for niche-adaptation purposes. Consistent with this model, ATP agonists promote NREMS, whereas ATP antagonists inhibit sleep.[110] Further, after sleep deprivation, mice lacking the P2X7 receptor have attenuated duration of NREMS and EEG δ wave power during NREMS compared with control mice.[110]

SUMMARY

IL-1 and TNF are well-characterized SRSs that form part of the sleep homeostat (see **Fig. 1**). Our knowledge of cytokine sleep mechanisms has led to a view of brain organization of sleep positing that sleep is a local property of neural networks being initiated, for example, within cortical columns. Cortical columns oscillate between functional states; the sleeplike state of cortical columns is promoted by TNF. Further, TNF is involved in glutamatergic AMPA receptor expression and in synaptic scaling mechanisms. Cytokine-mediated sleep mechanisms provide support for the hypothesis that sleep serves a synaptic-connectivity function and is tightly coupled to cerebral metabolism. IL-1 and TNF release from glia is enhanced by neuronal activity via ATP and, in turn, IL-1 and TNF activate NFκB, adenosine, and other downstream mechanisms.

REFERENCES

1. Ishimori K. True cause of sleep–a hypnogenic substance as evidenced in the brain of sleep-deprived animals. Tokyo Igakkai Zasshi 1909;23: 429–57.
2. Legendre R, Pieron H. Recherches sur le besoin de sommeil consécutif à une veille prolongée. Z Allg Physiol 1913;14:235–62.
3. Pappenheimer JR, Miller TB, Goodrich CA. Sleep-promoting effects of cerebrospinal fluid from sleep-deprived goats. Proc Natl Acad Sci U S A 1967;58:513–7.
4. Obal F Jr, Krueger JM. Biochemical regulation of non-rapid-eye-movement sleep. Front Biosci 2003;8:d520–50.
5. Borbely AA, Tobler I. Endogenous sleep-promoting substances and sleep regulation. Physiol Rev 1989;69:605–70.
6. Inoue S. Biology of sleep substances. Boca Raton (FL): CRC Press; 1989.
7. Jouvet M. Neuromédiateurs et facteurs hypnogènes. Rev Neurol (Paris) 1984;140:389–400.
8. Borbely AA, Tobler I. The search for an endogenous "sleep substance". Trends Pharmacol Sci 1980;1:356–8.
9. Krueger JM, Obal F. Sleep factors. In: Saunders NA, Sullivan CE, editors. Sleep and breathing. New York: Marcel Dekker; 1994. p. 79–112.
10. Krueger JM, Walter J, Dinarello CA, et al. Sleep-promoting effects of endogenous pyrogen (interleukin-1). Am J Physiol 1984;246:R994–9.
11. Shoham S, Davenne D, Cady AB, et al. Recombinant tumor necrosis factor and interleukin 1 enhance slow-wave sleep. Am J Physiol 1987; 253:R142–9.
12. Fang J, Wang Y, Krueger JM. Mice lacking the TNF 55 kDa receptor fail to sleep more after TNFalpha treatment. J Neurosci 1997;17:5949–55.
13. Fang J, Wang Y, Krueger JM. Effects of interleukin-1 beta on sleep are mediated by the type I receptor. Am J Physiol 1998;274:R655–60.
14. Krueger JM, Clinton JM, Winters BD, et al. Involvement of cytokines in slow wave sleep. Prog Brain Res 2011;193:39–47.
15. Vgontzas AN, Zoumakis E, Lin HM, et al. Marked decrease in sleepiness in patients with sleep apnea by etanercept, a tumor necrosis factor-alpha antagonist. J Clin Endocrinol Metab 2004; 89:4409–13.
16. Franklin CM. Clinical experience with soluble TNF p75 receptor in rheumatoid arthritis. Semin Arthritis Rheum 1999;29:172–81.
17. Taishi P, Davis CJ, Bayomy O, et al. Brain-specific interleukin-1 receptor accessory protein in sleep regulation. J Appl Physiol 2012;112:1015–22.
18. Baracchi F, Opp MR. Sleep-wake behavior and responses to sleep deprivation of mice lacking both interleukin-1 beta receptor 1 and tumor necrosis factor-alpha receptor 1. Brain Behav Immun 2008;22:982–93.
19. Lue FA, Bail M, Jephthah-Ochola J, et al. Sleep and cerebrospinal fluid interleukin-1-like activity in the cat. Int J Neurosci 1988;42:179–83.
20. Nguyen KT, Deak T, Owens SM, et al. Exposure to acute stress induces brain interleukin-1beta protein in the rat. J Neurosci 1998;18:2239–46.
21. Floyd RA, Krueger JM. Diurnal variation of TNF alpha in the rat brain. Neuroreport 1997;8:915–8.
22. Hansen MK, Taishi P, Chen Z, et al. Cafeteria feeding induces interleukin-1beta mRNA expression in rat liver and brain. Am J Physiol 1998;274: R1734–9.
23. Alt JA, Bohnet S, Taishi P, et al. Influenza virus-induced glucocorticoid and hypothalamic and lung cytokine mRNA responses in dwarf lit/lit mice. Brain Behav Immun 2007;21:60–7.
24. Kubota T, Li N, Guan Z, et al. Intrapreoptic microinjection of TNF-alpha enhances non-REM sleep in rats. Brain Res 2002;932:37–44.

25. Terao A, Matsumura H, Saito M. Interleukin-1 induces slow-wave sleep at the prostaglandin D2-sensitive sleep-promoting zone in the rat brain. J Neurosci 1998;18:6599–607.

26. De A, Churchill L, Obal F Jr, et al. GHRH and IL1-beta increase cytoplasmic Ca(2+) levels in cultured hypothalamic GABAergic neurons. Brain Res 2002;949:209–12.

27. Zhang J, Obal F Jr, Zheng T, et al. Intrapreoptic microinjection of GHRH or its antagonist alters sleep in rats. J Neurosci 1999;19:2187–94.

28. Peterfi Z, McGinty D, Sarai E, et al. Growth hormone-releasing hormone activates sleep regulatory neurons of the rat preoptic hypothalamus. Am J Physiol Regul Integr Comp Physiol 2010; 298:R147–56.

29. Alam MN, McGinty D, Bashir T, et al. Interleukin-1beta modulates state-dependent discharge activity of preoptic area and basal forebrain neurons: role in sleep regulation. Eur J Neurosci 2004;20:207–16.

30. De Sarro G, Gareri P, Sinopoli VA, et al. Comparative, behavioural and electrocortical effects of tumor necrosis factor-alpha and interleukin-1 microinjected into the locus coeruleus of rat. Life Sci 1997;60:555–64.

31. Nistico G, De Sarro G, Rotiroti D. Behavioral and electrocortical spectrum power changes of interleukins and tumor necrosis factor after microinjection into different areas of the brain. In: Smirne S, Francesch M, Ferini-Stambi L, editors. Sleep, hormones, and immunological system. Milan (Italy): Mason; 1992. p. 11–22.

32. Manfridi A, Brambilla D, Bianchi S, et al. Interleukin-1beta enhances non-rapid eye movement sleep when microinjected into the dorsal raphe nucleus and inhibits serotonergic neurons in vitro. Eur J Neurosci 2003;18:1041–9.

33. Brambilla D, Franciosi S, Opp MR, et al. Interleukin-1 inhibits firing of serotonergic neurons in the dorsal raphe nucleus and enhances GABAergic inhibitory post-synaptic potentials. Eur J Neurosci 2007;26:1862–9.

34. Serantes R, Arnalich F, Figueroa M, et al. Interleukin-1beta enhances GABAA receptor cell-surface expression by a phosphatidylinositol 3-kinase/Akt pathway: relevance to sepsis-associated encephalopathy. J Biol Chem 2006;281:14632–43.

35. Chen R, Yin Y, Zhao Z, et al. Elevation of serum TNF-α levels in mild and moderate Alzheimer patients with daytime sleepiness. J Neuroimmunol 2012;244:97–102.

36. Sookoian SC, Gonzalez C, Pirola CJ. Meta-analysis on the G-308A tumor necrosis factor alpha gene variant and phenotypes associated with the metabolic syndrome. Obes Res 2005;13:2122–31.

37. Gupta V, Gupta A, Jafar T, et al. Association of TNF-alpha promoter gene G-308A polymorphism with metabolic syndrome, insulin resistance, serum TNF-alpha and leptin levels in Indian adult women. Cytokine 2012;57:32–6.

38. Riha RL, Brander P, Vennelle M, et al. Tumour necrosis factor-alpha-308 gene polymorphism in obstructive sleep apnoea-hypopnoea syndrome. Eur Respir J 2005;26:673–8.

39. Zhang HF, Xie SL, Wang JF, et al. Tumor necrosis factor-alpha G-308A gene polymorphism and coronary heart disease susceptibility: an updated meta-analysis. Thromb Res 2011;127:400–5.

40. Mullington J, Korth C, Hermann DM, et al. Dose-dependent effects of endotoxin on human sleep. Am J Physiol Regul Integr Comp Physiol 2000; 278:R947–55.

41. Karadag O, Nakas D, Kalyoncu U, et al. Effect of anti-TNF treatment on sleep problems in ankylosing spondylitis. Rheumatol Int 2011;17:358–62.

42. Irwin MR, Olmstead R, Valladares EM, et al. Tumor necrosis factor antagonism normalizes rapid eye movement sleep in alcohol dependence. Biol Psychiatry 2009;66:191–5.

43. Arias MA, Garcia-Rio F, Alonso-Fernandez A, et al. CPAP decreases plasma levels of soluble tumour necrosis factor-alpha receptor 1 in obstructive sleep apnoea. Eur Respir J 2008;32:1009–15.

44. Steiropoulos P, Kotsianidis I, Nena E, et al. Long-term effect of continuous positive airway pressure therapy on inflammation markers of patients with obstructive sleep apnea syndrome. Sleep 2009; 32:537–43.

45. Eun YG, Kim MG, Kwon KH, et al. Short-term effect of multilevel surgery on adipokines and pro-inflammatory cytokines in patients with obstructive sleep apnea. Acta Otolaryngol 2010;130:1394–8.

46. Moldofsky H, Lue FA, Eisen J, et al. The relationship of interleukin-1 and immune functions to sleep in humans. Psychosom Med 1986;48:309–18.

47. Hohagen F, Timmer J, Weyerbrock A, et al. Cytokine production during sleep and wakefulness and its relationship to cortisol in healthy humans. Neuropsychobiology 1993;28:9–16.

48. Uthgenannt D, Schoolmann D, Pietrowsky R, et al. Effects of sleep on the production of cytokines in humans. Psychosom Med 1995;57:97–104.

49. Kubota T, Fang J, Guan Z, et al. Vagotomy attenuates tumor necrosis factor-alpha-induced sleep and EEG delta-activity in rats. Am J Physiol Regul Integr Comp Physiol 2001;280:R1213–20.

50. Hansen MK, Krueger JM. Subdiaphragmatic vagotomy blocks the sleep- and fever-promoting effects of interleukin-1beta. Am J Physiol 1997; 273:R1246–53.

51. Churchill L, Taishi P, Wang M, et al. Brain distribution of cytokine mRNA induced by systemic administration of interleukin-1beta or tumor necrosis factor alpha. Brain Res 2006;1120:64–73.

52. Hansen MK, Taishi P, Chen Z, et al. Vagotomy blocks the induction of interleukin-1beta (IL-1beta) mRNA in the brain of rats in response to systemic IL-1beta. J Neurosci 1998;18:2247–53.

53. Majde JA, Krueger JM. Links between the innate immune system and sleep. J Allergy Clin Immunol 2005;116:1188–98.

54. Kimura M, Majde JA, Toth LA, et al. Somnogenic effects of rabbit and recombinant human interferons in rabbits. Am J Physiol 1994;267:R53–61.

55. Knefati M, Somogyi C, Kapas L, et al. Acidic fibroblast growth factor (FGF) but not basic FGF induces sleep and fever in rabbits. Am J Physiol 1995;269:R87–91.

56. Brandt JA, Churchill L, Rehman A, et al. Sleep deprivation increases the activation of nuclear factor kappa B in lateral hypothalamic cells. Brain Res 2004;1004:91–7.

57. Chen Z, Gardi J, Kushikata T, et al. Nuclear factor-kappaB-like activity increases in murine cerebral cortex after sleep deprivation. Am J Physiol 1999; 276:R1812–8.

58. Basheer R, Rainnie DG, Porkka-Heiskanen T, et al. Adenosine, prolonged wakefulness, and A1-activated NF-kappaB DNA binding in the basal forebrain of the rat. Neuroscience 2001;104:731–9.

59. Kubota T, Kushikata T, Fang J, et al. Nuclear factor-kappaB inhibitor peptide inhibits spontaneous and interleukin-1beta-induced sleep. Am J Physiol Regul Integr Comp Physiol 2000;279:R404–13.

60. Luk WP, Zhang Y, White TD, et al. Adenosine: a mediator of interleukin-1beta-induced hippocampal synaptic inhibition. J Neurosci 1999;19: 4238–44.

61. Kapas L, Shibata M, Kimura M, et al. Inhibition of nitric oxide synthesis suppresses sleep in rabbits. Am J Physiol 1994;266:R151–7.

62. Rattenborg NC, Amlaner CJ, Lima SL. Behavioral, neurophysiological and evolutionary perspectives on unihemispheric sleep. Neurosci Biobehav Rev 2000;24:817–42.

63. Krueger JM, Obal F Jr. Sleep function. Front Biosci 2003;8:d511–9.

64. Krueger JM, Obal F. A neuronal group theory of sleep function. J Sleep Res 1993;2:63–9.

65. Tononi G, Cirelli C. Sleep and synaptic homeostasis: a hypothesis. Brain Res Bull 2003; 62:143–50.

66. Kavanau JL. Sleep and dynamic stabilization of neural circuitry: a review and synthesis. Behav Brain Res 1994;63:111–26.

67. Benington JH, Heller HC. Restoration of brain energy metabolism as the function of sleep. Prog Neurobiol 1995;45:347–60.

68. Schinder AF, Poo M. The neurotrophin hypothesis for synaptic plasticity. Trends Neurosci 2000;23: 639–45.

69. de Bock F, Dornand J, Rondouin G. Release of TNF alpha in the rat hippocampus following epileptic seizures and excitotoxic neuronal damage. Neuroreport 1996;7:1125–9.

70. De A, Krueger JM, Simasko SM. Glutamate induces the expression and release of tumor necrosis factor-alpha in cultured hypothalamic cells. Brain Res 2005;1053:54–61.

71. Schneider H, Pitossi F, Balschun D, et al. A neuromodulatory role of interleukin-1beta in the hippocampus. Proc Natl Acad Sci U S A 1998;95: 7778–83.

72. Yi PL, Tsai CH, Lin JG, et al. Kindling stimuli delivered at different times in the sleep-wake cycle. Sleep 2004;27:203–12.

73. Churchill L, Rector DM, Yasuda K, et al. Tumor necrosis factor alpha: activity dependent expression and promotion of cortical column sleep in rats. Neuroscience 2008;156:71–80.

74. Fix C, Churchill L, Hall S, et al. The number of tumor necrosis factor alpha-immunoreactive cells increases in layer IV of the barrel field in response to whisker deflection in the rats. Sleep 2006;29:A11.

75. Shibata M. Hypothalamic neuronal responses to cytokines. Yale J Biol Med 1990;63:147–56.

76. Tabarean IV, Korn H, Bartfai T. Interleukin-1beta induces hyperpolarization and modulates synaptic inhibition in preoptic and anterior hypothalamic neurons. Neuroscience 2006;141:1685–95.

77. Yasuda T, Yoshida H, Garcia-Garcia F, et al. Interleukin-1beta has a role in cerebral cortical state-dependent electroencephalographic slow-wave activity. Sleep 2005;28:177–84.

78. Yoshida H, Peterfi Z, Garcia-Garcia F, et al. State-specific asymmetries in EEG slow wave activity induced by local application of TNFalpha. Brain Res 2004;1009:129–36.

79. Taishi P, Churchill L, Wang M, et al. TNFalpha siRNA reduces brain TNF and EEG delta wave activity in rats. Brain Res 2007;1156:125–32.

80. Rector DM, Topchiy IA, Carter KM, et al. Local functional state differences between rat cortical columns. Brain Res 2005;1047:45–55.

81. Phillips DJ, Schei JL, Meighan PC, et al. Cortical evoked responses associated with arousal from sleep. Sleep 2011;34:65–72.

82. Walker JL, Walker BM, Fuentes FM, et al. Rat psychomotor vigilance task with fast response times using a conditioned lick behavior. Behav Brain Res 2011;216:229–37.

83. Strogatz SH, Stewart I. Coupled oscillators and biological synchronization. Sci Am 1993;269: 102–9.

84. Roy S, Krueger JM, Rector DM, et al. A network model for activity-dependent sleep regulation. J Theor Biol 2008;253:462–8.

85. Churchill L, Yasuda K, Yasuda T, et al. Unilateral cortical application of tumor necrosis factor alpha induces asymmetry in Fos- and interleukin-1beta-immunoreactive cells within the corticothalamic projection. Brain Res 2005;1055:15–24.

86. Yasuda K, Churchill L, Yasuda T, et al. Unilateral cortical application of interleukin-1beta (IL1beta) induces asymmetry in fos, IL1beta and nerve growth factor immunoreactivity: implications for sleep regulation. Brain Res 2007;1131:44–59.

87. Benington JH, Frank MG. Cellular and molecular connections between sleep and synaptic plasticity. Prog Neurobiol 2003;69:71–101.

88. Best J, Diniz Behn C, Poe GR, et al. Neuronal models for sleep-wake regulation and synaptic reorganization in the sleeping hippocampus. J Biol Rhythms 2007;22:220–32.

89. Krueger JM, Rector DM, Roy S, et al. Sleep as a fundamental property of neuronal assemblies. Nat Rev Neurosci 2008;9:910–9.

90. Tononi G, Cirelli C. Sleep function and synaptic homeostasis. Sleep Med Rev 2006;10:49–62.

91. Aton SJ, Seibt J, Dumoulin M, et al. Mechanisms of sleep-dependent consolidation of cortical plasticity. Neuron 2009;61:454–66.

92. Roffwarg HP, Muzio JN, Dement WC. Ontogenetic development of the human sleep-dream cycle. Science 1966;152:604–19.

93. Abbott LF, Nelson SB. Synaptic plasticity: taming the beast. Nat Neurosci 2000;3(Suppl):1178–83.

94. Krueger JM, Tononi G. Local use-dependent sleep; synthesis of the new paradigm. Curr Top Med Chem 2011;11:2490–2.

95. Krueger JM, Wisor JP. Local use-dependent sleep. Curr Top Med Chem 2011;11:2390–1.

96. De A, Krueger JM, Simasko SM. Tumor necrosis factor alpha increases cytosolic calcium responses to AMPA and KCl in primary cultures of rat hippocampal neurons. Brain Res 2003;981:133–42.

97. Beattie EC, Stellwagen D, Morishita W, et al. Control of synaptic strength by glial TNFalpha. Science 2002;295:2282–5.

98. Bazhenov M, Timofeev I, Steriade M, et al. Model of thalamocortical slow-wave sleep oscillations and transitions to activated states. J Neurosci 2002;22:8691–704.

99. Malinow R, Malenka RC. AMPA receptor trafficking and synaptic plasticity. Annu Rev Neurosci 2002;25:103–26.

100. Stellwagen D, Malenka RC. Synaptic scaling mediated by glial TNF-alpha. Nature 2006;440:1054–9.

101. Lai AY, Swayze RD, El-Husseini A, et al. Interleukin-1 beta modulates AMPA receptor expression and phosphorylation in hippocampal neurons. J Neuroimmunol 2006;175:97–106.

102. Czarnecki A, Birtoli B, Ulrich D. Cellular mechanisms of burst firing-mediated long-term depression in rat neocortical pyramidal cells. J Physiol 2007;578:471–9.

103. Farber K, Kettenmann H. Purinergic signaling and microglia. Pflugers Arch 2006;452:615–21.

104. Bianco F, Pravettoni E, Colombo A, et al. Astrocyte-derived ATP induces vesicle shedding and IL-1 beta release from microglia. J Immunol 2005;174:7268–77.

105. Hide I, Tanaka M, Inoue A, et al. Extracellular ATP triggers tumor necrosis factor-alpha release from rat microglia. J Neurochem 2000;75:965–72.

106. Suzuki T, Hide I, Ido K, et al. Production and release of neuroprotective tumor necrosis factor by P2X7 receptor-activated microglia. J Neurosci 2004;24:1–7.

107. Burnstock G. Physiology and pathophysiology of purinergic neurotransmission. Physiol Rev 2007;87:659–797.

108. Ferrari D, Pizzirani C, Adinolfi E, et al. The P2X7 receptor: a key player in IL-1 processing and release. J Immunol 2006;176:3877–83.

109. Duan S, Neary JT. P2X(7) receptors: properties and relevance to CNS function. Glia 2006;54:738–46.

110. Krueger JM, Taishi P, De A, et al. ATP and the purine type 2 X7 receptor affect sleep. J Appl Physiol 2010;109:1318–27.

Sleep Behavior and Sleep Regulation from Infancy Through Adolescence
Normative Aspects

Oskar G. Jenni, MD[a],*, Mary A. Carskadon, PhD[b]

KEYWORDS

- Normal sleep behavior • Sleep regulation • Sleep homeostasis • Circadian • Variability

KEY POINTS

- This article (1) describes normal sleep patterns in children and adolescents, (2) depicts sleep stages and sleep electrophysiology in children, and (3) identifies changes in sleep-wake (homeostatic) and circadian regulatory processes across early human development.
- Three basic principles should guide our consideration of sleep during childhood and adolescence: first, sleep patterns exhibit large variability among children; second, sleep behavior must be viewed within a biopsychosocial framework; and third, sleep may provide undisturbed insights into the developing brain.

INTRODUCTION

Biologic determinants of sleep and the ways in which sleep biology and environment interact play major roles in establishing behavioral and developmental norms and expectations regarding normal and problematic children's sleep.[1] Although the primary role of social, family, and cultural systems on children's sleep behavior are recognized, less is known about the physiologic and the bioregulatory nature of children's sleep. This article (1) describes normal sleep patterns in children and adolescents, (2) depicts sleep stages and sleep electrophysiology in children, and (3) identifies changes in sleep-wake (homeostatic) and circadian regulatory processes across early human development. Jenni and LeBourgeois[2] provided a conceptual framework for understanding and predicting sleep-wake patterns in infants, children, and adolescents. This article summarizes the research on sleep-wake mechanisms during development in the context of the 2-process model of sleep regulation, which was first articulated by Borbély[3] in 1982. The article also highlights another line of recent research the undisturbed recording of cortical activity during children's sleep, which may be a useful tool to study aspects of brain maturation, function, and morphology during development.

This article originally appeared in *Sleep Medicine Clinics Volume 2, Issue 3*.

Dr Jenni was supported by grants from The Swiss National Science Foundation (32473B-129956/1) and the Center for Integrative Human Physiology of the University of Zurich. Dr Carskadon was supported by grants from The National Institutes of Health (grant no. MH52415).

[a] Child Development Center, University Children's Hospital Zurich, Steinwiesstrasse 75, CH-8032 Zurich, Switzerland; [b] E. P. Bradley Hospital Chronobiology and Sleep Research Laboratory, Department of Psychiatry and Human Behavior, Warren Alpert Medical School of Brown University, 300 Duncan Drive, Providence, RI 02906, USA
* Corresponding author.
E-mail address: oskar.jenni@kispi.uzh.ch

sleep.theclinics.com

Three principles should guide our consideration of sleep during childhood:

- All aspects of children's sleep exhibit large variability among individuals and across cultures.
- Sleep behavior in children must be viewed within a biopsychosocial framework. Although sleep structure, organization, and regulation are primarily governed by intrinsic biologic processes, children's sleep is also shaped by cultural values, parental beliefs, and regulation of social systems.
- Sleep may provide undisturbed insights into the developing brain.

DEVELOPMENTAL PATTERNS OF HUMAN SLEEP BEHAVIOR
Newborn Period and Infancy

The sleep of newborns is distributed equally across day and night (**Fig. 1**). However, in the first few months of life, infants gain the ability to sustain longer episodes of sleep and waking[4,5]; as sleep becomes more and more consolidated toward the nighttime, nocturnal sleep duration increases, and daytime sleep declines (**Fig. 2**).[6] Although consolidated nocturnal episodes of sleep generally do not occur before 6 weeks of age, day-night differences in rest-activity behavior may be observed as early as in the first days of life in some babies.[7] The development of the 24-hour rhythm in sleep-wake behavior during infancy is driven by the emergence of both circadian and homeostatic sleep-wake processes (discussed later) as well as by parental daily activities (eg, feeding patterns). Most infants eventually begin sleeping through the night by the age of 6 to 9 months (ie, between 6–8 hours of nocturnal sleep without signaling).[8–10] A consolidated sleep episode throughout the nighttime is considered a major developmental milestone and is a central topic of infant care. In more than 70% of health supervision visits, infant sleep issues are discussed between parents and health care professionals.[11]

The average total sleep duration remains constant across the first year of life (see **Fig. 2**, mean 14 hours per day), although the most prominent feature of infant sleep is the large variability of sleep amount among individuals.[6] For example, at age 6 months, one infant may sleep as little as 10.5 hours, and another as much as 18 hours each day (at this age, the infant in **Fig. 1** slept 11.7 hours). This interindividual variability of sleep duration is never larger than in infancy (average standard deviation [SD] ± 1.9 hours during infancy

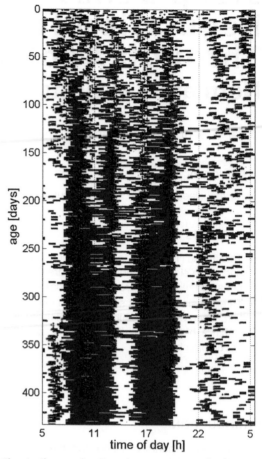

Fig. 1. Sleep-wake diurnal pattern across the first 425 days after birth in a healthy male infant recorded by daily sleep logs. Black and white areas represent waking and sleep, respectively. Red circles show feeding episodes.

compared with ± 0.8 hours SD from age 1–10 years), reflecting differences in the maturational tempo of early sleep-wake and circadian organization, although accuracy of parental observations and reports may also influence this apparent variation among the youngest children.

Early Childhood

Although the large differences of sleep duration among individuals remain a typical characteristic of children's sleep behavior, the decrease of the sleep length across early childhood (as a consequence of the reduction of daytime naps) becomes most obvious.[6] Nearly all children stop routine daily napping between the ages of 3 and 5 years, even though large cultural differences exist.[12] Furthermore, night wakings remain a common issue in toddlers/preschoolers and may be considered a typical developmental phenomenon (20% wake up at least once each night,

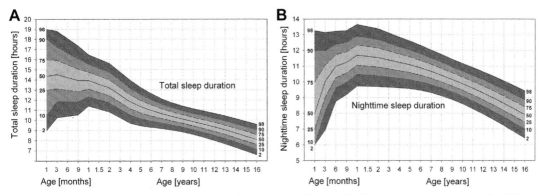

Fig. 2. Percentiles of total (*A*) and nighttime (*B*) sleep duration (time in bed) per 24 hours in 493 healthy children (Zurich Longitudinal Studies). (*From* Iglowstein I, Jenni OG, Molinari L, et al. Sleep duration from infancy to adolescence: reference values and generational trends. Pediatrics 2003;11:303, 304; with permission.)

50% at least 1 night per week).[8] Such awakenings are a consequence of nocturnal arousals driven by the ultradian rhythm of sleep cycles (50–90 minutes). Whether night wakings become a behavioral problem depends on the child's ability to fall back asleep without parental intervention (ie, the child as a self-soother).[9]

Major processes in child development influence sleep behavior of preschoolers[8]: (1) increased independent locomotion may result in parent-child bed sharing when a child awakens in the middle of the night (reactive cosleeping); (2) cognitive development may produce nighttime fears, as well as interests in transitional objects (sleep aids such as a pacifier, doll, or blanket) that facilitate children's transitions from waking into sleep; (3) attachment issues may emerge and manifest as separation anxiety leading to frequent night wakings and parent-child bed sharing; and (4) the toddler's drive for autonomy may be associated with frequent bedtime resistance. Whether these behaviors are considered problematic depends on parents' perceptions and expectations.[13] The bedtime routine (ie, a culturally specific set of activities such as dressing in a particular night dress, telling stories, and singing lullabies) is often an important part of the sleep-onset milieu in preschoolers. Although most Euro-American children sleep alone in separate rooms, the norm for children in many cultures is to sleep with an adult or with a sibling (lifestyle cosleeping). Climatic factors, family size, space availability, parental beliefs, and cultural preferences often condition sleeping arrangements (for a comprehensive review on children's sleep and culture, see Jenni and O'Connor[12]).

School Age

Preschool and school-aged children generally maintain their sleep duration in the course of

development at a similar position compared with other children of the same age.[14] Young children who are short sleepers during early childhood generally remain short sleepers as they grow into the teenage years, and the same is true for long sleepers. These findings from the Zurich Longitudinal Studies may indicate that the variability of sleep duration among children reflects, in part, traitlike characteristics of the individual. Thus, no optimal amount of sleep for the population of children can be determined; individual sleep need should be taken into account, which ideally will match parental expectations and school schedules. The child's individual sleep need may be approximated by the average amount of sleep in the course of a week with a self-selected sleep schedule and without imposition of externally driven daily activities.

School children usually begin to manifest an inherent circadian sleep phase preference (eg, evening type or so-called night owl in contrast with morning type or morning lark[15]). Again, determining the optimal bedtime for children at a specific age is not possible, considering the large biologically driven variation in the phase preference of the circadian timing system.[16] Rather, a goodness-of-fit approach should be encouraged in which a balance between the child's and the family's (and the society's) needs is achieved.[12,17] The emergence of large differences between sleep schedules on school days and weekends, with extended oversleeping on weekend mornings, may indicate a poor fit between a child's sleep need, circadian timing, and weekday schedules.

Adolescence

Although sleep duration decreases in the first 10 years of life, sleep need does not seem to decline in the course of adolescence (around 9 hours on average, with an increase of daytime sleep propensity).[18] The most notable change in adolescent sleep behavior is the delay of the sleep phase, although large differences exist among individuals (**Fig. 3**)[19]; thus, adolescents tend to stay up late at night and sleep late in the morning compared with preadolescents. This phase delay may result in insufficient sleep during the school week and catch-up sleep during weekends.[20] Explanations for the phase delay are easy to find in the changing adolescent psychosocial milieu, the teenage wishes for autonomy and independence, shifts in family configurations, peer culture and social expectations, academic demands, school culture, employment opportunities, and extracurricular activities.[21] However, maturational changes of biologic sleep processes are also related to sleep timing and amount during adolescence. Some investigators recently suggested that the biologic phase of the circadian timing system (as expressed by the chronotype) can mark the end of adolescence early in the second decade, when a reversal occurs in the trend for chronotype to delay (see **Fig. 3**).[22]

SLEEP STAGES AND SLEEP ELECTROPHYSIOLOGY DURING DEVELOPMENT

Two distinct sleep states are defined from polysomnography, which monitors brain activity (electroencephalography), eye movements (electrooculography), and muscle tone (electromyography): rapid eye movement (REM) and non-REM (NREM) sleep. In the first 6 months after birth,

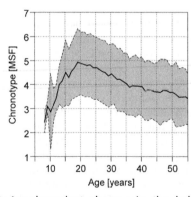

Fig. 3. Age-dependent changes in the behavioral phase marker (chronotype) from school age to middle adulthood. The black line represents the mean change (n = 25,000). Gray area illustrates the variability among individuals (standard deviation). MSF, midpoint of sleep on free days. (*From* Roenneberg T, Kuehnle T, Pramstaller PP, et al. A marker for the end of adolescence. Curr Biol 2004;14(24):R1039; with permission.)

cortical maturation and sleep electroencephalogram (EEG) organization are so different from the more mature brain patterns that different terms are used: REM sleep is called active sleep, whereas NREM sleep is termed quiet sleep. In newborns, quiet and active sleep are often disorganized and immature (called indeterminate or transitional sleep). NREM sleep is characterized by low-frequency, high-voltage EEG activity, low muscle tone, and absence of eye movements. An EEG pattern called tracé alternant with high-voltage slow activity interrupted by near electrical silence is common during quiet sleep in the very young. Respiration patterns and heart rate are regular in NREM sleep. After 6 months of age, NREM sleep can be divided into 4 stages from distinct EEG features. Stage 1 NREM sleep occurs at transitions of sleep and wakefulness. Stage 2 is characterized by frequent bursts of rhythmical EEG activity, so-called sleep spindles (first occurring after 4 weeks of age), and high-voltage slow spikes, so-called K-complexes (first appearing after 6 months). In stages 3 and 4, the EEG pattern comprises almost continuous high-voltage activity in the slowest (<2 Hz) frequency range. Newly announced sleep stage criteria include only 3 NREM sleep stages combining stages 3 and 4 into NREM sleep stage 3.[23] EEG voltage shows a significant increase in the first year, particularly evident in NREM sleep. Across ages 9 to 16 years, EEG voltages are markedly attenuated.

REM sleep is characterized by desynchronized cortical EEG activity (mixed frequencies, low voltage), absence of muscle tone, irregular heart rate and respiratory patterns, and episodic bursts of phasic eye movements, which is the hallmark of REM sleep. The term active sleep in young infants reflects frequent muscle twitches and body jerks that break through the muscle inhibition of infant REM sleep.

In the first few months of life, infants' sleep is divided evenly (50:50) between NREM sleep and REM sleep.[24] The proportion of REM sleep decreases throughout early childhood to the adolescent and adult level of about 20% to 25% of nocturnal sleep. When young infants fall asleep, the initial sleep episode is typically REM sleep; that is, sleep-onset REM periods. After 3 months, sleep-onset REM periods become replaced by the adult pattern of sleep-onset NREM periods. Slow wave sleep (SWS; NREM sleep stage 3) is greatest in preteens, declines abruptly in the course of puberty (60% decline between age 11 and 16 years,[25] see also **Fig. 4**), and further declines across the life span.[26,27] This developmental pattern of SWS reflects the changing EEG amplitude that may be related to the age-specific

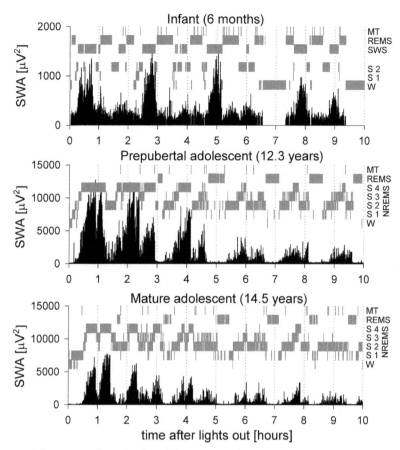

Fig. 4. Visually scored sleep stages (*gray bars*) and time course of slow wave activity (SWA; EEG power 0.6–4.6 Hz) during 10-hour sleep episodes at 3 different ages. At age 6 months, stages 3 and 4 were clustered as SWS. Note the different scaling of the y-axis at 6 months. The same girl was recorded longitudinally at ages 12.3 years (prepubertal stage Tanner 1) and 14.5 years (mature pubertal stage Tanner 5). MT, movement time. (*Data from* Jenni OG, Carskadon MA. Spectral analysis of the sleep electroencephalogram during adolescence. Sleep 2004;27(4):774–83; and Jenni OG, Borbély AA, Achermann P. Development of the nocturnal sleep electroencephalogram in human infants. Am J Physiol 2004;286:R528–38.)

programmed alterations in cortical synaptic density and connectivity among neurons and changes in neuronal, neurotransmitter, or neuroreceptor properties.[25,26]

NREM sleep and REM sleep alternate through the night in cycles (ultradian sleep rhythms) with a period of about 50 minutes in infancy. The period of this ultradian rhythm gradually lengthens through childhood, achieving mature period length of about 90 to 110 minutes around school age. SWS predominates in the sleep cycles early at night, whereas, in the last part of the night, the proportion of REM sleep is increased (see **Fig. 4**). An interesting sleep cycling pattern was recently observed in early infancy when SWS occurred in alternate NREM sleep episodes.[28,29] However, the mechanisms underlying this alternating SWS pattern remain unclear.

BASIC CONCEPTS OF SLEEP REGULATION DURING EARLY HUMAN DEVELOPMENT
The 2-Process Model of Sleep Regulation

Current theoretic models suggest that there are 2 interacting, but independent, regulatory processes that control the timing, intensity, and duration of sleep (as described in the 2-process model of sleep regulation, see **Fig. 5**): one is a homeostatic sleep process and the other is a circadian sleep process.[30–32]

The first regulatory process, sometimes called process S, represents a sleep-wake–dependent homeostatic component of sleep. Process S increases (or builds up) as a function of previous wakefulness and it decreases (or dissipates) over the course of a sleep episode. This process accounts for an increase of sleep pressure as

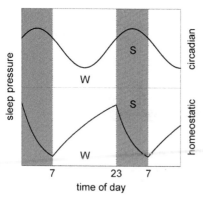

Fig. 5. Two-process model of sleep regulation. Circadian and homeostatic modulation of sleep pressure across the day and at night. The circadian process is a clocklike process, whereas the homeostatic sleep-wake–dependent process is an hourglass process. S, sleep; W, wake. (*Adapted from* Achermann P, Borbely AA. Mathematical models of sleep regulation. Front Biosci 2003;8:s684; with permission.)

waking is extended and seems to underpin a recovery or restorative process that occurs during sleep. The time course of the homeostatic process was initially derived from EEG slow wave activity (SWA; EEG power in the frequency range 0.75–4.5 Hz) during NREM sleep, which increases as a function of previous wakefulness and decreases in the course of sleep.[31] Recent research has indicated that the homeostatic sleep drive may be produced by sleep-promoting substances that accumulate during prolonged wakefulness and are depleted during sleep (such as adenosine or other somnogens).[33–35] Even more interesting from the perspective of developmental science is recent evidence that sleep homeostasis is critically involved in aspects of learning and neural plasticity (articulated in the synaptic homeostasis hypothesis of sleep, see also Refs.[36,37]).

The homeostatic process interacts with the other sleep-wake–independent circadian process. This clocklike daily oscillatory aspect of sleep regulation is often called process C and, under normal conditions, it is entrained to the light-dark cycle. The underlying circadian mechanisms have a distinct neuroanatomic locus in the nuclei suprachiasmatici of the hypothalamus (called the biologic clock), and various molecular and genetic components of the clock have been identified.[21,38]

Overall, the 2-process model of sleep regulation accounts well for the timing of sleep in humans (sleep and wake time) and their alertness during the day. When sleep-onset problems, frequent night wakings, or daytime sleepiness occur, an investigation of sleep-wake homeostatic and

circadian processes is needed. Understanding the 2 processes, how they interact with each other, and how they change across development is a basis for understanding normal and problematic sleep behavior during childhood.[2]

Development of the Circadian Timing System

The biologic clock, located in the bilateral suprachiasmatic nuclei of the anterior hypothalamus, seems to be functional in utero and thus may directly control fetal behavioral rhythms.[39] Immediately after birth, significant daily rhythms do not manifest; that is, episodes of sleeping and waking seem randomly distributed across day and night.[7] The circadian timing system undergoes major developmental changes within the first months after birth: at age 1 month, the 24-hour core body temperature rhythm emerges; at age 2 months, infants begin to sleep more at night than during the day; at age 3 months, endogenous production of the circadian-driven hormones melatonin and cortisol start to cycle in a 24-hour rhythm.[40] This early development of circadian rhythms is based on specific maturational processes of the brain interacting with social and environmental (light-dark cycle) time cues.

The circadian timing system becomes mature after around 6 months of age and seems to remain stable in the course of early and middle childhood, although research in this age range is limited (but see the recent article presenting the Children's ChronoType Questionnaire[15]). Several distinct changes of circadian regulation occur during puberty and influence the sleep phase delay common for most teenagers across many societies and cultures.[21,41] Three circadian timing mechanisms have been proposed to govern the adolescent sleep phase delay.[21] First, the intrinsic circadian phase undergoes a delay in association with puberty[16]; thus, the correlation of pubertal stage with the circadian phase marker melatonin shows that mature children show a late timing of melatonin secretion onset and offset phases. Second, the delay of the circadian phase may be related to a lengthening of the intrinsic period of the circadian clock.[21] Data suggest, but do not conclusively support, this hypothesis, showing longer intrinsic period in adolescents versus adults but not across adolescent development. Third, heightened sensitivity to evening light or decreased sensitivity to morning light across pubertal development may also drive a sleep phase delay, although data supporting this hypothesis are minimal. In contrast, a recent review provided supporting evidence for a juvenile phase delay in nonhuman mammals.[42] In addition to these proposed intrinsic changes to the circadian timing system, behaviorally guided changes in the timing of light exposure (eg, by TV watching late at night) may directly interact with the phase-resetting mechanism of the circadian timing system and reinforce or strengthen the phase delay tendency of teenagers.

Development of Sleep Homeostasis

Sleep is already homeostatically regulated early in human life[29,43,44]; brief episodes of sleep deprivation in young infants lead to compensatory increases of sleep time and intensity. Because sleep loss tolerance of newborns is low, infants cannot sustain consolidated periods of wakefulness. Several studies suggest that the accumulation rate of homeostatic sleep pressure with waking during the day and its dissipation during sleep are faster in infants than in adults.[29,44] Adult sleep pressure is indexed by SWA (EEG spectral power 0.5–4.5 Hz), whereas, in infants, θ activity (4.5–7 Hz) may be a marker for sleep homeostatic pressure.[29] The age at which SWA becomes the sleep homeostatic marker is not known. However, the effects of adolescent sleep deprivation on the sleep EEG are similar to those in young adults; the homeostatic response of SWA to sleep loss is manifested in 10-year-old children.[45] The increase rate of homeostatic sleep pressure during the day is slower in mature adolescents compared with prepubertal or early pubertal children, which may contribute to their differences in sleep timing (ie, the delay of the sleep phase[45]). However, the nocturnal dissipation of sleep pressure (reflecting recovery processes during sleep) does not differ between prepubertal and mature teenagers, which is in accordance with the notion that sleep need does not change in the course of pubertal maturation.[27]

These recent findings support the view that the dynamics of sleep homeostatic mechanisms slow down in the course of development (see also Jenni and LeBourgeois[2]). It is likely that younger children accumulate sleep pressure more quickly across the day than older children, thereby necessitating longer and more frequent daily daytime naps, and accounting for shorter nap sleep-onset latencies. If homeostatic sleep pressure accumulates more slowly across development, then older children should be able to sustain wakefulness for longer periods of time, resulting in fewer naps per week, shorter nap durations, and eventually a consolidated sleep-wake pattern. In addition, this developmental process may decrease the sensitivity to sleep loss in the course of puberty and increase the tolerance to sleep pressure, a prerequisite for adult lifestyles in modern societies.

Interaction of Circadian Processes and Sleep Homeostasis

Although sleep homeostatic and circadian processes are independent mechanisms, they interact in a complex way to control vigilance states and sleep timing. The increase of homeostatic sleep pressure during waking is opposed by the increasing circadian alertness in the course of the day, allowing adults to maintain constant levels of vigilance throughout the waking period. In contrast, during sleep, the increasing circadian sleep tendency counteracts the declining homeostatic sleep pressure, ensuring maintenance of sleep. The developing interaction of the 2 processes seems to be a key determinant for sleep-wake behavior in young humans. For example, adolescent development may result in a changed phase relationship between these 2 processes, as proposed by Carskadon and Acebo.[41]

In the well-slept pubertal child, the alignment of the 2 processes fully supports sustained waking alertness during the day and sleep during the night. However, with adolescent development, the delay of the circadian phase reorganizes the alignment such that, even in a well-slept adolescent, the circadian evening increase in alertness occurs later and contributes to developmental augmentation of daytime sleepiness at midday **(Fig. 6)**[18] and difficulty falling asleep at a reasonable

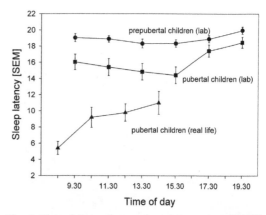

Fig. 6. Sleep latency (mean sleep latency test [MSLT]) profiles in well-slept prepubertal (*circles*) and pubertal (*squares*) adolescents under laboratory conditions and from pubertal adolescents under real life situations (*triangles*). SEM, standard error of mean (*Data from* Carskadon MA, Harvey K, Duke P, et al. Pubertal changes in daytime sleepiness. Sleep 1980;2:453–60; and Carskadon MA, Wolfson AR, Acebo C, et al. Adolescent sleep patterns, circadian timing, and sleepiness at a transition to early school days. Sleep 1998;21(8):871–81.)

time (vis-à-vis school demands) in the circadian evening wake-promoting zone. Furthermore, this rearranged adolescent phase alignment also contributes to severe difficulty waking up and intense sleepiness in morning hours when teens get too little sleep. One study showed short sleep latencies and sleep-onset REM episodes in adolescents with an early school start.[20]

In infant development, neither the interaction of the homeostatic and the circadian processes nor the nature of their sleep regulatory organization have been well studied. Nevertheless, it is likely that such an interaction contributes to the organization and timing of sleep and waking in early development. Thus, the development of a strong clock-dependent alerting signal in the absence of the opposing sleep homeostatic process during the first few months after birth may underlie the tendency for some infants to express crying behavior preferentially at certain times of day (ie, in the evening hours).

In conclusion, a misalignment of the 2 processes may lead to problems at sleep onset, nocturnal wakings, difficulties awakening in the morning, or daytime sleepiness, which are the 4 most common sleep problems during childhood.

THE SLEEP EEG DURING CHILDHOOD AND ADOLESCENCE: A WINDOW INTO THE DEVELOPING BRAIN

Several recent studies highlighted that sleep may be an undisturbed window into the developing brain.[46–51] For instance, the topographic distribution of SWA was shown to parallel cortical maturation during childhood and adolescence.[49] High-density EEG recordings between 2 and 20 years of age showed a shift of maximal SWA from posterior to anterior regions, reaching frontal derivations only during adolescence (**Fig. 7**).

The local SWA maxima parallels the time course of postmortem synaptic density,[52] cortical gray matter,[53,54] and behavioral maturation.[55] These findings may indicate that SWA is not only a good marker for sleep homeostasis, but also for cortical plasticity during development. This interpretation is in agreement with an increasing number of reports showing a direct relationship between sleep slow waves and plastic processes.[37,56] In the synaptic sleep homeostasis hypothesis, sleep slow waves were proposed to directly reflect changes in synaptic strength.[37] The close relationship between synaptic strength and sleep was shown in vitro,[57] in *Drosophila melanogaster*,[58] rats,[59] and also in humans.[60] Thus, we suggest that the functional relationship between sleep slow waves and synaptic strength explains the close correspondence between cortical maturation, including massive changes in synaptic strength and the topography of sleep SWA.

Another line of research is the examination of traitlike characteristics of the sleep EEG during development. Two recent studies indicated that, despite the massive changes in brain architecture and function discussed earlier, traitlike features can be detected in the sleep EEG of children and

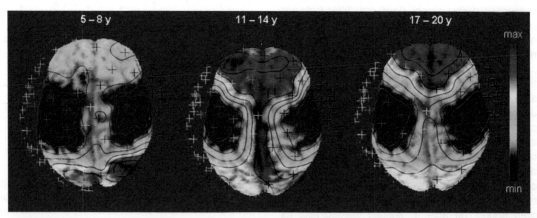

Fig. 7. Maps of SWA during NREM sleep. Topographic distribution of SWA (EEG power 1–4.5 Hz) for 3 age groups (5–8 years, n = 6; 11–14 years, n = 9; 17–20 years, n = 5). Maps are based on 109 electrodes (indicated by colored crosses) from the first 60 minutes of NREM sleep stages 2 and 3. Maps were normalized for each individual and then averaged for each age group. Values are color coded (maxima in red, minima in blue) and plotted on the planar projection of the hemispheric scalp model. Each map was proportionally scaled, and values between the electrodes were interpolated. (*Courtesy of* Reto Huber, PhD; and *Data from* Kurth S, Ringli M, Geiger A, et al. Mapping of cortical activity in the first two decades of life: a high-density sleep electroencephalogram study. J Neurosci 2010;30(40):13211–9.)

adolescents.[61,62] These finding suggest that the brain oscillators responsible for generating the sleep EEG signal remain stable across childhood and adolescence. Biologic endophenotypes are closer to gene function than behavioral measures and, thus, the sleep EEG represents a reliable biologic endophenotype during adolescent development.

We conclude from theses studies that the undisturbed recording of cortical activity during NREM sleep may be a useful tool to uncover aspects of brain maturation, function, and morphology in normal healthy children but also in children with developmental disorders. We eagerly await further developments in this area of research.

REFERENCES

1. Jenni OG, Werner H. Cultural issues in children's sleep: a model for clinical practice. Pediatr Clin North Am 2011;58(3):755–63.
2. Jenni OG, LeBourgeois MK. Understanding sleep-wake behavior and sleep disorders in children: the value of a model. Curr Opin Psychiatry 2006;19(3): 282–7.
3. Borbély AA. A two process model of sleep regulation. Hum Neurobiol 1982;1(3):195–204.
4. Kleitmann N, Engelmann TG. Sleep characteristics of infants. J Appl Physiol 1953;6:269–82.
5. Parmelee A. Sleep patterns in infancy. A Study of one infant from birth to eight months of age. Acta Paediatr 1961;50:160–70.
6. Iglowstein I, Jenni OG, Molinari L, et al. Sleep duration from infancy to adolescence: reference values and generational trends. Pediatrics 2003;11:302–7.
7. Jenni OG, DeBoer T, Achermann P. Development of the 24-h rest-activity pattern in human infants. Infant Behav Dev 2006;29:143–52.
8. Jenni OG, Fuhrer HZ, Iglowstein I, et al. A longitudinal study of bedsharing and sleep problems among Swiss children in the first 10 years of life. Pediatrics 2005;115:233–40.
9. Anders TF, Keener M. Developmental course of nighttime sleep-wake patterns in full-term and premature infants during the first year of life. Sleep 1985;8(3):173–92.
10. Lohr B, Siegmund R. Ultradian and circadian rhythms of sleep-wake and food-intake behavior during early infancy. Chronobiol Int 1999;16(2):129–48.
11. Olson LM, Inkelas M, Halfon N, et al. Overview of the content of health supervision for young children: reports from parents and pediatricians. Pediatrics 2004;113(Suppl 6):1907–16.
12. Jenni OG, O'Connor BB. Children's sleep: an interplay between culture and biology. Pediatrics 2005; 115:204–16.
13. Sadeh A, Mindell J, Rivera L. "My child has a sleep problem": a cross-cultural comparison of parental definitions. Sleep Med 2011;12(5):478–82.
14. Jenni OG, Molinari L, Caflisch JA, et al. Sleep duration from age 1 to 10 years: variability and stability in comparison with growth. Pediatrics 2007;120(4): e769–76.
15. Werner H, LeBourgeois MK, Geiger A, et al. Assessment of chronotype in four- to eleven-year-old children: reliability and validity of the Children's Chronotype Questionnaire (CCTQ). Chronobiol Int 2009;26(5):992–1014.
16. Carskadon MA, Acebo C, Richardson GS, et al. An approach to studying circadian rhythms of adolescent humans. J Biol Rhythms 1997;12(3):278–89.
17. Werner H, Jenni OG. Do parental expectations play a role in children's sleep and mothers' distress? an exploration of the goodness of fit concept in 54 mother-child dyads. Sleep Disorders 2011. http://dx.doi.org/10.1155/2011/104832.
18. Carskadon MA, Harvey K, Duke P, et al. Pubertal changes in daytime sleepiness. Sleep 1980;2:453–60.
19. Carskadon MA, Vieira C, Acebo C. Association between puberty and delayed phase preference. Sleep 1993;16(3):258–62.
20. Carskadon MA, Wolfson AR, Acebo C, et al. Adolescent sleep patterns, circadian timing, and sleepiness at a transition to early school days. Sleep 1998;21(8):871–81.
21. Carskadon MA, Acebo C, Jenni OG. Regulation of adolescent sleep: implications for behavior. Ann N Y Acad Sci 2004;1021:276–91.
22. Roenneberg T, Kuehnle T, Pramstaller PP, et al. A marker for the end of adolescence. Curr Biol 2004;14(24):R1038–9.
23. Grigg-Damberger M, Gozal D, Marcus CL, et al. The visual scoring of sleep and arousal in infants and children: development of polygraphic features, reliability, validity, and alternative methods. J Clin Sleep Med 2007;3(2):201–40.
24. Roffwarg HP, Muzio JN, Dement WC. Ontogenetic development of the human sleep-dream cycle. Science 1966;152(3722):604–19.
25. Campbell IG, Feinberg I. Longitudinal trajectories of non-rapid eye movement delta and theta EEG as indicators of adolescent brain maturation. Proc Natl Acad Sci U S A 2009;106(13):5177–80.
26. Feinberg I, Thode HC Jr, Chugani HT, et al. Gamma distribution model describes maturational curves for delta wave amplitude, cortical metabolic rate and synaptic density. J Theor Biol 1990;142(2):149–61.
27. Jenni OG, Carskadon MA. Spectral analysis of the sleep electroencephalogram during adolescence. Sleep 2004;27(4):774–83.
28. Bes F, Schulz H, Navelet Y, et al. The distribution of slow-wave sleep across the night: a comparison for infants, children, and adults. Sleep 1991;14(1):5–12.

29. Jenni OG, Borbély AA, Achermann P. Development of the nocturnal sleep electroencephalogram in human infants. Am J Physiol 2004;286:R528–38.

30. Achermann P, Borbély AA. Sleep homeostasis and models of sleep regulation. In: Kryger M, Roth T, Dement W, editors. Principles and practices of sleep medicine. 5th edition. St. Louis, MO: Elsevier Saunders; 2011. p. 431–44.

31. Borbély AA, Baumann F, Brandeis D, et al. Sleep deprivation: effect on sleep stages and EEG power density in man. Electroencephalogr Clin Neurophysiol 1981;51:483–93.

32. Daan S, Beersma DG, Borbély AA. Timing of human sleep: recovery process gated by a circadian pacemaker. Am J Physiol 1984;246(2 Pt 2): R161–83.

33. Kong J, Shepel PN, Holden CP, et al. Brain glycogen decreases with increased periods of wakefulness: implications for homeostatic drive to sleep. J Neurosci 2002;22(13):5581–7.

34. Porkka-Heiskanen T, Alanko L, Kalinchuk A, et al. Adenosine and sleep. Sleep Med Rev 2002;6(4): 321–32.

35. Porkka-Heiskanen T, Strecker RE, Thakkar M, et al. Adenosine: a mediator of the sleep-inducing effects of prolonged wakefulness. Science 1997;276(5316): 1265–8.

36. Tononi G, Cirelli C. Sleep and synaptic homeostasis: a hypothesis. Brain Res Bull 2003;62:143–50.

37. Tononi G, Cirelli C. Sleep function and synaptic homeostasis. Sleep Med Rev 2006;10:49–62.

38. Albrecht U, Eichele G. The mammalian circadian clock. Curr Opin Genet Dev 2003;13(3):271–7.

39. Rivkees SA. Developing circadian rhythmicity in infants. Pediatrics 2003;112(2):373–81.

40. Allen RP. Development of the human circadian cycle. In: Loughlin GM, Caroll JL, Marcus CL, editors. Sleep and Breathing in Children, vol. 147. New York: Marcel Dekker; 2000. p. 313–32.

41. Carskadon MA, Acebo C. Regulation of sleepiness in adolescents: update, insights, and speculation. Sleep 2002;25(6):606–14.

42. Hagenauer MH, Perryman JI, Lee TM, et al. Adolescent changes in the homeostatic and circadian regulation of sleep. Dev Neurosci 2009;31(4): 276–84.

43. Peirano P, Algarin C, Uauy R. Sleep-wake states and their regulatory mechanisms throughout early human development. J Pediatr 2003;143(Suppl 4): S70–9.

44. Salzarulo P, Fagioli I. Post-natal development of sleep organization in man: speculations on the emergence of the 'S process'. Neurophysiol Clin 1992;22(2):107–15.

45. Jenni OG, Achermann P, Carskadon MA. Homeostatic sleep regulation in adolescents. Sleep 2005; 28(11):1446–54.

46. Buchmann A, Ringli M, Kurth S, et al. EEG sleep slow-wave activity as a mirror of cortical maturation. Cereb Cortex 2011;21(3):607–15.

47. Feinberg I, Campbell IG. Sleep EEG changes during adolescence: an index of a fundamental brain reorganization. Brain Cogn 2010;72(1):56–65.

48. Feinberg I, de Bie E, Davis NM, et al. Topographic differences in the adolescent maturation of the slow wave EEG during NREM sleep. Sleep 2011; 34(3):325–33.

49. Kurth S, Ringli M, Geiger A, et al. Mapping of cortical activity in the first two decades of life: a high-density sleep electroencephalogram study. J Neurosci 2010;30(40):13211–9.

50. Tarokh L, Carskadon MA. Developmental changes in the human sleep EEG during early adolescence. Sleep 2010;33(6):801–9.

51. Tarokh L, Carskadon MA, Achermann P. Developmental changes in brain connectivity assessed using the sleep EEG. Neuroscience 2010;171(2):622–34.

52. Huttenlocher PR, Dabholkar AS. Regional differences in synaptogenesis in human cerebral cortex. J Comp Neurol 1997;387(2):167–78.

53. Gogtay N, Giedd JN, Lusk L, et al. Dynamic mapping of human cortical development during childhood through early adulthood. Proc Natl Acad Sci U S A 2004;101(21):8174–9.

54. Sowell ER, Thompson PM, Leonard CM, et al. Longitudinal mapping of cortical thickness and brain growth in normal children. J Neurosci 2004;24(38): 8223–31.

55. Luna B, Sweeney JA. The emergence of collaborative brain function: FMRI studies of the development of response inhibition. Ann N Y Acad Sci 2004;1021: 296–309.

56. Vyazovskiy VV, Olcese U, Lazimy YM, et al. Cortical firing and sleep homeostasis. Neuron 2009;63(6): 865–78.

57. Liu ZW, Faraguna U, Cirelli C, et al. Direct evidence for wake-related increases and sleep-related decreases in synaptic strength in rodent cortex. J Neurosci 2010;30(25):8671–5.

58. Bushey D, Tononi G, Cirelli C. Sleep and synaptic homeostasis: structural evidence in *Drosophila*. Science 2011;332(6037):1576–81.

59. Vyazovskiy VV, Cirelli C, Pfister-Genskow M, et al. Molecular and electrophysiological evidence for net synaptic potentiation in wake and depression in sleep. Nat Neurosci 2008;11(2):200–8.

60. Huber R, Ghilardi MF, Massimini M, et al. Local sleep and learning. Nature 2004;430(6995):78–81.

61. Geiger A, Huber R, Kurth S, et al. The sleep EEG as a marker of intellectual ability in school age children. Sleep 2011;34(2):181–9.

62. Tarokh L, Carskadon MA, Achermann P. Trait-like characteristics of the sleep EEG across adolescent development. J Neurosci 2011;31(17):6371–8.

Sleep in Normal Aging

Michael V. Vitiello, PhD

KEYWORDS

- Aging • Older adults • Sleep • Normal • Circadian rhythms • Sleep disorders • Napping
- Excessive daytime sleepiness

KEY POINTS

- Sleep in an older adult should not be assumed to be disturbed or of poor quality; many high-functioning older adults are satisfied with their sleep, even though it is of objectively poorer quality compared with younger adults.
- When screened for various factors that disrupt the sleep, such as health burden, primary sleep disorders, and poor sleep hygiene practice, aging adults can expect to undergo little change in their sleep, relative to those in the early to middle adult life span.
- Nevertheless, older adults can expect on average to be earlier to bed and to rise, and to be less tolerant of circadian phase shifts such as those induced by jet lag, than younger similarly healthy adults.

INTRODUCTION

As of 2006, persons 65 years of age or older comprise approximately 12% of the United States population, but by 2030 the proportion of older adults will increase to 20%. This older portion of the national population is increasing twice as fast as other age groups, so that by 2030 the number of persons 65 years or older in the United States will effectively double to 72 million. In this rapidly expanding older portion of the national population, one of the major changes that commonly accompany the aging process is an often profound disruption of an individual's daily sleep-wake cycle. As many as 50% of older individuals complain about sleep problems, including disturbed or "light" sleep, frequent awakenings, early-morning awakenings, and undesired daytime sleepiness.[1–3] Such disturbances can lead to impaired daytime function and seriously compromise quality of life.

The most striking change in sleep in older adults is the repeated and frequent interruption of sleep by long periods of wakefulness, possibly the result of an age-dependent intrinsic lightening of homeostatic processes of sleep.[4,5] Furthermore, older adults are more easily aroused from nighttime sleep by auditory stimuli, suggesting that they may be more sensitive to environmental stimuli.[6] Both of these changes indicate impaired sleep maintenance and depth, and contribute to the characterization of the sleep of older adults as "lighter," or more fragile, than that of younger adults.

These age-associated increases of nighttime wakefulness are mirrored by increases in daytime fatigue, excessive daytime sleepiness, and increased likelihood of napping or falling asleep during the day. Aging is also associated with a tendency to both fall asleep and awaken earlier (eg, Ref.[7]); that is, a tendency for older individuals to be "larks" rather than "owls." Older individuals also tend to be less tolerant of phase shifts in time of the sleep-wake schedule such as those produced by jet lag and shift work.[8,9] These changes suggest an age-related breakdown of the normal adult circadian sleep/wake cycle.

Even carefully screened older adults who do not complain of sleep disturbance and with minimal medical burdens show the changes described

This article originally appeared in *Sleep Medicine Clinics, Volume 1, Issue 2.*
Supported by PHS grants AG025515, HP70139, AT002108, MH072736, and NR04101.
Department of Psychiatry and Behavioral Sciences, University of Washington, Room BB-1520D, Box 356560, 1959 Northeast Pacific Street, Seattle, WA 98195-6560, USA
E-mail address: vitiello@u.washington.edu

Sleep Med Clin 7 (2012) 539–544
http://dx.doi.org/10.1016/j.jsmc.2012.06.007
1556-407X/12/$ – see front matter © 2012 Elsevier Inc. All rights reserved.

above when compared with the younger adults.[10,11] This finding suggests that at least some of the sleep disturbance seen in older adults is part of the aging process per se, apparently independent of any medical or psychiatric illnesses or primary sleep disorders, and often referred to as age-related sleep change.[12-14] A 60-year-old generally does not expect to be able to do all things as well as when he or she was 20. Similarly, the ability to sleep need not be the same. Just as older individuals can no longer run a 100-yard dash with the speed of youth because of the physiologic changes that accompany the aging process, so too can they no longer sleep with the relatively undisturbed length and depth of the sleep of their younger years. Whether this age-related decline in the ability to generate sleep equates with a decreased need for sleep in the later years of the human life span remains unclear. Nevertheless, the available scientific evidence suggests that it is important to remember that as we age it might be best to modify our expectations about our "inalienable rights" to life, liberty, and ... 8 hours of sound, uninterrupted sleep.

SLEEP IN NORMAL AGING

Clearly sleep changes with advancing age, but the question remains, exactly when do these changes occur? Since the publication of the classic article by Roffwarg and colleagues in 1966,[14] the accepted wisdom has been that the age-related sleep changes that characterize the sleep of older adults begin to appear in early adulthood and progress steadily across the full continuum of the adult human life span, including the older adult years. Nearly 50 years of regular republication of the sleep change across the human life span described by Roffwarg and colleagues,[14] by the current author among many others, essentially reified this assumption.

However, more recent findings call this assumption into serious question. The results of an extensive meta-analysis of objective sleep measures across the human life span by Ohayon and colleagues[15] in 2004 demonstrated that the bulk of the changes seen in adult sleep patterns occur between early adulthood, beginning at age 19 and age 60, and that after age 60 changes in sleep macroarchitecture effectively asymptote, declining only minimally from age 60 to 102 years.

The adult life span sleep changes reported by Ohayon and colleagues[15] are summarized in **Table 1**. These results are based on meta-analyses conducted on data from 2391 adults aged 19 to 102 years. When the full adult life span was examined, the investigators confirmed

Table 1
Summary of significant findings from meta-analyses examining the associations between various sleep measures and age across both the full adult life span (19–102 years) and the older adult life span (60–102 years)

	Adults 19–102 y	Older Adults 60–102 y
Total sleep time	⇩	⇔
Sleep latency	⇔	⇔
WASO	⇧	⇔
Sleep efficiency	⇩	⇩
Percent Stage 1	⇧	⇔
Percent Stage 2	⇧	⇔
Percent SWS	⇩	⇔
Percent REM	⇩	⇔
REM latency	⇔	⇔

Abbreviations: REM, rapid eye movement sleep; SWS, slow-wave sleep; WASO, wake after sleep onset; ⇔, unchanged; ⇩, decreased; ⇧, increased.
From Ohayon MM, Carskadon M, Guilliminault C, et al. Meta-analysis of quantitative sleep parameters from childhood to old age in healthy individuals: developing normative sleep values across the human lifespan. Sleep 2004;27(7):1255–73; with permission.

the 4 consistently reported age-related changes in polysomnographic studies of sleep macroarchitecture: decreases in total sleep time (TST), sleep efficiency (SE), and slow-wave sleep (SWS); and increases in wake after sleep onset (WASO). Ohayon and colleagues further demonstrated that less consistently reported age-related sleep changes were all observed in their meta-analyses: increases in Stage 1 (S1) and Stage 2 (S2) sleep; and decreases in rapid eye movement (REM) stage sleep. However, they also reported that age-related changes in either sleep latency or REM latency were minimal.

However, all of these significant age changes in objectively assessed sleep architecture were found only when the full adult life span was examined. When the sleep of only older (>60 years) adults was examined, meta-analyses demonstrated that only SE declined significantly from ages 60 to 70 to ages 70 years or older, and even then at a modest rate of approximately 3% per decade. None of the other 8 sleep measures showed any significant age-related change within the older adult portion of the study sample. It is also of interest that these findings were comparable for both older men and older women.

These findings seem counterintuitive, and fly against the wind of our commonly held concepts of sleep changes with aging. However, it is important to remember that Ohayon and colleagues used very rigorous selection criteria in choosing the study subjects for their meta-analyses. The approximately 2400 subjects were not representative of the older population, but rather were in excellent health and more likely represent individuals who are "optimally" or "successfully" aging. That is, the findings report "normative" sleep-architecture data representing only those older adults who are in very good health, and not average data for the overall older adult population, an extremely important distinction.

To better illustrate this crucial point, it is informative to contrast the findings of Ohayon and colleagues with those of a recent large (2685 subjects) cross-sectional study of objective sleep measures of adults (age 37–92 years), the Sleep Heart Health Study (SHHS) cohort.[16] In this large and well-conducted study, Redline and colleagues concluded, among other things, that "…sleep architecture varies with sex, [and] age…" and that "men, but not women, show evidence of poorer sleep with aging…" These conclusions seem at odds with those of Ohayon and colleagues; however, several important differences in the two studies need to be considered, beyond the obvious one of Ohayon and colleagues' being a meta-analysis and Redline and colleagues' being the report of a prospective cohort study. First, and perhaps most important, the SHHS cohort was "…recruited from 9 existing epidemiological studies in which data on cardiovascular risk factors had been collected…" forming a cohort which "…met the inclusion criteria (age ≥40 years), no history of sleep apnea, no tracheotomy, and no current home oxygen therapy…" This relatively mild screening is in marked contrast to the extensive screening criteria used to develop the study sample of Ohayon and colleagues.[15] Second, Redline and colleagues, when examining possible age effects, did not break down their sample to see if there were any age effects in the older half of their sample, but rather examined such effects across the full age range available.[16]

Essentially the two studies are complementary, with Ohayon and colleagues reporting on the impact of age in individuals who are aging "successfully" while Redline and colleagues, with their much more liberal selection criteria, are reporting on the impact of age in a group of individuals who are likely much more representative of the older population as a whole; in other words they are reporting on "average" aging. It is of particular interest that Redline concludes that men, but not women, tend to show poorer sleep with aging.[16] Likely this is the result of excess subclinical morbidity in men, because when such morbidity is screened out, as in the case of Ohayon and colleagues,[15] there are minimal sex differences in the sleep of men and women across the adult life span.

What all of these finding suggest is that sleep clearly changes significantly across the human life span. However, when the comorbidities that typically accompany the aging process are controlled for and optimal aging examined, the bulk of age-related sleep changes occurs in early and middle adulthood (years 19–60) and after age 60, assuming one is in good health, further age-related sleep changes are, at most, modest. Conversely, if co-morbidities are present, it is clear that normal age-related sleep changes may well be exacerbated.

CIRCADIAN RHYTHMS IN NORMAL AGING

Not only does the quality of sleep change across the human life span as already described, but the timing of that sleep also changes with aging. Circadian rhythms are those that occur within a period of 24 hours (from the Greek "about {circa} a day {dies}"), such as the adult human sleep/wake cycle. The impact of aging on human circadian rhythms has recently been comprehensively reviewed by Monk.[17] As with sleep, there is a considerable disparity regarding the conventional wisdom concerning circadian rhythms and aging, as well as the evidence supporting or not supporting such conventionally held beliefs. Monk summarizes the conventional wisdom regarding what happens to human circadian processes with aging as: (1) circadian amplitude is reduced; (2) there is a circadian phase advance, that is, the circadian rhythm moves earlier relative to the environment; (3) there is a shortening of the circadian free-running period (tau); and (4) the ability to tolerate rapid phase shifts, such as shift work or rapid transmeridian travel (jet lag), declines.[17]

However, the available evidence convincingly supports only 2 of these assumptions: older people tend to have earlier circadian phases, with a corresponding tendency to go to and rise from bed earlier than younger adults (eg, Ref.[7]); and, have more trouble than younger adults adjusting to the rapid phase shifts of shift work and jet lag, at least in terms of sleep quality, subjective complaint and performance measures (eg, Refs.[8,9]). It is interesting that the data in support of diminished circadian amplitudes and shortened circadian taus in healthy older adults are, at best, equivocal.[17]

NAPPING AND EXCESSIVE DAYTIME SLEEPINESS IN NORMAL AGING

Two other commonly held assumptions about sleep and aging are that older adults typically nap more than younger adults and report more excessive daytime sleepiness (EDS). While numerous community-based epidemiologic studies have reported prevalence rates for sleep disturbances, daytime sleep-related complaints such as EDS, and possibly undiagnosed sleep disorders among older adults to be as high as 20% to 30%,[1,18,19] few of these have reported the prevalence of regular napping and its association with sleep complaints and other mental and physical health problems, especially in relation to EDS.[18] Perhaps surprisingly, while epidemiologic studies typically show a significant increase in the prevalence of regular napping with advancing age, a similar increase in the prevalence of EDS among older adults is not demonstrated.[18,20] Consistent with the aforementioned findings for nighttime sleep measures, more recent findings indicate that the presence of comorbidities (medical illness, depression, and so forth) is highly associated with the likelihood of an older adult reporting regular napping or EDS.[21,22] That is, healthy older adults, even those complaining of significant nighttime sleep disturbance, are much less likely to report regular napping or EDS than their more health-burdened cohorts.

Regarding napping behavior, there is also considerable debate as to whether regular napping among older adults, particularly those in good health, may be beneficial to daytime wakefulness or perhaps detrimental to their nighttime sleep propensity.[23–25] The two studies that examined the impact of daytime napping on the nighttime sleep quality of healthy older adults found that napping had only a mild to moderate impact on nighttime sleep quality[24,25]; one of them further demonstrated that such napping resulted in improved cognitive performance post nap.[24] However, these results need to be interpreted with caution, as it must be emphasized that the subjects involved were healthy older adults without significant sleep complaints, and neither older adults unhappy with their sleep quality nor geriatric insomniacs. It is unclear whether similar results would be obtained, for example, with a sample of older insomniacs.

CAUSES OF DISTURBED SLEEP IN OLDER ADULTS

Much has been made of the often repeated fact that epidemiologic studies report that as much as 50% of older adults complain of significant, chronic sleep disturbance. However, it is important to keep in mind that 50% of older adults do not! Ohayon and colleagues[15] demonstrated that the bulk of age-related sleep changes occur in early to middle adulthood and that the sleep of very healthy older adults changes only very slowly across the later human life span. It has

Table 2
Causes of poor sleep in older adults

Cause/Problem	Examples
Physiologic	Age-related sleep change Age-related circadian rhythm change (phase advance)
Medical illnesses	Arthritis or other conditions causing chronic or intermittent pain Chronic cardiac or pulmonary disease Gastroesophageal reflux disorder
Psychiatric illnesses	Depression
Medications	Diuretics (leading to nocturnal awakenings) Inappropriate use of over-the-counter medications
Primary sleep disorders	Sleep-disordered breathing (sleep apnea) Restless legs syndrome REM behavior disorder
Behavioral/social	Retirement/lifestyle change reducing need for regular bed and rise times Death of a family member or friend Inappropriate use of social drugs Transmeridian air travel Napping
Environmental	Bedroom environment (eg, ambient noise, temperature, light, bedding) Moving to a new home, or downsizing to a smaller space or a retirement community or related facility Institutionalization

correspondingly been demonstrated that older adults who do not complain of any sleep problems nevertheless have objective sleep quality that is markedly compromised (eg, less TST, SE, and SWS, and more WASO) compared with that of healthy, non–sleep-complaining, younger adults. Nevertheless, there are many factors over and above age-related sleep (both sleep homeostatic and circadian) changes that can and do contribute to the significant sleep disturbance reported by nearly half of all older adults. These factors can include: (1) medical and psychiatric comorbidities and their treatments, such as cardiovascular disease, arthritis, gastroesophageal reflux, or depression, and many of the drugs used to treat them; (2) primary sleep disorders, many of which such as sleep apnea, restless legs syndrome, and REM behavior disorder, tend to occur with increasing frequency in older adults; (3) the many behavioral, environmental, and social factors, often collectively referred to as sleep hygiene, which can maximize or compromise an individual's sleep quality; or (4) some combination of these factors.[12,13,26] A more comprehensive list of these factors is given in **Table 2**, and many of these issues are explored in the articles that follow this one.

SUMMARY

There is no reason to assume, a priori, that the sleep of an older adult is necessarily disturbed or of poor quality; in fact, many high-functioning older adults are satisfied with their sleep, even though it is of objectively poorer quality compared with that of younger adults. It further appears that, when the various factors that can disrupt sleep (health burden, primary sleep disorders, poor sleep hygiene practices, and so forth) are screened out, optimally or successfully aging adults can expect to undergo little change in their sleep, relative to those in the early to middle adult life span, and not be likely to experience excessive daytime sleep and the concomitant need to nap regularly during the day. Nevertheless, even successfully aging older adults can expect on average to be earlier to bed and to rise, and to be less tolerant of circadian phase shifts, such as those induced by jet lag, than younger similarly health adults.

REFERENCES

1. Foley DJ, Monjan AA, Brown SL, et al. Sleep complaints among older persons: an epidemiological study of three communities. Sleep 1995;18:425–32.

2. Foley DJ, Monjan A, Simonsick EM, et al. Incidence and remission of insomnia among elderly adults: an epidemiologic study of 6,800 persons over three years. Sleep 1999;2(Suppl 22):S366–72.

3. Vitiello MV, Foley D, Stratton KL, et al. Prevalence of sleep complaints and insomnia in the Vitamins And Lifestyle (VITAL) Study cohort Of 77,000 older men and women [abstract]. Sleep 2004;27(Suppl):A120.

4. Dijk DJ, Duffy JF, Riel E, et al. Ageing and the circadian and homeostatic regulation of human sleep during forced desynchrony of rest, melatonin and temperature rhythms. J Physiol 1999;516(Pt 2):611–27.

5. Dijk DJ, Duffy JF, Czeisler CA. Age-related increase in awakenings: impaired consolidation of nonREM sleep at all circadian phases. Sleep 2001;24(5):565–77.

6. Zepelin H, McDonald CS, Zammit GK. Effects of age on auditory awakening thresholds. J Gerontol 1984; 39(3):294–300.

7. Duffy JF, Zeitzer JM, Rimmer DW, et al. Peak of circadian melatonin rhythm occurs later within the sleep of older subjects. Am J Physiol Endocrinol Metab 2002;282(2):E297–303.

8. Harma MI, Hakola T, Akerstedt T, et al. Age and adjustment to night work. Occup Environ Med 1994;51(8):568–73.

9. Bonnefond A, Harma M, Hakola T, et al. Interaction of age with shift-related sleep-wakefulness, sleepiness, performance, and social life. Exp Aging Res 2006;32(2):185–208.

10. Buysse DJ, Reynolds CF 3rd, Monk TH, et al. Quantification of subjective sleep quality in healthy elderly men and women using the Pittsburgh Sleep Quality Index (PSQI). Sleep 1991;14(4):331–8.

11. Vitiello MV, Larsen LH, Moe KE. Age-related sleep change: gender and estrogen effects on the subjective-objective sleep quality relationships of healthy, non-complaining older men and women. J Psychosom Res 2004;56(5):503–10.

12. Vitiello MV. Normal versus pathological sleep changes in aging humans. In: Kuna ST, Suratt PM, Remmers JE, editors. Sleep and respiration in aging adults. New York: Elsevier; 1991. p. 71–6.

13. Vitiello MV. Effective treatment of sleep disturbances in older adults. Clin Cornerstone 2000;2(5):16–27.

14. Roffwarg HP, Muzio JN, Dement WC. Ontogenetic development of the human sleep-dream cycle. Science 1966;152:604–19.

15. Ohayon MM, Carskadon MA, Guilleminault C, et al. Meta-analysis of quantitative sleep parameters from childhood to old age in healthy individuals: developing normative sleep values across the human lifespan. Sleep 2004;27(7):1255–73.

16. Redline S, Kirchner HL, Quan SF, et al. The effects of age, sex, ethnicity, and sleep-disordered breathing on sleep architecture. Arch Intern Med 2004;164(4):406–18.

17. Monk TH. Aging human circadian rhythms: conventional wisdom may not always be right. J Biol Rhythms 2005;20(4):366–74.

18. Young TB. Epidemiology of daytime sleepiness: definitions, symptomatology, and prevalence. J Clin Psychiatry 2004;65(Suppl 16):12–6.

19. Ohayon MM. Epidemiology of insomnia: what we know and what we still need to learn. Sleep Med Rev 2002;6:97–111.

20. Metz ME, Bunnell DE. Napping and sleep disturbances in the elderly. Fam Pract Res J 1990;10: 47–56.

21. Vitiello MV, Larsen LH, Bliwise DL, et al. Relationship of regular napping to health and self-reported sleep quality in older adults: results from the 2003 NSF Sleep in America poll [abstract]. Sleep 2004; 27(Suppl):A126.

22. Foley DJ, Vitiello MV, Bliwise DL, et al. Frequent napping is associated with excessive daytime sleepiness, depression, pain and nocturia in older adults: findings from the National Sleep Foundation "2003 Sleep in America" poll. Am J Geriatr Psychiatry 2007;15:344–50.

23. Tamaki M, Shirota A, Tanaka H, et al. Effects of a daytime nap in the aged. Psychiatry Clin Neurosci 1999;53:273–5.

24. Campbell SS, Murphy PJ, Stauble TN. Effects of a nap on nighttime sleep and waking function in older subjects. J Am Geriatr Soc 2005;53:48–53.

25. Monk TH, Buysse DJ, Carrier J, et al. Effects of afternoon "siesta" naps on sleep, alertness, performance, and circadian rhythms in the elderly. Sleep 2001;24(6):680–7.

26. Vitiello MV, Moe KE, Prinz PN. Sleep complaints co-segregate with illness older adults: clinical research informed by and informing epidemiological studies of sleep. J Psychosom Res 2002;53:555–9.

Neurobiological Mechanisms in Chronic Insomnia

Michael Perlis, PhD[a],*, Wil Pigeon, PhD[b],
Phil Gehrman, PhD[a], Jim Findley, PhD[a],
Sean Drummond, PhD[c]

KEYWORDS

• Insomnia • Neurobiology • VLPO • ARAS • Homeostasis • Inhibition of wakefulness

KEY POINTS

- This article states that insomnia can or should be defined in physiologic terms; insomnia is better understood from a neurobiological perspective.
- A review of the neurobiology of sleep and wakefulness is provided with a special emphasis on the implications for insomnia.
- A complete understanding of insomnia requires the neurobiological characterization of insomnia be informed by modern cognitive concepts and methods.

INTRODUCTION

Insomnia has long been conceptualized in psychologic and physiologic terms[1]; hence, the primary diagnostic classification of "psychophysiologic" insomnia. This diagnostic category[2] was adopted to indicate that this form of sleep disturbance was primary (a disorder vs. a symptom) and determined by both psychologic and physiologic factors. Psychological factors were thought to be related to cognitive phenomena, such as worry and rumination, and behavioral processes, such as instrumental and classical conditioning. Physiologic factors were thought to be related to elevated heart rate, respiration rate, muscle tone, and so on (ie, elevated end organ tone and/or increased metabolic rate). The term psychophysiologic insomnia (as opposed to the alternative construction physiopsychological insomnia) implies that this form of insomnia occurs primarily as a physiologic phenomenon. This conceptualization not only questions the primacy of cognition[3] in insomnia but also leads one to wonder whether somatic hyperarousal (or elevated metabolic rate) is appropriately identified as the primary cause. The emphasis on physiology seems to be a historical precedent than the likely possibility that somatic arousal is sufficiently elevated in patients with chronic insomnia to directly interfere with sleep initiation and maintenance.

The alternative perspective is, if "sleep is of the brain, by the brain, and for the brain,"[4] that insomnia is better conceptualized in terms of abnormal neurobiology. This perspective is supported by the information provided regarding (1) the brain structures that are implicated in sleep-wake regulation and how abnormal function within these areas may lead to specific insomnia complaints and (2) the neurophysiologic control of sleep and wakefulness and how dysregulation at the system level may contribute to the incidence and severity of insomnia. Following this review, information is provided regarding insomnia in terms of neurobiological abnormalities as assessed with

This article originally appeared in *Sleep Medicine Clinics Volume 4, Issue 4*.
[a] Behavioral Sleep Medicine Program, Department of Psychiatry, University of Pennsylvania, Suite 670, 3535 Market Street, Philadelphia, PA 19104, USA; [b] Sleep and Neurophysiology Research Laboratory, Department of Psychiatry, University of Rochester, 300 Crittenden Boulevard, Rochester, NY 14642, USA; [c] Laboratory of Sleep & Behavioral Neuroscience, UCSD and VA San Diego Healthcare System, 3350 La Jolla Village Drive, MC 151B, Building 13, 3rd Floor, San Diego, CA 92161, USA
* Corresponding author.
E-mail address: mperlis@upenn.edu

Sleep Med Clin 7 (2012) 545–554
http://dx.doi.org/10.1016/j.jsmc.2012.06.005
1556-407X/12/$ – see front matter © 2012 Elsevier Inc. All rights reserved.

neurophysiological, neuroendocrine, and neuroimaging measures. This overview concludes with a comment on the dual nature of psychophysiologic insomnia.

STRUCTURES IMPLICATED IN SLEEP-WAKE REGULATION AND DYSREGULATION

Although this article does not review every brain structure that is thought to play a role in sleep-wake regulation, a short review illustrates the role of functional neurobiology in understanding the clinical entity of insomnia. Information regarding the role of the following brain regions is provided: the pons, the thalamus, the frontal cortex, and the basal ganglia.

Pons

The pons is located in the brain stem and contains nuclei that are related to the coordination of eye and facial movements, facial sensation, hearing, balance, respiration, and the genesis of REM sleep. Because pons is mostly dedicated to the performance of nonautonomic functions, the behavioral quiescence of NREM sleep is paralleled by the global deactivation within this region. An equally important consideration is the extent to which the aminergic and cholinergic components of the ascending reticular activating system (ARAS) (see below) reside within, or traverse through, the pons. The most straightforward consequence of hyperarousal in the pons on NREM sleep would be a direct link to the inability to initiate and maintain sleep. At the level of patient report, this condition would translate as the complaint of feeling alert while desiring to fall asleep.

Thalamus

The thalamus contains a variety of nuclei that are believed to process and relay sensory information to various parts of the cerebral cortex. For example, visual information from the eyes travels to the thalamus on the way to the occipital cortex. The thalamus also contains structures (the reticular nuclei) that actively inhibit sensory flow from the thalamus to the cortex. Increased thalamic activation in the nuclei related to sensory processing and/or decreased activity within the reticular nuclei during sleep could lead to more sensory information reaching the cortex and thus greater sensory processing perisleep onset or during sleep. Presumably, this mechanism would be related to the tendency of patients with insomnia to be hyper-responsive to environmental stimuli, which may account for patients' difficulties falling and staying asleep and/or the perception of shallow sleep. This mechanism might be the neurobiological basis of patients' reports of being light sleepers.

Frontal Cortex

The frontal lobes contain many subregions involved in cognitive processes related to, among other things, working memory, problem solving, the planning of goal-directed activity, and evaluative judgment.[5] Thus, abnormal activity in the frontal cortex will depend on the specific subregion involved and whether the area or circuit is inhibitory or excitatory. An example of excitatory subregions would be the dorsolateral prefrontal and left limbic areas. Activation within these areas is associated with anticipatory anxiety.[6] In insomnia, increased activation within this region is associated with the worry and rumination that may interfere with sleep initiation and possibly sleep maintenance. An example of inhibitory subregions would be the orbital frontal cortex and the cortical-striatal-thalamic-cortical loops.[7] Reduced activation in this region/circuit is associated with behavioral, and likely, cognitive disinhibition of subcortical structures. In this instance, hypoactivation may be associated with the tendency of patients with insomnia to be highly ruminative and their complaint of being unable to turn their minds off.[8–10]

Basal Ganglia

The primary structures of the basal ganglia (caudate, putamen, globus pallidus, substantia nigra, and subthalamic nucleus) and the striatum have major projections from the motor cortex and are known to play a well-defined role in the execution of voluntary movement. In addition, the basal ganglia has been (1) implicated in neurobiological models of obsessive compulsive disorder[11] and (2) found to play a role in the homeostatic regulation of sleep.

Regarding sleep homeostasis, Braun and colleagues[12] have hypothesized that the basal ganglia may be actively involved in the regulation of slow wave sleep because of their ability to modulate cortical arousal.[13] Structures within the basal ganglia may, in feed forward fashion, modulate the activity of the reticular nucleus of the thalamus and contribute to the homeostatic regulation of sleep.[14] The basal ganglia may not only be involved in the homeostatic regulation of sleep but also be the sleep homeostat itself because they are responsible for the execution of voluntary movement and potentially the modulation of cortical arousal. Thus, it is uniquely situated to modulate cortical arousal based on diurnal activity levels.

At the level of symptom complaint, abnormal metabolism within the basal ganglia during sleep may be associated with a variety of clinical phenomena. To the extent that the circuits are related to inhibition and disinhibition, abnormal activity within these regions may be associated with a patient's tendency to ruminate and worry. Alternatively, abnormal activity in the basal ganglia may be related to the homeostatic dysregulation that seems to occur with insomnia. To the extent that the basal ganglia are related to sleep homeostasis, it may account for the occurrence of sleep initiation and maintenance problems on a given night and for the cyclic pattern of symptoms across time.

NEUROPHYSIOLOGIC CONTROL OF SLEEP AND WAKEFULNESS

Based on the early work of Von Economo[15] and Moruzzi,[16–18] cortical arousal is regulated by the ARAS). This system originates in the brain stem with 2 major branches. One branch originates from cholinergic cell groups in the upper pons (including the pedunculopontine and the laterodorsal tegmental nuclei), inputs into the thalamus, and activates the thalamic relays that densely innervate the cortex. This system and its source neurons fire maximally during wakefulness and REM sleep and lowest during NREM sleep.[6,19–21] The other branch originates in the lower pons from a series of

neurons, including the locus coeruleus (norepinephrine), dorsal and medial raphe (serotonin), and tuberomammillary cells (histamine) to innervate neurons in the lateral hypothalamic area, the basal forebrain, and throughout the cortex. The ascending aspect of this system is monoaminergic and the end target neurons are cholinergic or γ-aminobutyric acid (GABA) -mediated. Neurons within this system fire maximally during wakefulness, more slowly during NREM sleep, and are relatively silent during REM sleep. This description of cortical arousal as it is modulated by the cholinergic and monoaminergic systems was, in 2000, significantly amended with the discovery of orexin (also called hypocretin).[22–25] This neurotransmitter seems to augment activity within the monoaminergic branch of the ARAS (particularly the output from the lateral hypothalamus) and is thought to act in concert with the circadian system to promote the consolidation of wakefulness during the diurnal phase of the 24-hour day. **Fig. 1** provides a schematic representation of the aforementioned arousal systems.

Although the above description serves to delineate the pathways within the ARAS and their relative degree of activation across the wake, NREM, and REM states, the characterization does not suggest how sleep is initiated, maintained, and terminated in favor of new episodes of wakefulness. To comprehend this mechanism, it is necessary to posit that there is either a gating system or

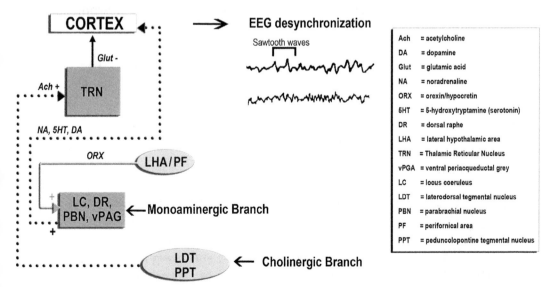

Fig. 1. Ascending pathways that lead to cortical desynchronization (activation). Although the cholinergic and monoaminergic branches of this system have been well characterized, orexinergic component (and its contribution to the consolidation of wakefulness) is relatively new. One of the many important aspects of this system is that this arousal system is not the same as the ARAS (the Ascending Reticular Activation System [the fight or flight system]) anatomically of functionally. With respect to the latter, the orexin system appears to be under the control of, or intimately related to, the circadian system.

a related descending system that influences the structures that initiate cortical arousal. In the cholinergic branch of the ARAS, there is substantial evidence to suggest that the reticular nucleus of the thalamus serves to block ascending inputs and thereby permit cortical synchronization (ie, sleep). In the monoaminergic branch of the ARAS, investigators during the 1980s and 1990s found a mechanism that might serve as the switch for a descending de-arousal system; the switch being the ventrolateral preoptic area (VLPO).[6,21] The VLPO is maximally active during sleep; has major *outputs* to most, if not all, the hypothalamic and brain stem components of the monoaminergic branch of the ARAS; and contains inhibitory neurotransmitters (ie, galanin and GABA). Thus, the VLPO seems to be uniquely positioned to function as an "off switch" (to inhibit arousal). This putative function was confirmed by Saper and colleagues,[6,21] who have shown that lesions within this region reduce NREM and REM sleep by more than 50%.

Saper and colleagues[6,21] have also demonstrated that the VLPO also has major *inputs* from the hypothalamic and brain stem components of the monoaminergic branch of the ARAS and that the VLPO is strongly inhibited by noradrenaline and serotonin. The existence of such inputs and neurotransmitter effects suggests that the VLPO not only inhibits wakefulness but also inhibited by

wakefulness. Saper and colleagues[6,21] compared this reciprocal relationship between the VLPO and the ARAS with the functioning of a "flip flop circuit." This analogy is taken from electrical engineering and provides a framework for conceptualizing how the wake-promoting and sleep-promoting halves of the circuit are mutually influential. Each half of the circuit strongly inhibits the other and creates a bistable feedback loop. When the brain is in a state of wakefulness, sleep is inhibited so that there is a consolidated period of wakefulness. When the switch moves in the sleep direction, wake is inhibited, producing a consolidated period of sleep. This pattern prevents frequent transitions between sleep and wake and the presence of intermediate states characterized by features of both wakefulness and sleep. **Fig. 2** represents the VLPO's inhibitory influence on the cortex and its "bi-stable" configuration.

Although elegant, this conceptualization also does not explain how sleep is initiated and terminated (ie, it only serves to explain how sleep and wakefulness tend to occur in a consolidated fashion). To initiate and terminate sleep, there must also be a system that impinges on the circuit and allows for homeostasis and allostasis.

In the case of sleep/wake homeostasis, there must be a process that represents the accumulation of wakefulness and/or sleep that can act to "trip the switch." The concept of sleep/wake homeostasis

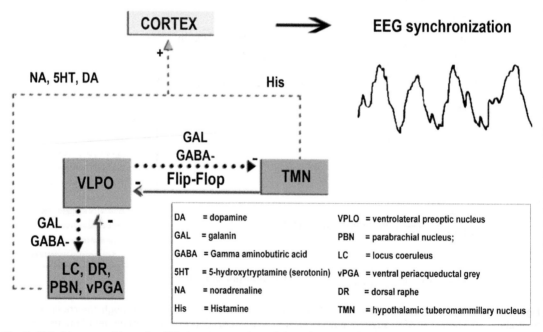

Fig. 2. This figure provides a simplified representation of the "Sleep Switch," ie, the circuit and ascending pathways that lead to cortical synchronization (deactivation). One of the many important aspects of this system is the mutually inhibitory functioning between the VLPA and the TMN. For a thorough review of this system the reader is referred to Saper and colleagues.[21]

(and its interaction with the circadian system) has been described theoretically and tested empirically by Borbely and colleagues.[26–29] In this model, the accumulation of wakefulness is represented by "Process S" and is measured in terms of the relationship between the duration of wakefulness and the discharge of slow wave activity during NREM sleep. To date, the neurobiological structures that comprise the sleep homeostat are unknown. The accumulation of adenosine within the basal forebrain may represent the duration of wakefulness. Experimental work with this hypothesis has shown that (1) adenosine levels increase in proportion to the duration of wakefulness and (2) when injected into the basal forebrain, adenosine induces sleep and promotes activity within the VLPO.

In the case of sleep/wake allostasis, it has been proposed that orexin neurons within the posterior half of lateral hypothalamus serve to reinforce wakefulness (promote sustained wakefulness) and thereby act as a "finger" on the flip-flop switch that prevents unwanted transitions into sleep[1].

NEUROBIOLOGICAL IMPLICATIONS FOR INSOMNIA

The above description of the normal regulation of sleep and wakefulness suggests that insomnia may occur in association with one of several neurobiological abnormalities. First, the switch itself may be malfunctioning. Saper and colleagues[6] describe this as follows

> ...mathematical models show that when either side of a flip-flop neural circuit is weakened, homeostatic forces cause the switch to ride closer to its transition point during both states. As a result, there is an increase in transitions, both during the wake and the sleep periods, regardless of which side is weakened. This is certainly seen in animals with VLPO lesions, which fall asleep about twice as often as normal animals, wake up much more often during their sleep cycle and, on the whole, only sleep for about one-quarter as long per bout - in other words, they wake up and are unable to fall back asleep during the sleep cycle, but also are chronically tired, falling asleep briefly and fitfully during the wake cycle....[6]

This description seems to characterize, not so much psychophysiologic insomnia, sleep as it occurs in neonates/infants and insomnia as it occurs in the elderly (ie, polyphasic sleep with middle and/or late insomnia), and/or in patients with narcolepsy. A malfunctioning switch could also produce an intermediate state characterized by aspects of both sleep and wakefulness. This malfunctioning can be seen in several studies of individuals with insomnia who, compared with good sleepers, show evidence of wakefulness in terms of increased beta electroencephalogram (EEG) activity while otherwise appearing to be asleep.

Chronic activation of the monoaminergic branch of the ARAS might lead to some form of desensitization and/or a compensatory down-regulation, which results in insufficient "force" to trip the switch and a switch that tends to favor the "wake on" position (ie, there is a failure to inhibit wakefulness and/or substantially more wakefulness is required to flip the switch to the sleep position.) In this instance, a decreased activation within the nuclei that input to the VLPO (eg, locus coeruleus, the dorsal and/or medial raphe, and/or the tuberomammillary cells) is expected. From a neuroendocrine point of view, however, continued evidence of hyperarousal in parallel with the neurobiological down-regulation is expected, that is, patients with chronic insomnia would exhibit hypercortisolemia, and/or excessive secretion of the monoamines and/or even hypocretin/orexin, despite diminished activity of the central nervous system . Evidence for some of these possibilities, which are presaged by the Psychobiological Inhibition Model,[30] are reviewed in the sections entitled Neuroendocrine Measures of Insomnia and Neuroimaging Measures of Insomnia.

The neurobiological abnormalities that occur with insomnia may occur within the cholinergic branch of the ARAS and appear as altered functioning within the thalamus, basal forebrain, and cortex. For example, one might expect

1. A reduction in activity during wakefulness within the adenosinergic regions of the basal forebrain
2. An overall decrease in cortical arousal during wakefulness
3. An increase in activity during the sleep period within the thalamic nuclei related to sensory processing and reduced activity within the sensory gating nuclei (ie, the reticular nucleus)
4. An overall increase in cortical arousal during sleep.

Alterations within this system may be relevant to sleep, not only for continued disturbance but also

---

[1] A second possible, albeit highly speculative, candidate mechanism for sleep wake homeostasis is noted in the above discussion regarding the Basal Ganglia.

the phenomenon of sleep state misperception as it is known to occur in psychophysiologic insomnia and paradoxical insomnia, and perhaps in all forms of primary insomnia (PI). The evidence for these possibilities, which are presaged by the Neurocognitive Model,[31] are also reviewed in the sections entitled Neurophysiologic Measures of Insomnia, neuroendocrine Measures of Insomnia, and Neuroimaging Measures of Insomnia.

EVIDENCE FOR NEUROBIOLOGICAL ABNORMALITIES IN INSOMNIA
Neurophysiologic Measures of Insomnia

To date, several studies have shown that patients with PI exhibit more cortical arousal than either good sleepers or patients with insomnia comorbid with major depression.[32–38] These studies show that patients with PI exhibit more high-frequency EEG activity (beta and gamma frequencies) at sleep onset and during NREM sleep. These EEG frequencies are associated with the active processing of mental information during wakefulness, suggesting that patients with insomnia have a failure to terminate mental processing while otherwise asleep. There is also evidence that (1) patients with sleep state misperception (ie, paradoxical insomnia) exhibit more beta EEG activity than good sleepers or patients with PI[38] and (2) beta EEG activity is negatively associated with the perception of sleep quality[39,40] and positively associated with the degree of subjective-objective discrepancy.[37] These data suggest that cortical arousal may occur uniquely in association with PI (ie, one or more of the types of PI, including psychophysiologic insomnia, paradoxical insomnia, idiopathic insomnia, etc.) and may be associated with the tendency toward sleep state misperception.

Comment

Although the data acquired from this measurement strategy strongly support cortical arousal as a biomarker for insomnia (and this is theoretically appealing to the extent that the increased occurrence of beta and gamma activity is thought to be permissive of increased sensory and information processing), the lack of replication across larger scale contemporary investigations[41] and unpublished studies (Buysse D, personal communication, 2005; Perlis M, unpublished work, 2005) suggests that this approach has some limitations. According to the authors, the occurrence of beta and gamma activity varies not only with trait considerations (diagnostic category) but also appears to be mediated/moderated by a variety of factors including first night effects,[42] prior sleep debt, degree of circadian dysrhythmia, type of

insomnia, technical considerations, and the extent of environmental noise. There is also recent evidence that beta and gamma activity varies by sex.[43]

Neuroendocrine Measures of Insomnia

Several studies have begun to examine the activation of stress response system in patients with insomnia, focusing on the hypothalamic-pituitary-adrenal (HPA) axis. These studies provide evidence that insomnia involves, or results from, chronic activation of the stress response system. Other neuroendocrine measures, including norepinephrine, melatonin, and, most recently, GABA have also been examined as potential correlates of insomnia.

Urinary measures

An early study of urinary free 11-hydroxycorticosteriods (11-OHCS), which are metabolites of HPA axis activity, in young adult good and poor sleepers found that the mean 24-hour rate of 11-OHCS excretion over 3 days was significantly higher in the poor sleepers.[44] A subsequent study of urinary cortisol and epinephrine in middle-aged good and poor sleepers found no significant differences although poor sleepers showed higher urinary cortisol and epinephrine secretion.[45,46] More recently, Vgontzas and colleagues[45,46] collected 24-hour urine specimens for urinary free cortisol (UFC), catecholamine metabolites (3,4-dihydroxyphenylglycol [DHPG] and 3,4-dihydroxyphenylacetic acid [DOPAC]), and growth hormone and correlated these measures with polysomnographic measures of sleep continuity and sleep architecture in subjects with PI. UFC levels were positively correlated with total wake time, and DHPG and DOPAC measures were positively correlated with percent stage 1 sleep and wake after sleep onset time. Although not statistically significant, norepinephrine levels tended to correlate positively with Stage 1 and wake after sleep onset, and negatively with percentage of slow wave sleep. These data suggest that HPA axis and sympathetic nervous system activity are associated with objective sleep disturbance.

Plasma measures

Plasma measures of corticotropin (ACTH) and cortisol have also been compared among patients with PI and matched with good sleepers. In one study, patients with insomnia had significantly higher mean levels of ACTH and cortisol over the course of the 24-hour day, with the largest group differences observed in the evening and first half of the night.[45,46] Patients with a high degree of sleep disturbance (sleep efficiency <70%)

secreted higher amounts of cortisol than patients with less sleep disturbance. In contrast to these findings, a recent study of patients with PI and age and gender matched good sleepers found no differences in the mean amplitude or area under the curve for cortisol secretion over a 16-hour period (19:00 to 09:00 hours).[47]

Comment

Some of the variability of neuroendocrine findings in insomnia may be explained by the intrusion of wakefulness into the measured sleep period. This intrusion is a particular concern for studies using urinary measures, which integrate biological activity over a long period. This possibility is important when considering causality, that is, whether increased HPA activity leads to insomnia or whether insomnia leads to increased HPA activity. However, there is a certain degree of face validity in the association between insomnia and HPA axis activity given the presumed relationship between stress and insomnia. A recent study investigating a possible animal model of acute insomnia demonstrated that activity in the amygdala, a key brain region for activation of the stress response, is critically necessary for stress-induced insomnia to occur.[48,49] There is evidence that the VLPO contains receptors for the stress hormone ACTH-releasing factor, suggesting that stress may have direct effects on the sleep switch.[6] Although the findings from various studies are not entirely consistent, the elevations in ACTH and cortisol levels before and during sleep in insomnia patients may help to shed light on the intimate association between insomnia and major depression, which is also associated with HPA axis activation. Specifically, insomnia is a risk factor for,[11,50–57] a prodromal symptom of,[58] and a ubiquitous[59,60] and persistent symptom of major depression.[60] The common link may be that acute stress leads to both an activation of the HPA axis and insomnia, and that chronic insomnia in turn leads to a persistent activation of the HPA axis.

Neuroimaging Measures of Insomnia

To date 2 studies on brain activity, which evaluate sleep in patients with insomnia have been undertaken: 1 using technetium hexamethylpropyleneamine oxime single-photon emission computed tomography (Tc 99 HMPAO SPECT) and the other using positron emission tomography (PET) with fludeoxyglucose F 18. In the Tc 99 HMPAO SPECT study, imaging was conducted around the sleep onset interval in patients with PI and good sleepers. Contrary to expectation, patients with insomnia exhibited a consistent pattern of reduced activity across 8 preselected regions of interest, with the

most prominent effect observed in the basal ganglia.[61] The frontal medial, occipital, and parietal cortices also showed significant decreases in blood flow compared with good sleepers. In the PET study, imaging data were acquired from patients with chronic insomnia and participants in the control group for an interval during wakefulness and during consolidated NREM sleep. Patients with insomnia exhibited increased global cerebral glucose metabolism during wakefulness and NREM sleep.[62] In addition, patients with insomnia exhibited smaller declines in relative glucose metabolism from wakefulness to sleep in wake-promoting regions, including the ARAS, hypothalamus, and thalamus. A smaller decrease was also observed in areas associated with cognition and emotion including the amygdala, hippocampus, insular cortex, and in the anterior cingulate and medial prefrontal cortices.

In addition to the brain activity studies, Winkelman and colleagues[63] used proton magnetic resonance spectroscopy to assess brain GABA levels in 16 patients with PI andcompared it with 16 good sleepers. GABA was measured in terms of global activity within the basal ganglia, thalamus, and the temporal, parietal, and occipital cortical areas. Average brain GABA levels were nearly 30% lower in patients with PI. Given that GABA is the primary inhibitor neurotransmitter in the brain, this finding suggests that there was less inhibition (ie, more activation) in the insomnia group. Further, GABA levels were negatively correlated with wake after sleep onset measures. This data suggest that (1) GABA deficiency may be a neurobiological characteristic of insomnia and (2) the efficacy of benzodiazepine hypnotics may reside in their potential to increase GABA secretion/activity within the brain.

Comment

Although results from the 2 studies on brain activity seem to be inconsistent, numerous methodological differences may help to explain differences in the findings. For example, the SPECT study with its short time resolution may have captured a more transient phenomenon that occurs when subjects with chronic and severe insomnia first achieve persistent sleep. The PET study with its longer time resolution may have captured a more stable phenomenon that occurs throughout NREM sleep in subjects with moderately chronic and severe insomnia. In addition to the temporal resolution issues, the PET study used a sample of insomnia patients who did not show objective sleep continuity disturbances in the laboratory, whereas the SPECT study included patients with objective sleep continuity disturbances. Thus, the samples may have differed with respect to the type of insomnia, the degree of partial sleep deprivation, and the degree of sleep state misperception. Although further studies are needed, these preliminary investigations clearly demonstrate the feasibility of using functional neuroimaging methods in the study of insomnia, and suggest that insomnia complaints may indeed have a basis in altered brain activity. For additional information on how imaging may be informative regarding the neurobiology of insomnia, the reader is referred to an article by Drummond and colleagues.[64]

SUMMARY

Although it is provocative and intellectually challenging to claim, in essence, that insomnia is "of the brain and by the brain...",[4] the causes and consequences of insomnia are not likely to be so narrowly circumscribed.

First, if chronic insomnia occurs because of the abnormal functioning of specific brain regions or the sleep-wake systems, it is still likely that the changes in brain function are permissive of cognitive processes that independently contribute to problems with initiating and maintaining sleep (and/or perceiving sleep as sleep). For example, if the insomnia occurs in relation to altered thalamic activation, the consequent increase in sensory processing (via either increased sensory flow or reduced sensory inhibition) likely independently contributes to insomnia because the individual experiences an increased sensitivity to external stimuli.

Second, if it is demonstrated that insomnia is neurobiological condition, it is still likely to be true that insomnia frequency, severity, and/or chronicity are mediated/moderated by cognitive and behavioral factors. For example, one may not be awake during the preferred sleep phase because of, for example, worry or attention bias, but these factors are nevertheless likely to exacerbate the condition in ways that make it more serve, more frequent, and more chronic.

Third, irrespective of the mechanisms that cause insomnia, it is likely that the condition interferes with many, if not, all the putative functions of sleep. Thus, in the end, the causes of insomnia may be primarily related to the brain, but the effects of insomnia may span many domains including both the psychological (eg, mood, daytime fatigue and/or sleepiness, cognitive capacity from executive function to long term memory) and the physiologic domains (eg, immunity, the capacity to recover from traumatic injury, and even longevity in the absence of illness).

In the final analysis, insomnia may be precisely, as it has been classically defined: a psychophysiologic condition. Perhaps the only difference between the original concept and the current one is a matter of scope. Originally, it may have been the case that (1) psychological factors were construed only in terms of mental phenomena like worry and rumination and behavioral phenomena, such as sleep extension and poor stimulus control, and (2) physiologic factors were construed only in terms of metabolic rate. At present, psychological factors include sensory and information processing abnormalities and attentional bias, and physiologic factors include not only end organ function and tone but also the brain abnormalities that may directly cause the insomnia condition. Expanding existing frames of reference in this manner may allow us to abandon the mind-brain dichotomies and longstanding discipline-specific research agendas (eg, psychology vs neuroscience) that have long plagued mind-brain research and specifically insomnia research. Further, expanding existing frames of reference in this manner may lead us to a new approach to the problem of insomnia, one that is more integrative and synthetic.

REFERENCES

1. Perlis ML, Smith MT, Pigeon WR. Etiology and pathophysiology of insomnia. In: Kryger M, Roth T, Dement WC, editors. Principle and practice of sleep medicine. Philadelphia: Elsevier Saunders; 2005. p. 714–25.
2. American Academy of Sleep Medicine. International classification of sleep disorders. Diagnostic and coding manual. Second edition. Westchester (IL): American Academy of Sleep Medicine; 2005.
3. Lazarus RS. On the primacy of cognition. Am Psychol 1984;39:124–9.
4. Hobson JA. Sleep is of the brain, by the brain and for the brain. Nature 2005;437:1254–6.
5. Eric Kandel, James Schwartz, Thomas Jessell. Principles of neural science. 4th edition. New York: McGraw-Hill; 2000.
6. Saper CB, Scammell TE, Lu J. Hypothalamic regulation of sleep and circadian rhythms. Nature 2005; 437:1257–63.
7. Tekin S, Cummings JL. Frontal-subcortical neuronal circuits and clinical neuropsychiatry–an update. J Psychosom Res 2002;53:647–54.
8. Lichstein KL, Rosenthal TL. Insomniacs' perceptions of cognitive versus somatic determinants of sleep disturbance. J Abnorm Psychol 1980;89:105–7.
9. Freedman RR, Sattler HL. Physiological and psychological factors in sleep-onset insomnia. J Abnorm Psychol 1982;91:380–9.

10. Nicassio PM, Mendlowitz DR, Fussell JJ, et al. The phenomenology of the pre-sleep state: the development of the pre-sleep arousal scale. Behav Res Ther 1985;23:263–71.

11. Chang PP, Ford DE, Mead LA, et al. Insomnia in young men and subsequent depression. The Johns Hopkins Precursors Study. Am J Epidemiol 1997; 146:105–14.

12. Braun AR, Balkin TJ, Wesenten NJ, et al. Regional cerebral blood flow throughout the sleep-wake cycle. An H2(15)O PET study. Brain 1997;120(Pt 7): 1173–97.

13. Lavin A, Grace AA. Modulation of dorsal thalamic cell activity by the ventral pallidum: its role in the regulation of thalamocortical activity by the basal ganglia. Synapse 1994;18:104–27.

14. Steriade M, Timofeev I, Durmuller N, et al. Dynamic properties of corticothalamic neurons and local cortical interneurons generating fast rhythmic (30-40 Hz) spike bursts. J Neurophysiol 1998;79:483–90.

15. Von Economo C. Sleep as a problem of localization. J Nerv Ment Dis 1949;71:249–59.

16. Moruzzi G. Sleep mechanisms. Summary statement. Prog Brain Res 1965;18:241–3.

17. Moruzzi G. Reticular influences on the EEG. Electroencephalogr Clin Neurophysiol 1964;16:2–17.

18. Moruzzi G, Magoun HW. Brain stem reticular formation and activation of the EEG. 1949. J Neuropsychiatry Clin Neurosci 1995;7:251–67.

19. Jones BE. The organization of central cholinergic systems and their functional importance in sleep-waking states. Prog Brain Res 1993;98:61–71.

20. Jones BE. Toward an understanding of the basic mechanisms of the sleep-waking cycle. Behav Brain Sci 1978;1:495.

21. Saper CB, Chou TC, Scammell TE. The sleep switch: hypothalamic control of sleep and wakefulness. Trends Neurosci 2001;24:726–31.

22. George CF, Singh SM. Hypocretin (orexin) pathway to sleep. Lancet 2000;355:6.

23. Kilduff TS, Peyron C. The hypocretin/orexin ligand-receptor system: implications for sleep and sleep disorders. Trends Neurosci 2000;23:359–65.

24. Siegel JM. Narcolepsy: a key role for hypocretins (orexins). Cell 1999;98:409–12.

25. Takahashi JS. Narcolepsy genes wake up the sleep field. Science 1999;285:2076–7.

26. Borbely AA, Achermann P. Sleep homeostasis and models of sleep regulation. J Biol Rhythms 1999; 14:557–68.

27. Borbely AA. Processes underlying sleep regulation. Horm Res 1998;49:114–7.

28. Borbely AA, Achermann P. Sleep homeostasis and models of sleep regulation. In: Kryger M, Roth T, Dement WC, editors. Principals and practice of sleep medicine. 3rd edition. Philadelphia: W.B. Saunders; 2000. p. 377–90.

29. Borbely AA. A two process model of sleep regulation. Hum Neurobiol 1982;1:195–204.

30. Espie CA, Broomfield NM, MacMahon KM, et al. The attention-intention-effort pathway in the development of psychophysiologic insomnia: an invited theoretical review. Sleep Med Rev 2006;10:215–45.

31. Perlis ML, Giles DE, Mendelson WB, et al. Psychophysiological insomnia: the behavioural model and a neurocognitive perspective. J Sleep Res 1997;6: 179–88.

32. Freedman R. EEG power in sleep onset insomnia. Electroencephalogr Clin Neurophysiol 1986;63: 408–13.

33. Merica H, Gaillard JM. The EEG of the sleep onset period in insomnia: a discriminant analysis. Physiol Behav 1992;52:199–204.

34. Merica H, Blois R, Gaillard JM. Spectral characteristics of sleep EEG in chronic insomnia. Eur J Neurosci 1998;10:1826–34.

35. Lamarche CH, Ogilvie RD. Electrophysiological changes during the sleep onset period of psychophysiological insomniacs, psychiatric insomniacs, and normal sleepers. Sleep 1997;20:724–33.

36. Jacobs GD, Benson H, Friedman R. Home-based central nervous system assessment of a multifactor behavioral intervention for chronic sleep-onset insomnia. Behav Ther 1993;24:159–74.

37. Perlis ML, Smith MT, Orff HJ, et al. Beta/Gamma EEG activity in patients with primary and secondary insomnia and good sleeper controls. Sleep 2001;24: 110–7.

38. Krystal AD, Edinger JD, Wohlgemuth WK, et al. NREM sleep EEG frequency spectral correlates of sleep complaints in primary insomnia subtypes. Sleep 2002;25:630–40.

39. Hall M, Buysse DJ, Nowell PD, et al. Symptoms of stress and depression as correlates of sleep in primary insomnia. Psychosom Med 2000;62: 227–30.

40. Nofzinger EA, Price JC, Meltzer CC, et al. Towards a neurobiology of dysfunctional arousal in depression: the relationship between beta EEG power and regional cerebral glucose metabolism during NREM sleep. Psychiatry Res 2000;98:71–91.

41. Bastien CH, LeBlanc M, Carrier J, et al. Sleep EEG power spectra, insomnia, and chronic use of benzodiazepines. Sleep 2003;26:313–7.

42. Curcio G, Ferrara M, Piergianni A, et al. Paradoxes of the first-night effect: a quantitative analysis of antero-posterior EEG topography. Clin Neurophysiol 2004;115:1178–88.

43. Buysse DJ, Germain A, Hall ML, et al. EEG spectral analysis in primary insomnia: NREM period effects and sex differences. Sleep 2008;31:1673–82.

44. Johns MW. Relationship between sleep habits, adrenocortical activity and personality. Psychosom Med 1971;33:499–508.

45. Vgontzas AN, Tsigos C, Bixler EO, et al. Chronic insomnia and activity of the stress system: a preliminary study. J Psychosom Res 1998;45:21–31.

46. Vgontzas AN, Bixler EO, Lin HM, et al. Chronic insomnia is associated with nyctohemeral activation of the hypothalamic-pituitary-adrenal axis: clinical implications. J Clin Endocrinol Metab 2001;86:3787–94.

47. Riemann D, Klein T, Rodenbeck A, et al. Nocturnal cortisol and melatonin secretion in primary insomnia. Psychiatry Res 2002;113:17–27.

48. Cano G, Saper CB. Mechanisms underlying stress-induced insomnia. 35rd Annual Meeting of the Society for Neuroscience. Washington, November 12–16, 2005.

49. Cano G, Mochizuki T, Saper CB. Neural circuitry of stress-induced insomnia in rats. J Neurosci 2008; 28:10167–84.

50. Ford DE, Kamerow DB. Epidemiologic study of sleep disturbances and psychiatric disorders. An opportunity for prevention? [see comments]. JAMA 1989;262:1479–84.

51. Dryman A, Eaton WW. Affective symptoms associated with the onset of major depression in the community: findings from the US National Institute of Mental Health Epidemiologic Catchment Area Program. Acta Psychiatr Scand 1991;84:1–5.

52. Breslau N, Roth T, Rosenthal L, et al. Sleep disturbance and psychiatric disorders: a longitudinal epidemiological study of young adults. Biol Psychiatry 1996;39:411–8.

53. Livingston G, Blizard B, Mann A. Does sleep disturbance predict depression in elderly people? A study in inner London [see comments]. Br J Gen Pract 1993;43:445–8.

54. Mallon L, Broman JE, Hetta J. Relationship between insomnia, depression, and mortality: a 12-year follow-up of older adults in the community. Int Psychogeriatr 2000;12:295–306.

55. Roberts RE, Shema SJ, Kaplan GA, et al. Sleep complaints and depression in an aging cohort: a prospective perspective [In Process Citation]. Am J Psychiatry 2000;157:81–8.

56. Vollrath M, Wicki W, Angst J. The Zurich study. VIII. Insomnia: association with depression, anxiety, somatic syndromes, and course of insomnia. Eur Arch Psychiatry Neurol Sci 1989;239:113–24.

57. Weissman MM, Greenwald S, Nino-Murcia G, et al. The morbidity of insomnia uncomplicated by psychiatric disorders. Gen Hosp Psychiatry 1997; 19:245–50.

58. Perlis ML, Giles DE, Buysse DJ, et al. Self-reported sleep disturbance as a prodromal symptom in recurrent depression. J Affect Disord 1997;42:209–12.

59. Perlis ML, Giles DE, Buysse DJ, et al. Which depressive symptoms are related to which sleep electroencephalographic variables? Biol Psychiatry 1997;42: 904–13.

60. Thase ME. Antidepressant treatment of the depressed patient with insomnia. J Clin Psychiatry 1999;60(Suppl 17):28–31.

61. Smith MT, Perlis ML, Chengazi VU, et al. Neuroimaging of NREM sleep in primary insomnia: a Tc-99-HMPAO single photon emission computed tomography study. Sleep 2002;25:325–35.

62. Nofzinger EA, Buysee DJ, et al. Insomnia: functional imaging evidence for hyperarousal. Am J Psychiatry 2004;161:2126–8.

63. Winkelman JW, Buxton OM, Jensen JE, et al. Reduced brain GABA in primary insomnia: preliminary data from 4T proton magnetic resonance spectroscopy (1H-MRS). Sleep 2008;31:1499–506.

64. Drummond SP, Smith MT, Orff HJ, et al. Functional imaging of the sleeping brain: review of findings and implications for the study of insomnia. Sleep Med Rev 2004;8:227–42.

Neurologic Basis of Sleep Breathing Disorders

Aman A. Savani, MD[a], Christian Guilleminault, MD, DBiol[b],*

KEYWORDS

- Obstructive sleep apnea syndrome • Upper airway muscles • Snoring neurogenic factors

KEY POINTS

- Evidence suggests that Obstructive sleep apnea syndrome (OSAS) is associated with local neurologic impairment and that some of the impairment may persist despite adequate treatment.
- The number of local neurogenic lesions that exist in a given subject is never well appreciated in the work-up of a patient with OSAS, despite the impact of such lesions on long-term results of therapeutic efforts.
- Development of specific tools to explore the severity and extension of the neurogenic impairment should be a clinical goal.
- Dentists and orthodontists should clearly incorporate an assessment of the upper airway in their general evaluation of the oral and dental development of young individuals as well as the routine dental examination of adults.

INTRODUCTION

Obstructive sleep apnea syndrome (OSAS) is a disorder resulting from partial or complete repetitive collapse of the pharynx occurring during sleep. OSAS is a common problem affecting about 2%–4% of the adult population in the United States.[1] The diagnosis is made when 5 or more such events, lasting a minimum of 10 seconds, are observed per hour of sleep on a polysomnogram. Patients with sleep apnea are variably symptomatic from the disease. Snoring is a commonly reported symptom of OSAS, but is neither necessary nor sufficient for the diagnosis. Waking up gasping, choking, drooling or with a dry mouth and bruxism are also commonly associated nocturnal symptoms of OSAS. Disturbed nighttime sleep can be associated with excessive daytime sleepiness, impaired concentration, cognitive deficits, increased irritability, depression, and anxiety.

There are several risk factors for the disease, including increasing age, obesity, postmenopausal state, and positive family history.[2] Several anatomic factors that are associated with obstructive sleep apnea include neck circumference of 17 in or greater, turbinate hypertrophy, narrow mandible and maxilla, retrognathia, and dental mal-occlusion. Dempsey and colleagues[3] showed that the severity of sleep apnea is predicted by the horizontal dimension of the maxilla. The role of gender in the development of sleep-disordered breathing has also been evaluated. Men may have inherent structural and functional differences in their airways making them more vulnerable to collapse and obstruction.[4] Based on these observations, obstructive sleep apnea is often approached as a purely mechanical problem or a structural disorder, which leads to increased respiratory effect and sleep fragmentation.

The evolution of sleep medicine into a multidisciplinary specialty has enhanced our understanding of OSAS. Advances in neuroscience are increasing our understanding of OSAS as a more complex problem with sensory impairment, motor

A version of this article originally appeared in *Sleep Medicine Clinics Volume 1, Issue 4*.
a Neurology center, 5454 Wisconsin Avenue Suite 1720, Chevy Chase, MD 20815, USA; b Sleep Medicine Program, Stanford University, 450 Broadway Street M/C 5704, Redwood City, CA 94063, USA
* Corresponding author.
E-mail address: cguil@stanford.edu

dysfunction, and altered cortical processing all playing a role in the underlying pathogenesis of the disease, in addition to the observed structural abnormalities. Younes[5] suggested that 2 of 3 patients with OSAS are attributable to neurologic factors. This article reviews the evidence supporting a neurologic basis for obstructive sleep apnea and the anatomy of normal upper airway as well as discusses the sensory impairment, abnormal cortical processing, motor dysfunction, and histopathological derangements associated with OSAS.

UPPER AIRWAY ANATOMY

The upper airway is separated into 3 separate regions: the nasopharynx, the oropharynx, and the hypopharynx. The nasopharynx is the path from the nasal turbinates to the hard palate. The oropharynx is further subdivided into the retropalatal region, which extends from the hard palate to the caudal border of the soft palate, and the retroglossal region, which extends from the caudal border of the soft palate to the base of the epiglottis. The hypopharynx is defined as the region from the base of the tongue to the larynx. The soft palate and the tongue form the anterior wall of the oropharynx whereas the posterior wall comprises superior, middle, and inferior constrictor muscles. The lateral walls are formed by several structures, including the hypoglossus, styloglossus, stylohyoid, stylopharyngeus, palatoglossus, palatopharyngeus, and pharyngeal constrictors. The pharyngeal airway is largely unsupported by bony structures, leaving it susceptible to collapse under the negative pressures generated during inspiration. Obesity influences airway collapsibility by increasing the amount of soft tissue surrounding the pharyngeal airway.[6] Body position can also affect airway collapsibility. Obstructive breathing events occur more frequently in the supine position. The upper airway assumes more of an elliptical shape when supine as opposed to a more circular shape when in the lateral recumbent position without changing the cross-sectional area. Thus, the closer opposition of the pharyngeal walls may make the upper airway more susceptible to collapse.[7] The muscles surrounding the pharyngeal airway can influence its patency by actively dilating and opening the airway or stiffening to reduce susceptibility to negative pressure collapse, as is seen in OSAS. The most active and relevant of these muscles is an extrinsic tongue muscle, the genioglossus.

The genioglossus is the largest of the upper airway dilator muscles and is often modified in sleep apnea surgery. Anterior movement of the tongue and widening of the oropharyngeal airway is facilitated by contraction of this muscle. The genioglossus is innervated by the medial branch of the hypoglossal nerve and receives input from the pre-Botzinger complex as well as the neurons that regulate sleep-wake states.[8] Recent evidence from single motor unit recordings indicates that the genioglossus consists of motor units with a variety of firing patterns. The activity of individual units can be divided into 6 classes based on their discharge patterns. One study showed that 29% of sampled units discharged tonically without phasic respiratory control, 16% increased their firing during expiration, and 50% increased firing during inspiration. Adjacent units had differing respiratory and tonic drives suggesting a complex interaction of tonic and phasic activities at the hypoglossal motor nucleus.[9] Wilkinson and colleagues[10] studied sampled motor units from healthy patients at sleep onset and found that 50% of units ceased activity entirely at sleep onset. The different units likely have different functional roles. Inspiratory motor units may be phasically active to compensate for negative pressures generated during inspiration whereas inspiratory/expiratory units tonically discharge to maintain tongue position.[11] The genioglossus also receives input from the negative pressure receptors within the upper airway. Consequently, genioglossus activity is increased during inspiration to prevent negative pressure collapse. Genioglossus also remains active during expiration although to a lesser degree. Thus, genioglossus activity is increased in response to respiratory drive through its connection to neurons that generate respiratory rhythm and in response to negative airway pressure. This increased activity has been demonstrated through the application of brief negative pressure pulses to the upper airway. However, the genioglossus reflex to negative pressure seems to be inhibited at during REM sleep, potentially explaining why the upper airway is more susceptible to collapse during this stage of sleep.[12] Increased genioglossus muscle tone is also associated with spontaneous periods of stable flow limited breathing in patients with obstructive sleep apnea.[13] The mechanism behind this observation could be long-term facilitation of genioglossus activity due to repeated hypoxia. A recent study of anesthetized, spontaneously breathing rats showed increases in peak genioglossus activity after 8 hypoxic episodes measured by electromyography (EMG) 1 hour after the last episode, demonstrating a long-term facilitatory change.[14]

The stiffness and position of the palate, tongue, and pharynx, as well as the shape of the uvula are determined by the palatal muscles (tensor palatine, levator veli palatine, palatoglossus, palatopharyngeus, and musculus uvulae). These muscles are important in maintenance of upper airway patency. McWhorter and colleagues[15] showed that tensor veli palatini stimulation in cats decreases upper airway collapsibility. The pharyngeal branch of the vagus nerve innervates all these muscles with the exception of the tensor veli palatine, which is innervated by the trigeminal nerve. Another study showed that vagal nerve stimulation in patients with epilepsy can adversely affect respiration during sleep.[16]

There are 3 pharyngeal constrictor muscles: superior, middle, and inferior. These muscles may play a role in stiffening the posterior pharyngeal wall and are innervated by the vagus nerve. Kuna and colleagues showed that the activation of the pharyngeal constrictor muscles constricts the airway at relatively high airway volumes but dilates the airway at relatively low volumes.[17] Thus activation of the pharyngeal constrictor muscle at the end of an apneic episode, when airway volumes are low, could help restore airway patency in individuals with obstructive sleep apnea. However, there is little evidence supporting the role of these muscles in apnea pathogenesis.

The hyoid arch and its muscle attachments, including the geniohyoid, mylohyoid, sternohyoid, stylohyoid, and thyrohyoid, strongly influence hypopharyngeal airway patency and resistance. These muscles are innervated by the hypoglossal nerve (geniohyoid and thyrohyoid), trigeminal nerve (mylohyoid), facial nerve (stylohyoid), and ansa cervicalis (sternohyoid). The geniohyoid and mylohyoid act to pull the hyoid bone forward and upward while the sternohyoid and thyrohyoid pull the bone caudally. Tandem activation of both muscle groups results in ventral/caudal movement of the hyoid, facilitating airway dilation.[18]

SENSORY DYSFUNCTION

There are multiple different types of sensory receptors in the upper airway. They respond to a variety of stimuli including pressure, cold, heat, irritants, and respiratory muscle drive. Among the various types of receptors, mechanoreceptors have been well studied.

The upper airway reflex opposes the negative pressure collapsing forces generated during inhalation. This reflex is accomplished through activation of pharyngeal dilator muscles, which can increase the airway patency. The sensory input for this reflex comes from the mechanosensory receptors of the upper airway through the central respiratory centers, which represents a true reflex because increase in pharyngeal dilator activity can be demonstrated with a shorter latency than would be expected with voluntary activation.[19]

Proprioceptive feedback from the thoracic and upper airway receptors can alter motor output to the pharyngeal muscles. Studies in animal models have shown that negative pressure generation in the upper airway can increase activity in the genioglossus. This response can be blocked by transecting the superior laryngeal nerve or by applying topical anesthesia. Diversion of tidal volume away from the mechanosensory receptors in the upper airway through a tracheostomy tube also induces pharyngeal closure in animal models, which was reversible on restoration of normal flow.[20] Because topical anesthesia can block this response, the receptors mediating this reflex are believed to be located superficially in the airway wall. Most of these receptors seem to be located in the upper trachea and transmit information through the superior laryngeal nerve as well as the glossopharyngeal and trigeminal nerves.

During apneas and hypopneas, receptors distal to the obstruction sense and transmit information about the resultant pressure changes. Abnormalities in the sensory component of the airway reflex can be primary, secondary, or both, as contributing factors to obstructive sleep apnea.[21] Primary sensory deficitspreexisting factors that increase the threshold for the negative pressure reflex making the airway more collapsible in certain individuals. Secondary deficits are the result of accumulated damage over time caused by local trauma in the setting of snoring and obstructive sleep apnea, creating a vicious cycle that perpetuates the disease.

As mentioned earlier, snoring is a common symptom associated with obstructive sleep apnea. Snoring is a manifestation of airway resistance, which creates turbulent flow and vibrates distensible tissues. Repetitive snoring and upper airway occlusion has been shown to lead to edema of the upper airway soft tissue structures, which further narrows the airway and increases resistance to normal airflow. Snoring also causes damage to mechanosensory receptors. Prior occupational and environmental health studies have shown that repetitive use of vibrating tools can lead to localized nerve lesions. In the vibration-induced white finger syndrome, 3 characteristic pathologic changes were found: First, the muscular layer of arteries showed thickening with significant hypertrophy of muscle cells. Second, a demyelinating peripheral neuropathy was noted with marked loss of nerve fibers. Third, connective tissues with collagen were increased.[22,23] Similarly, continuous snoring produces low-frequency vibration. Vibration from chronic snoring represents repetitive trauma to the palate and other upper airway structures. A recent study showed the mechanical stimulus of vibration triggers an early proinflammatory process in the upper airway of rats. Specifically, vibration–induced significant overexpression of tumor necrosis factor alpha, and macrophage inflammatory protein-2.[24] This inflammation seems to be related to contractile dysfunction, loss of sensory afferents, and impaired vascular reactivity in pharyngeal structures, which further compromises the negative pressure reflex and increases the likelihood of partial or complete closure of the airway.[25]

The importance of sensory feedback in the upper airway reflex has been demonstrated in studies of sleep and awake patients when selective anesthetization of various upper airway structures with topical lidocaine resulted in diminished upper airway patency. Similar studies in snorers have shown an increase in the frequency of abnormal breathing events (hypopneas and sometime even apneas) with the application of topical lidocaine and bupivacaine to the oropharynx.[26] These findings suggest that nasal receptors sensitive to airflow may be important in maintaining breathing rhythmicity during sleep.[27] Other studies that support this theory have shown reduced temperature thresholds for the sensation of heat and cold on the tonsillar pillars of snorers compared with participants in the control group, with exaggerated vasodilation and vascular reactivity. There is also evidence that 2-point discrimination and vibratory sensation are impaired in patients who snore and with obstructive sleep apnea[28] as is mucosal sensory function at multiple points in the upper airway.[29] Two-point palatal discrimination has also been evaluated in normal individuals and compared with individuals with upper airway resistance syndrome (UARS) and individuals with obstructive sleep apnea. Patients with OSAS had a clear impairment of their palatal sensory response with a decrement in 2-point discrimination compared with the patients with UARS, suggesting that they are less capable of transmitting sensory inputs.[30] Upper airway sensory impairment also contributes to altered swallowing function in patients with OSAS, measured by prolongation of the respiratory cycle after swallowing.[31] There is also evidence that a history of sleep apnea increases the arousal threshold to upper airway occlusion and prolongs the duration of apneic events.[32]

It is not clear whether upper airway sensory dysfunction represents a cause or an effect of obstructive sleep apnea. However, these findings emphasize the importance of recognizing the disease early to avoid further damage and perpetuation of the disorder.

IMPAIRED CORTICAL PROCESSING

One of the principal features of obstructive sleep apnea is the presence of electroencephalographic (EEG) arousals associated with hypopneas, apneas, and increased respiratory effort. The EEG arousal can be considered an important part of the neural mechanism that is required to abort an abnormal breathing event and restore normal airway patency. However, arousals are state changes that result in sleep fragmentation. In obstructive sleep apnea, cortical arousability is diminished, suggesting that arousal thresholds are blunted. This condition would increase the duration of apneas as well as the likelihood of additional events.

Neurogenic activity can be recorded in the somatosensory area of the cortex in relation to respiratory occlusion. The respiratory-related evoked potential (RREP) is a cortical response to the rapid application of resistive loads to breathing.[33] During wakefulness, RREP's are formed of early and late components. P1 and Nf are the early positive and negative responses occurring 40 and 80 seconds after the inspiratory resistive load is applied as recorded in the parietal and frontal scalp regions, respectively. The potentials are present bilaterally but diminished over midline sites.[34] Additional components of the RREP during wakefulness include N1 and P300 components, which are related to attention and perception of the respiratory sensitivity and effort.[35]

Patients with obstructive sleep apnea have a significantly increased inspiratory effort–related arousal threshold when compared with controls. Thus, more stimulus is required to produce an arousal during an obstructive breathing event. This abnormality could be attributed to differences in afferent processing caused by focal neuropathic lesions. Studies of RREP's in both asleep and awake patients have been performed in patients with OSAS to further investigate this finding. During wakefulness cortical processing of airway occlusion related afferents is abnormal in untreated patients with obstructive sleep apnea. Specifically, N1 latencies, and P2 and N2 were significantly delayed despite no significant differences in P1 latencies.[36] However, this finding has been disputed by studies. Gora and colleagues[37] found that the RREP waveform is broadly similar in patients with obstructive sleep apnea when awake but differed significantly during stage 2 non-rapid eye movement (NREM) sleep. Specifically, fewer K-complexes were elicited in response to occlusion stimuli in the OSAS group. To determine whether these observations reflect a sleep-specific dampening of inspiratory effort related stimuli, Afifi and colleagues[38] performed both respiratory and auditory evoked potentials in NREM sleep and wakefulness patients with OSAS and individuals in the control group. The amplitude of the N550 potential and the proportion of elicited K-complexes did not differ between the 2 groups in response to auditory stimuli presented during stage 2 NREM sleep. However, in response to respiratory stimuli presented during stage 2 sleep, the N550 amplitude and K-complex elicitation rate was significantly reduced in patients with OSAS compared with controls. These results confirm a sleep-specific blunted cortical response to inspiratory occlusions. The sleep-related differences in patients with OSAS specific to the processing of inspiratory stimuli is highlighted by the absence of a significant difference in response to auditory stimuli between the 2 groups.[38]

The natural question that follows is whether or not the changes in cortical processing are reversible with continuous positive airway pressure (CPAP) treatment. Sangal and Sangal[39] performed auditory and visual P300 testing in patients with severe obstructive sleep apnea (defined as a respiratory disturbance index greater than 40) before and after CPAP therapy for 2 to 4 months. Although there was significant symptomatic improvement with therapy, there was no significant change in the P300 latencies. Patients with severe obstructive sleep apnea had prolonged P300 latencies before and after treatment.[39] These results suggest that the changes in cortical processing associated with severe sleep apnea are irreversible and reinforce the importance of early diagnosis and treatment of this disorder.

MOTOR DEFICITS

Airway patency during wakefulness and sleep is determined by the pharyngeal motor control, which requires an intact neural response. Hence not all patients with predisposing anatomic features have obstructive sleep apnea, and why not all patients with obstructive sleep apnea have obvious anatomic abnormalities. Patients with obstructive sleep apnea are able to maintain sufficient airway patency during wakefulness, suggesting that a compensatory mechanism must be functioning to prevent collapse. Failure of these mechanisms compromises airway patency and leads to collapse under negative inspiratory pressure and obstruction.

Pharyngeal dilator muscle activity is influenced by inputs from the central respiratory center in the medulla, mechanoreceptor feedback from the pharynx itself, vagal input from the lungs, and by the drive for wakefulness.[13] These muscles function to keep the airway open against the negative pressures generated during inhalation. The action of the genioglossus, palatopharyngeus, levator palatine, and tensor palatine represents the final common pathway of the negative pressure airway reflex. Dysfunction in the genioglossus and tensor palatine has been well described in patients with obstructive sleep apnea.

Impaired electromyographic activation of the levator palatini and palatoglossus in response to negative pressure pulses was described in awake patients with OSAS compared with controls. Patients showed improved responses with chronic nightly CPAP therapy.[40]

Unlike the palatal muscles, the genioglossus seems to be more active during wakefulness in patients with sleep apnea compared with controls, and has a well-preserved response to negative pressure, possibly representing a compensatory mechanism for a more collapsible airway.[41,42] Single motor unit recordings from the genioglossus of awake patients with severe OSAS showed larger area and longer duration action potentials with earlier recruitment, and higher discharge frequencies. Patients with obstructive sleep apnea also have a greater reduction in genioglossus muscle tone at sleep onset compared with controls even when airway resistance is controlled for by application of CPAP.[43] These findings suggest that neurogenic changes have occurred in patients with severe obstructive sleep apnea with possibly altered output from the hypoglossal nucleus.[44]

HISTOPATHOLOGICAL CORRELATES

Several studies have demonstrated the associated pathologic changes associated with OSAS. There is evidence that motor neuron lesions and damage to airway musculature can lead to weakness of the pharyngeal muscles, making the airway more susceptible to collapse. The results of muscle biopsies from the palatopharyngeal muscle of patients with obstructive sleep apnea performed during uvulopalatopharyngoplasty showed atrophy with a fascicular distribution, increased number of angulated atrophic fibers, and an abnormal distribution of fiber types in many muscle fascicles.[45] There is also evidence of hypertrophy of the salivary glands as well as congestion and dilation of the thin-walled vessels along with lymphocytic infiltrates reflective of inflammatory changes.[46] Normal vasodilation in response to electrical stimulation is also exaggerated in habitual snorers and patients with mild OSAS in comparison to normal individuals.[47] Light microscopy of both apneics and snorers has revealed mucous gland hypertrophy with ductal dilation and focal squamous metaplasia, disruption of muscle bundles by infiltrating mucous glands, focal atrophy of muscle fibers, and significant edema of the lamina propria. Electron microscopy of pharyngeal tissues in severe apneics has shown focal degeneration of myelinated nerve fibers and axons.[48] Confirmatory digital analysis of uvular specimens from patients with obstructive sleep apnea has demonstrated an increase in the total muscle bulk of the palatine muscles when compared with patients who snore, but do not meet the diagnostic for OSAS. This finding suggests that muscular hypertrophy may also underlie the pathophysiology of the disease.[49] Biopsy results of palatopharyngeal muscle from patients with habitual snoring and different degrees of upper airway obstruction showed numerous morphologic abnormalities, including neurogenic signs (eg, type grouping). The extent of the abnormality was significantly increased in patients compared with controls and correlated to the severity periodic obstructive breathing but not to oxygen desaturation. Analyses of the individual fiber-size spectra have demonstrated a significantly increased number of hypertrophied and/or atrophied fibers in patients compared with controls.[50]

The genioglossus is a well-studied muscle in patients with obstructive sleep apnea. The results of Biopsy of this muscle in patients with OSAS have shown an increase in the percentage of type II ("fast twitch") fibers compared with controls. Analysis of these muscle fibers also demonstrated increased fatigability compared with controls.[51] These changes are present to a greater extent in patients with OSASS who are obese, potentially making the airway of this group of patients even more collapsible.[52]

These studies support the hypothesis that upper airway efferent nerve lesions are present in patients with OSAS. However, it is still unclear whether these lesions represent a cause or an effect of obstructive sleep apnea.

Reversal of Neurologic Lesions with Treatment

A growing body of evidence suggests that upper airway neurologic lesions are associated with obstructive sleep apnea. Nasal CPAP therapy is recognized as an effective means of treating sleep-related obstructive breathing events. Studies have shown improvement of the symptoms associated with obstructive sleep apnea, including excessive daytime sleepiness, snoring, and cognitive impairment. However, improvement in the associated neurologic lesions has not been as demonstrated as consistently with the use of CPAP. Carrera and colleagues[51] showed that pathologic and physiologic alterations in the genioglossus of patients with OSAS improved after treatment with CPAP. Guilleminault and colleagues[53] evaluated healthy, nonobese, patients for 5 years. Despite compliance with CPAP therapy and maintenance of body mass index, pressure had to be increased by at least 2 cm of H_2O in two-thirds of the participants in the study. In addition, abnormal 2-point palatal discrimination during wakefulness was present at the conclusion the study when compared with controls. Both of these observations suggest that the neurologic lesions persist despite effective treatment with CPAP.[53]

However, as with larger muscle groups that are weakened by underlying neurologic lesions, the muscles of the pharyngeal airway may be amenable to rehabilitation with physical therapy. A recent study evaluated the effectiveness of a set of oropharyngeal exercises involving the tongue, soft palate, and lateral pharyngeal wall compared with that of sham therapy in patients with moderate obstructive sleep apnea. After 3 months of daily exercise for approximately 30 minutes, reduction in OSAS severity and symptoms was noted in the treatment group, suggesting some degree of improvement in the targeted muscles.[54]

SUMMARY

Evidence suggests that OSAS is associated with local neurologic impairment and that some of the impairment may persist despite adequate treatment. The number of local neurogenic lesions that exist in a given subject is never well appreciated in the work-up of a patient with OSAS, despite the impact of such lesions on long-term results of therapeutic efforts. Development of specific tools to explore the severity and extension of the neurogenic impairment should be a clinical goal. Furthermore, the philosophy of how to recognize, diagnose, and treat individuals with known risk factors for a collapsible airway should be an important question to visit. Opening the upper airway should be a primary goal in young individuals with high-risk anatomic features to prevent the development, progression, and irreversible sequelae of associated neurologic lesions. Dentists and orthodontists should clearly incorporate an assessment of the upper airway in their general evaluation of the oral and dental development of young individuals as well as the routine dental examination of adults.

REFERENCES

1. Young T, Palta M, Dempsey J, et al. The occurrence of sleep disordered breathing among middle-aged adults. N Engl J Med 1993;328:1230–5.

2. Young T, Peppard PE, Gottlieb DJ. Epidemiology of obstructive sleep apnea: a population health perspective. Am J Respir Crit Care Med 2002; 165(9):1217–39.

3. Dempsey JA, Skatrud JB, Jacques AJ, et al. Anatomic determinants of sleep-disordered breathing across the spectrum of clinical and nonclinical male subjects. Chest 2002;122(3):840–51.

4. Mohsenin V. Gender differences in the expression of sleep-disordered breathing: role of upper airway dimensions. Chest 2001;120(5):1442–7.

5. Younes M. Role of respiratory control mechanisms in the pathogenesis of obstructive sleep disorders. J Appl Physiol 2008;105:1389–405.

6. Kryger MH, Roth T, Dement WC. Principles and practice of sleep medicine. Elsevier Saunders; 2005. p. 983–8.

7. Walsh JH, Leigh MS, Paduch A, et al. Effect of posture on pharyngeal shape and size in adults with and without obstructive sleep apnea. Sleep 2008;31(11):1543–9.

8. Phillipson EA. Regulation of breathing during sleep. Am Rev Respir Dis 1977;115:217–24.

9. Sabiosky JP, Butler JE, Fogel RB, et al. Tonic and phasic respiratory drives to human genioglossus motoneurons during breathing. J Neurophysiol 2006;95(4):2213–21.

10. Wilkinson V, Malhotra A, Nicholas CL, et al. Discharge patterns of human genioglossus motor units during sleep onset. Sleep 2008;31(4):525–33.

11. Tsuiki S, Ono T, Ishiwata Y, et al. Functional divergence of human genioglossus motor units with respiratory-related activity. Eur Respir J 2000;15(5): 906–10.

12. Shea SA, Edwards JK, White DP. Effect of wake-sleep transitions and rapid eye movement sleep on pharyngeal muscle response to negative pressure in humans. J Physiol 1999;520:897–908.

13. Jordan AS, White DP, Wellman A, et al. Airway dilator muscle activity and lung volume during stable breathing in obstructive sleep apnea. Sleep 2009; 32(3):361–8.

14. Ryan D, Nolan P. Episodic hypoxia induces long-term facilitation of upper airway muscle activity in spontaneously breathing anaesthetized rats. J Physiol 2009; 587(Pt 13):3329–42 [Epub 2009 Mar 30].

15. McWhorter AJ, Rowley JA, Eisele DW. The effect of tensor veli palatini stimulation on upper airway patency. Arch Otolaryngol Head Neck Surg 1999; 125(9):937–40.

16. Marzec M, Edwards J, Sagher O, et al. Effects of vagus nerve stimulation on sleep related breathing disorders in epilepsy patients. Epilepsia 2003; 44(7):930–5.

17. Kuna ST. Respiratory-related activation and mechanical effects of the pharyngeal constrictor muscles. Respir Physiol 2000;119(2–3):155–61.

18. Van de Graaff WB, Gottfried SB, Mitra J, et al. Respiratory function of the hyoid muscles and the hyoid arch. J Appl Physiol 1984;57(1):197–204.

19. Horner RL, Innes JA, Murphy K, et al. Evidence for reflex upper airway dilator muscle activation by sudden negative airway pressure in man. J Physiol 1991;436:15–29.

20. Abu-Osba YK, Mathew OP, Thach BT. An animal model for airway sensory deprivation producing obstructive sleep apnea with postmortem findings of sudden infant death syndrome. Pediatrics 1981; 68:796–801.

21. Broderick M, Guilleminault C. Neurological aspects of obstructive sleep apnea. Ann N Y Acad Sci 2008;1142:44–57.

22. Sauni R, Paakkonen R, Virtema P. Vibration-induced white finger syndrome and carpal tunnel syndrome among Finnish metal workers. Int Arch Occup Environ Health 2009;82(4):445–53.

23. Takeuchi T, Futatsuka M, Imanishi H, et al. Pathological changed observed in the finger biopsy of patients with vibration-induced white finger. Scand J Work Environ Health 1986;12:280–3.

24. Almendros I, Acerbi I, Puig F. Upper-airway inflammation triggered by vibration in a rat model of snoring. Sleep 2007;30(2):225–7.

25. Ramar K, Guilleminault C. Obstructive sleep apnea: a neurologic disease? Sleep Med Clin 2008.

26. Chadwick GA, Crowley P, Fitzgerald MX, et al. Obstructive sleep apnea following topical oropharyngeal anesthesia in loud snorers. Am Rev Respir Dis 1991;143(4):810–3.

27. White DP, Cadieux RJ, Lombard RM, et al. The effects of nasal anesthesia on breathing during sleep. Am Rev Respir Dis 1985;132(5):972–5.

28. Kimoff RJ, Sfozra E, Champagne V, et al. Upper airway sensation in snoring and obstructive sleep apnea. Am J Respir Crit Care Med 2001;164(2):250–5.

29. Nguyen AT, Jobin V, Payne R, et al. Laryngeal and velopharyngeal sensory impairment in obstructive sleep apnea. Sleep 2005;28(5):585–93.

30. Guilleminault C, Li K, Poyares D. Two-point palatal discrimination in patients with upper airway resistance syndrome, OSASS, and normal control subjects. Chest 2002;122(3):866–70.

31. Jobin V, Champagne V, Beauregard J, et al. Swallowing function and upper airway sensation in obstructive sleep apnea. J Appl Physiol 2007; 102(4):1587–94.

32. Berry RB, Kouchi KG, Der DE, et al. Sleep apnea impairs the arousal response to airway occlusion. Chest 1996;109(6):1490–6.

33. Davenport PW, Friedman WA, Thompson FJ. Respiratory-related evoked potentials evoked by inspiratory occlusion in humans. J Appl Physiol 1986; 60(6):1843–8.

34. Davenport PW, Colrain IM, Hill PM. Scalp topography of the short-latency components of the respiratory-related evoked potential in children. J Appl Physiol 1996;80(5):1785–91.

35. Webster KE, Colrain IM. The relationship between respiratory-related evoked potentials and the perception of inspiratory resistive loads. Psychophysiology 2000;37(6):831–41.

36. Donzel-Raynaud C, Redolfi S, Arnulf I, et al. Abnormal respiratory-related evoked potentials in untreated awake patients with severe obstructive sleep apnoea syndrome. Clin Physiol Funct Imaging 2009;29(1):10–7.

37. Gora J, Trinder J, Pierce R, et al. Evidence of a sleep specific blunted cortical response to inspiratory occlusions in mild OSASS. Am J Respir Crit Care Med 2002;166(9):1225–34.

38. Afifi L, Guilleminault C, Colrain IM. Sleep and respiratory stimulus specific dampening of cortical responsiveness in OSASS. Respir Physiol Neurobiol 2003;136(2–3):221–34.

39. Sangal RB, Sangal JM. Abnormal visual P300 latency in obstructive sleep apnea does not change acutely upon treatment with CPAP. Sleep 1997;20(9):702–4.

40. Mortimore IL, Douglas NJ. Palatal muscle EMG response to negative pressure in awake sleep apneic and control subjects. Am J Respir Crit Care Med 1997;156:867–73.

41. Fogel RB, Malhotra A, Pillar G, et al. Genioglossal activation in patients with obstructive sleep apnea versus control subjects: mechanisms of muscle control. Am J Respir Crit Care Med 2001;164(11):2025–30.

42. Berry RB, White DP, Roper J, et al. Awake negative pressure reflex response of the genioglossus in OSAS patients and normal subjects. J Appl Physiol 2003;94(5):1875–82.

43. Fogel RB, Trinder J, White DP, et al. The effect of sleep onset on upper airway muscle activity in patients with sleep apnoea versus controls. J Physiol 2005;564:549–62.

44. Sabiosky JP, Butler JE, McKenzie DK, et al. Neural drive to human genioglossus in obstructive sleep apnoea. J Physiol 2007;585(1):135–46.

45. Edstrom L, Larsson J, Larsson L. Neurogenic effects on the palatopharyngeal muscle in patients with obstructive sleep apnoea: a muscle biopsy study. J Neurol Neurosurg Psychiatr 1992;55(10): 916–20.

46. Namyslowski G, Scierski W, Zembala-Nosynska E, et al. Histopathologic changes of the soft palate in snoring and OSASS patients. Otolaryngol Pol 2005;59(1):13–9.

47. Friberg D, Gazelius B. Evaluation of the vascular reaction in pharyngeal mucOSAS. Acta Otolaryngol 1998;118(3):413–8.

48. Woodson BT, Garancis JC, Toohill RJ. Histopathological changes in snoring and OSASS. Laryngoscope 1991;101:1318–22.

49. Bassiouny A, Mashaly M, Nasr S, et al. Quantitative analysis of uvular muscles in cases of simple snoring and obstructive sleep apnea: an image analysis study. Eur Arch Otorhinolaryngol 2008; 265(5):581–6.

50. Friberg D, Ansved T, Borg K, et al. Histological indications of a progressive snorer's disease in an upper airway muscle. Am J Respir Crit Care Med 1998;157(2):586–93.

51. Carrera M, Barbe F, Sauleda J, et al. Patients with obstructive sleep apnea exhibit genioglossus dysfunction that is normalized after treatment with continuous positive airway pressure. Am J Respir Crit Care Med 1999;159(6):1960–6.

52. Carrera M, Barbe F, Sauleda J, et al. Effects of obesity upon genioglossus structure and function in obstructive sleep apnoea. Eur Respir J 2004; 23(3):425–9.

53. Guilleminault CG, Huang YS, Kirisoglu C, et al. Is OSASS a neurological disorder? a continuous positive pressure follow-up study. Ann Neurol 2005; 58(6):880–7.

54. Guimaraes KC, Drager LF, Genta PR. Effects of oropharyngeal exercises on patients with moderate OSASS. Am J Respir Crit Care Med 2009;179(10): 962–6.

Cyclic Alternating Pattern (CAP) and Sleep-Disordered Breathing in Young Women
History of the Validation of CAP Scoring and a Translational Study

Christian Guilleminault, MD, DM, DBiol*,
Agostinho da Rosa, PhD, Chad C. Hagen, MD,
Olga Prilipko, MD, PhD

KEYWORDS

- Sleep-disordered breathing • Cyclic alternating pattern • NREM sleep disruption

KEY POINTS

- There is poor correlation between daytime complaints of patients with sleep-disordered breathing (SDB) and visual scoring of sleep disruption. However, the cyclic alternating pattern (CAP) brings forth new information on non–rapid eye movement sleep disturbances.
- CAP is an important adjunct in the investigation of sleep disturbance in SDB patients. The CAP automatic scoring system tested is sufficiently accurate to aid in CAP scoring.
- Current respiratory scoring criteria to evaluate the severity of SDB in premenopausal women may be inadequate.

INTRODUCTION

Sleep disruption defined by changes in sleep stages scored according to the international criteria of Rechtschaffen and Kales[1] has correlated poorly with common complaints such as fatigue and decrements in alertness. The American Sleep Disorders Association (ASDA) addition of scoring electroencephalograph (EEG) arousals of 3 seconds or longer[2] has improved the detection of sleep disruption but remains insensitive to more subtle EEG changes. Correlating sleep disruptions

This article originally appeared in *Sleep Medicine Clinics Volume 1, Issue 4*.
The validation of the CAP automatic analysis program was performed without any commercial financial support. The Parma and Stanford meetings of the CAP Consensus Group members were supported by an educational unrestricted grant from Sanofi-Avantis.
Stanford Outpatient Medical Center, 450 Broadway, Redwood City, CA 94603, USA
* Corresponding author.
E-mail address: cguil@stanford.edu

Sleep Med Clin 7 (2012) 563–569
http://dx.doi.org/10.1016/j.jsmc.2012.06.004
1556-407X/12/$ – see front matter © 2012 Published by Elsevier Inc.

with subjective complaints is complicated by the occurrence of patients with a high apnea-hypopnea index (AHI; ie, number of apneas and hypopneas per hour of sleep) in the absence of excessive sleepiness complaints. This finding may be related to the fact that breathing events may terminate with brainstem activation and not with an EEG arousal. Conversely, patients may also complain of tiredness and fatigue or cognitive impairment during the daytime while demonstrating a low number of EEG arousals that again fails to correlate with the severity of the daytime symptoms.

Visual EEG sleep analysis by current scoring approaches may fail to adequately reflect the disturbances associated with sleep-disordered breathing (SDB), thereby contributing to these discrepancies. Analysis of the cyclic alternating pattern (CAP) during nocturnal sleep has been used as a more sensitive investigation of sleep fragmentation in sleep disorders.[3–6] This article reports on the development and validation of CAP scoring, and presents a translational research application of CAP analysis to a case-control series of fatigued young women with mild obstructive sleep apnea.

WHAT IS CAP?

CAP is formed by electrocortical events that recur at regular intervals, in the range of seconds, during NREM sleep. These cortical events have been seen during the transition between sleep onset and establishment of consolidated delta sleep or spindle sleep during non–rapid eye movement (NREM) sleep segments. These events are clearly distinguishable from the background EEG rhythms and are identified by abrupt frequency shifts or amplitude changes.[7–9] Two adjacent phases (A and B) form a CAP cycle and recur within 2 to 60 seconds. When neither of the 2 phases is identifiable, sleep has reached a new stable state. Phase A is identified by transient events typically observed in NREM sleep. This phase includes EEG patterns of predominantly higher voltage and slower frequency, with a simultaneous faster frequency lower voltage in the background EEG. This increase in amplitude represents an activation phase that by definition is at least one-third higher than the background EEG, and lasts 2 to 60 seconds. Phase B follows phase A and is the interval between 2 A phases. It has a duration of 2 to 58 seconds, and has been defined by decreased EEG amplitude with EEG evidence of NREM sleep stages 1 to 2.

Phase A has been subdivided into 3 subtypes.[8] Subtype A1 is marked by a predominance of synchronized EEG activity with less than 20% de- and low

amplitude). This subtype appears as waveforms such as delta bursts, K-complex sequences, vertex waves, and polyphasic bursts of slow and fast EEG rhythms. Subtype A2 is scored in the presence of 20% to 50% desynchronized EEG activity with a predominance of polyphasic bursts. Subtype A3 is scored when at least 50% of the EEG activity comprises low-amplitude fast rhythms such as K-alpha complexes, ASDA-defined arousals,[2] and polyphasic bursts.

THE DEVELOPMENT OF CAP SCORING

More than 40 years ago, "trace alternant" was defined in NREM sleep of infants in France. Since then, extensive research on cyclic EEG patterns occurring during NREM sleep in children and adults has produced broadening clinical applications. Much of the seminal work was performed in Italy over the past 20 years. The definition of CAP and different components was the result of pioneering work performed by the Parma University sleep laboratory, with investigation in normal subjects and in patients with sleep abnormalities.[3,4,7–18]

The proposed definitions of CAP were originally based on visual scoring of EEG involving simultaneous analysis of at least 4 differently located EEG leads, 1 of which must be a central lead. The proposed definitions were reviewed and tested by a CAP Consensus Workgroup led by Dr Terzano, which met several times at the University of Parma. Early results of the workgroup included publication of the atlas, rules, and recording techniques for the scoring of CAP in human sleep, which outlined how to visually score CAP and present results.[8]

The CAP consensus group recognized early that the different EEG patterns analyzed when scoring CAP could easily be identified and quantified with computerized analysis. The development of automated computerized CAP scoring had obvious advantages for both research and clinical applications. Consistent with the clinical practice of scoring sleep and wake stages on a single central EEG lead, automated scoring has also been based on data from a single central lead. The biomedical engineering laboratory of the University of Lisbon in Portugal, led by Dr Agostinho da Rosa, a member of the CAP Consensus Workgroup, initiated the pursuit of an automated CAP scoring method. Several segments of the project were portions of Masters or PhD theses. Continuous interaction between the Lisbon and Parma academic laboratories led to the development of an analytical computerized system. Publications on reliability between automatic CAP scoring systems and arousal and CAP phase A[12,19–26] were published, using different tracings and segments from different parts of the night.

This analytical system was tested for accuracy in Europe, then financed in part by a sleep system company, which permitted integration into a sleep-scoring program. This user-friendly product was tested at 2 sites not involved in the development of the program (Federal University of Sao Paolo and Stanford University). Once tested and modified, the product was presented to members of the CAP Consensus Workgroup at a working meeting lasting several days. The workgroup reviewed sleep recordings from normal subjects and patients with data collected in European Data Format (EDF)[27] from different commercially available sleep systems. Short segments of polysomnograms with an EEG sampling frequency of 128 Hz and C3/A2, C4/A1, Fp1-Fp2, and O1-O2 leads were presented to the panel of experts with the request to indicate presence or absence of CAP. If CAP was judged present, the exact beginning and end of phases A and B were placed by one of the experts until the CAP sequence was over. This analysis was then presented to the panel of experts, and reconsideration of scoring and rationale for changes were written down. Once consensus from experts was obtained, spectral analysis with relative and absolute EEG power calculated per 1-second window was displayed below each identified CAP phase for each EEG segment. The automated system's scoring was displayed on a third channel to allow visual inspection of agreement between the automated scoring system and the visual scoring of the expert consensus.

The experts reviewed the consensus and automated data evaluating discrepancies between the different methods. Some findings were expected. The human eye is poor at recognizing low alpha frequencies in the absence of associated mixtures of alpha and beta frequencies. Visual scoring also failed to recognize short bursts of low alpha power lasting up to 2 seconds. In addition, visual scoring was not as sensitive as automated scoring for recognizing significant delta power of up to 50% in the presence of beta surges of up to 20% of the total reliable power for 1 or 2 seconds. This finding is particularly relevant, as it hinders the visual recognition of phase A or phase A1 termination. A discrepancy between the human eye and automated systems' recognition of subtle midline crossing and wave amplitude was also shown. Because of these discrepancies, the computer interpreted the high amplitude segments to last longer than did the visual scorers; this was a systematic discrepancy. As CAP is based on

visual scoring, the Consensus Workgroup made a specific modification to the automated system's rule for ending phase A1 that was more consistent with the human eye's recognition of EEG amplitude and visual scoring. These default parameters were implemented at the first meeting day of the analytical program. Further investigation indicated much better agreement between experts and automated scoring after the modification.

Although the number of CAP cycles was in agreement between automated and expert scorers, interexpert scorer and expert-automated system disagreement related to duration of some CAP phases remained. These discrepancies were again related to the discriminative capabilities of the human eye, as shown by simultaneous EEG power analysis of the considered EEG segment. This human-computer scoring confrontation indicated, not surprisingly, that computer scoring was much more consistent over time. It also showed that automated scoring was better than the eye at overall recognition of mean EEG frequencies during 1 second. Throughout the confrontation, at least one expert scorer scored as the computer did for each considered segment. Of importance, whereas the addition of other EEG leads for expert-scorer analysis improved their interscorer agreement, it did not affect the automated versus visual scoring agreement. Following this meeting, selected parameters for CAP and CAP-phase scoring were communicated to the company programmers and were implemented in the Somnologica Science 3.3 CAP automated analysis program.

SUBSEQUENT VALIDATION OF AUTOMATED VERSUS VISUAL SCORING

Sixteen hours of single-channel EDF format recordings were obtained from 4 different laboratories with either C4/A1 or C3/A2 channels and with different sampling frequencies (100, 128, or 256 Hz). Two 1-hour epochs of NREM sleep, one at the beginning of the night and one during the second half of the night, were extracted from each recording to obtain 16 files. The files were all scored by 7 visual scorers, the proprietary system, and one automatic wavelet CAP scoring system implemented on MatLab 6.0.[28]

Analysis of the agreement between the 9 conditions was performed using an event-related analysis whereby an agreement is scored whenever 2 events have intersection longer than 0.5 seconds, which is designated as a hit. This type of analysis allows identification of a hit, miss (negative), or false-positive result. Comparing one scoring method with another, this analysis can calculate the sensitivity of scoring A versus scoring B, and the positive predictive value. Likewise, scoring B is compared with scoring A and similar descriptive values obtained. If neither A nor B is considered as a reference, a Mutual Agreement (MA) score can be obtained. In addition, a number of disagreement, which includes false negatives and false positives, can be derived.

Using this approach, all 9 scoring conditions were compared file by file (results of this analysis will be presented in a specific report; Rosa and colleagues, personal communication). An interscorer sensitivity was calculated with one outlier scorer at 49.06, but all other scorers, the proprietary program, and the CAP-Lisbon automatic oscillated between 72.36 and 84.69. The automated proprietary program obtained the highest interscorer sensitivity. The next highest sensitivity was a visual scorer from the University of Parma laboratory from which the visual CAP scoring system originated and the automated method was developed. The average MA oscillated between 60.35% and 73.82%, again with the highest score for the automated system, one outlier visual scorer, and the other scorers remaining around 70% to 71%. Investigation of the MA between all files visually scored by the most experienced and most knowledgable CAP scoring laboratory had a mean percentage of around 71%.

The results of this extensive process indicate that commercially available automatic algorithms can identify A phases (and therefore CAP cycle and CAP time) with precision that equals or exceeds that of traditional human scorers. It must be emphasized that this scoring was performed using only one EEG channel. Research protocols may have additional EEG channels, possibly improving scoring and agreement rates. Advantages of automated systems are their sensitivity to EEG changes and consistent scoring, which decreases variability when an analysis of a group of subjects (normal or patients) is performed. Even the most experienced scorers, as shown here, can have much larger scoring variability.

TRANSLATIONAL RESEARCH USING CAP ANALYSIS IN WOMEN WITH A COMPLAINT OF FATIGUE AND SLEEP-DISORDERED BREATHING
Methods

Patients
Participants were 40 women aged 18 to 38 years referred to the Stanford Sleep Medicine Clinic with sleep-related complaints (**Table 1**). All

Table 1
Patients and control subjects: clinical presentation

Variables	Patient Group (n = 40)	Control Group (n = 20)
Complaints		
Daytime fatigue	12	–
Sleep-maintenance insomnia	18	–
Sleep-onset insomnia	10	–
Ethnicity		
Caucasian	22	9
Far-East Asian	12	8
South Indian	9	1
African American	2	1
Hispanic	1	1
Mean body mass index (kg/m²)	22.4 ± 1.1	23 ± 1.1
Past Medical History		
Past adenotonsillectomy	18	4
Past orthodontic treatment	28	5
Wisdom-teeth extraction early in life	22	–
Bruxism	17	–
Childhood asthma	5	–
Nasal allergies	25	–

subjects were otherwise healthy and took no medications except for birth-control tablets.

Clinical evaluation of the upper airway indicated that 10 had tonsil scores greater than 2 using scales of Friedman and colleagues,[29] and 27 had a Mallampati scale score of 3 or 4.[30] Nasal evaluation indicated asymmetric external nasal valve in 21 subjects with presence of deviated septum in 20, enlarged inferior nasal turbinates in 29, and internal nasal valve collapse in 33. All presented evidence of a narrow upper airway, with a high and narrow hard palate in 29 patients and mandibular retroposition of greater than 2.2 mm in 13.[31] Nasopharyngoscopy demonstrated the presence of a small upper airway involving the base of the tongue in 18 patients and nasopalatal impairment in 22.

Measures
All participants completed the Epworth Sleepiness Scale (ESS) and a visual analog scale (VAS) for daytime fatigue (ranging from 0 for no fatigue

to 100 indicating "extreme fatigue to the point of not moving").[32] The following variables were monitored during nocturnal polysomnography: 4 EEG leads (C3/A2, C4/A1, Fp3-Fp4, O1-O2), 2 electro-oculograms, chin and leg electromyographs, 1 electrocardiograph lead (modified V2 derivation), nasal cannula pressure transducer, mouth thermistor, neck microphone, chest and abdominal piezoelectric bands, finger pulse oximetry, transcutaneous CO_2 electrode, and a position sensor. Lights out was determined by the subject's usual bedtime. A minimum of 7.5 hours of bedtime was requested.

Control subjects

Twenty women aged 20 to 40 years (mean 29 ± 6 years) were recruited from the community. None reported health or sleep problems and all were considered in good health, with absence of chronic medication intake except birth-control tablets. All had a clinical examination (see **Table 1**). None had wisdom-teeth extraction and all had an upper airway scored as normal size on physical evaluation. One subject had deviation of the nasal septum. All individuals completed the ESS and VAS scales. Subjects underwent nocturnal polysomnography with monitoring of same variables and following the same protocol as the patients.

Analysis

Recordings were scored for sleep and waking status using international criteria. Abnormal breathing was scored using the definitions for apnea and hypopnea. As the nasal cannula pressure transducer was used, hypopnea was defined as a decrease of nasal flow by 30% of prior normal recording. An associated decrease in oxygen saturation (SaO_2) of 3% or an EEG arousal was required to score hypopneas. Flow limitation was scored based on a nasal cannula pressure transducer indicating abnormal breathing characterized by a decrease of basal flow by 5% to 30% of prior normal breathing associated with a specific pattern of the nasal flow curve ("flattening" or "abrupt drop" at the beginning of inspiration).[33] Four successive breaths with the pattern were needed to score a flow-limitation event. Also, 30-second epochs with tachypnea (defined as respiratory rate >20 breaths per minute during 30 seconds) were noted. The addition of flow limitation to the AHI yielded the respiratory disturbance index (RDI). The lowest SaO_2 during the night and the number of 30-second epochs with snoring events were also tabulated.

All NREM sleep periods for both patients and control subjects were transformed to EDF format and transferred to CD-ROM. Each CD-ROM was numbered to permit blinding of the scorers, then analyzed for CAP. Two separate investigators performed the analysis. The CAP analysis was first performed based on EEG leads C3/A2 or C4/A1, with selection of the lead based on the investigator's choice after inspecting the tracings. The analysis was also performed using the Somnologica Science 3.3 automated program. Then each recording was analyzed visually by the investigators using the 4 EEG leads available. Changes in the computer analysis could be done at this stage, and each investigator change was marked.

Comparison of results between controls and patients was performed using the Mann-Whitney test ($P = .05$ for significance). Correlation between CAP parameters and clinical variables were performed using the Pearson correlation test. Percentages were analyzed by χ^2 statistics.

Results

There were 40 patients and 20 controls. The mean age of patients was 28.6 ± 6 years and 27.9 ± 7 years for controls (not significant). The mean ESS score was 5 ± 2 and 4.5 ± 2 for patients and controls, respectively (not significant). All patients presented complaints of fatigue, and the mean VAS score for fatigue was 58 ± 10 for patients and 16 ± 5 for controls ($P = .0001$). Polysomnography indicated that both groups had a relatively low AHI of 9 ± 3 and 1.1 ± 0.6 for patients and controls, respectively. Usage of RDI indicated a score of 22 ± 5 for patients and 1.5 ± 0.7 for controls. Both AHI and RDI were significantly different ($P = .0001$) between the groups. The mean lowest SaO_2 was 92% ± 2.5% for patients and 97% ± 1% for controls. (χ^2, $P = .001$). Analysis of EEG arousals 3 seconds or longer indicated a mean arousal index of 14 ± 3.1 for patients and 8.9 ± 4.6 for controls ($P = .001$).

The CAP rate was 59% ± 10% for patients versus 32% ± 5% for controls ($P = .01$). The mean CAP time for patients versus controls was 190 ± 37 and 73 ± 26 seconds, respectively ($P = .01$). There was a mean of 382 ± 104 (patients) versus 135 ± 75 (controls) CAP cycles ($P = .01$).

These numbers were derived from comparison of the scores given by the 2 independent scorers. For patients, the CAP scores from automated and visual scoring were very close, with a mean difference of 0.3 for CAP rate and 1.1 for CAP cycle. Of note, the automatic scoring mean was between the mean for each of the 2 visual scorers.

Phase A1 in patients was calculated as 57 ± 14 by automatic scoring, 56 ± 15 by scorer A, and 59 ± 12 by scorer B. After conjoint review it was concluded to be at 57.8 ± 13.6. Phase A2 was calculated at 26 ±10 by automatic analysis, 21 ± 11 by scorer A, and 27.6 ± 11 by scorer B. Opposing this trend, phase A3 was calculated at 15.3 ± 7 by automatic analysis, 19.8 ± 10 by scorer A, and 14.3 ± 9 by scorer B.

For controls, there was a greater discrepancy. Mean CAP rate was still between that for the 2 visual scorers but was 34% ± 7% for one scorer and 31% ± 6% for the other scorer, while automatic scoring yielded 31.9% ± 8%. The presented score is the result of the review performed jointly by the 2 investigators to reconcile discrepancies. The initial scoring of the 2 investigators showed a large variation between the amount of phase A2 and phase A3. There were fewer discrepancies between scorers for controls, after joint scoring index of phase A2 was scored at 25.8 ± 11.5 and index of phase A3 at 15.7 ± 7.5. The percentage of CAP phase A1 was 68.3 ± 17 with automatic analysis, 69 ± 18 for scorer A, and 68 ± 16 for scorer B. Percentage of CAP phase A2 was 19.5 ± 13 for automatic analysis, 20 ± 14 for scorer A, and 19 ± 12.6 for scorer B. Percentage of CAP phase A3 was 10.5 ± 7 for automatic scoring, 10 ± 6.5 for scorer A, and 10.9 ± 7.7 for scorer B.

Pearson correlation coefficient indicated a positive correlation ($r = 0.59$, $P = .0001$) between CAP rate and fatigue VAS score while usage of arousal index did not reach significance.

Comments

This study shows that young women with a low AHI present a remarkably higher RDI when attention is paid to less obvious breathing abnormalities rather than the AHI. This finding is an important one, as many women may not be appropriately identified and treated if these more subtle respiratory abnormalities are not taken into consideration. Sleepiness was not the major complaint among the patient group and the low, equivalent ESS scores between groups demonstrate this well, whereas fatigue was the primary feature. In practice it is often difficult to articulate the nuances of fatigue and sleepiness with patients; however, subjects clearly dissociated the "sleepiness" assessed with ESS from what they scored as "fatigue" using the VAS.

The study demonstrates an important correlation between the CAP rate and the fatigue VAS score. The CAP rate was clearly different for patients in comparison with controls. The arousal index was also significantly different but much less so than the CAP rate. Clearly the CAP rate allows investigation of changes in sleep architecture that are

adequately detected with tabulation of short EEG arousals. There is an overlap between these EEG arousals and phase A3 of CAP, but there is no equivalent to the scoring of phase A2 of CAP to indicate a change in sleep architecture. Further work is needed to better understand what physiologic changes occur when such patterns are seen, but they clearly indicate a change from normal sleep architecture when present in large amounts.

Accurate quantification of CAP is dependent on sensitive recognition of these patterns. The definition of phases A2 and A3 call on recognition of EEG frequency changes and determination of dominant EEG frequencies. This task is a difficult one for the human eye. Training may improve results, but there will always be interrater discrepancies. The superior consistency of automated CAP scoring suggests that computers may arguably provide better CAP scoring than humans. However, the rules forming the basis of the automated programs are critical, and human scorers must always be able to overrule the computerized score. Efforts have been made over several years to develop and validate an automated scoring program. Use of this automatic program has highlighted the difficulty in visually scoring CAP phases A2 and A3 even when using multiple EEG leads. It has also shown that an automatic CAP scoring program provides valid information on sleep architecture and can be helpful when investigating sleep under both normal and pathologic conditions.

ACKNOWLEDGMENTS

The Somnologica Science 3.3 program was the product of combined efforts from the Bioengineering Department, University of Lisbon (Portugal) and the Flaga-Embla research and development team (Reykjavik, Iceland). It is currently the property of Medicare Inc (USA).

The CAP consensus group was created by M.G. Terzano, MD, and involved the following individuals: R.D. Chevron, S. Chokroverty, B. Consens, R. Ferri, C. Guilleminault, M. Hirshkovitz, Y.S. Huang, M.C. Lopes, M. Mahowald, H. Moldosky, L. Parrino, T. Roerhs, A. Rosa, R. Thomas, M. Zucconi, A. Walters.

REFERENCES

1. Rechtschaffen A, Kales A. Manual of standardized terminology: techniques and scoring system for sleep stages of human subjects. Los Angeles (CA): UCLA Brain Information Service/Brain Research Institute; 1968.

2. American Sleep Disorders Association. EEG arousals: scoring rules and examples. A preliminary report from sleep disorders atlas task force of the American Sleep Disorder Association. Sleep 1992; 15:173–84.

3. Terzano MG, Mancia D, Salati MR, et al. The cyclic alternating pattern as a physiologic component of normal NREM sleep. Sleep 1985;8:137–45.

4. Terzano MG, Parrino L. Clinical applications of cyclic alternating pattern. Physiol Behav 1993;54:807–13.

5. De Gennaro L, Ferrara M, Spadini V, et al. The cyclic alternating pattern decreases as a consequence of total sleep deprivation and correlates with EEG arousals. Neuropsychobiology 2002;45:95–8.

6. Zucconi M, Oldani A, Ferini-Strambi L, et al. Arousal fluctuations in non-rapid eye movement parasomnias: the role of cyclic alternating pattern as a measure of sleep instability. J Clin Neurophysiol 1995;12:147–54.

7. Terzano MG, Parrino L, Spaggiari MC. The cyclic alternating pattern sequences in the dynamic organization of sleep. Electroencephalogr Clin Neurophysiol 1988;69:437–47.

8. Terzano M, Parrino L, Smerieri A, et al. Atlas, rules, and recording techniques for the scoring of cyclic alternating pattern (CAP) in human sleep. Sleep Med 2002;3:187–99.

9. Ferrillo F, Gabarra M, Nobili L, et al. Comparison between visual scoring of cyclic alternating pattern (CAP) and computerized assessment of slow EEG oscillations in the transition from light to deep non-REM sleep. J Clin Neurophysiol 1997;14:210–6.

10. Parrino L, Boselli M, Spaggiari MC, et al. Cyclic alternating pattern (CAP) in normal sleep: polysomnographic parameters in different age groups. Electroencephalogr Clin Neurophysiol 1998;107:439–50.

11. Terzano MG, Parrino L, Boselli M, et al. Polysomnographic analysis of arousal responses in OSAS by means of the cyclic alternating pattern (CAP). J Clin Neurophysiol 1996;13:145–55.

12. Rosa AC, Parrino L, Terzano M. Automatic detection of cyclic alternating pattern (CAP) sequences in sleep: preliminary results. Electroencephalogr Clin Neurophysiol 1999;110:585–92.

13. Ferri R, Parrino L, Smerieri A, et al. Cyclic alternating pattern and spectral analysis of heart rate variability during normal sleep. J Sleep Res 2000;9:13–8.

14. Terzano MG, Parrino L, Rosa A, et al. CAP and arousals in the structural development of sleep: an integrative perspective. Sleep Med 2002;3:221–2.

15. Ferri R, Parrino L, Smerieri A, et al. Non-linear EEG measures during sleep: effects of the different sleep stages and cyclic alternating pattern. Int J Psychophysiol 2002;43:273–86.

16. Ferri R, Rundo F, Bruni O, et al. Dynamics of the EEG slow-wave synchronization during sleep. Clin Neurophysiol 2005;116:2783–95.

17. Ferri R, Bruni O, Miano S, et al. All-night EEG power spectral analysis of the cyclic alternating pattern components in young adult subjects. Clin Neurophysiol 2005;116:2429–40.

18. Bruni O, Ferri R, Miano S, et al. Sleep cyclic alternating pattern in normal preschool-age children. Sleep 2005;28:220–30.

19. Rosa AC, Allen Lima J. Fuzzy classification of microstructural dynamics of human sleep. Proceedings of the 1996 IEEE International Conference on Systems, Man and Cybernetics—Information, Intelligence and Systems, SMC '96, vol. 2;1996:1108–13.

20. Allen Lima J, Rosa AC. Maximum likelihood based classification for the microstructure of human sleep. ACM SigBio Newslett 1997;17(3):2–6.

21. Navona C, Barcaro U, Bonanni E, et al. An automatic method for the recognition and classification of the A-phases of the cyclic alternating pattern. Clin Neurophysiol 2002;113:1826–31.

22. Largo R, Rosa A. Wavelets based detection of a phases in sleep EEG. Proc IEEE Int Conf Comput Bioeng 2005;2:1105–15 ISBN 972-8469-37-3, IST Press.

23. Largo R, Munteanu C, Rosa A. CAP event detection by wavelet and GA tuning. Proceedings of IEEE-WISP Evolutionary Computation 2005. CD-Rom.

24. Ferri R, Bruni O, Miano S, et al. Inter-rater reliability of sleep cyclic alternating pattern (CAP) scoring and validation of a new computer-assisted CAP scoring method. Clin Neurophysiol 2005;116:696–707.

25. Ferri R, Rundo F, Bruni O, et al. Regional scalp EEG slow-wave synchronization during sleep cyclic alternating pattern A1 subtypes. Neurosci Lett 2006;404: 352–7.

26. Ferri R, Bruni O, Miano S, et al. The time structure of the sleep cyclic alternating pattern. Sleep 2006;29:693–9.

27. Kemp B, Varri A, Rosa A, et al. A simple format for exchange of digitized polygraphic recordings. Electroencephalogr Clin Neurophysiol 1992;82:391–3.

28. MatLab v6.0 from Matwork Inc. Available at: http://www.mathworks.com. Accessed November 10, 2006.

29. Friedman M, Tanyeri H, La Rosa M, et al. Clinical predictors of obstructive sleep apnea. Laryngoscope 1999;109:1901–7.

30. Mallampatti SR, Gatt SP, Gugino LD, et al. A clinical sign to predict difficult tracheal intubation: a prospective study. Can Anaesth Soc J 1985;32:429–34.

31. Kolar JC, Salter EM. Craniofacial anthropometry. Practical measurement of the head and face for clinical, surgical and research use. Springfield (IL): Charles C Thomas; 1997.

32. Johns MW. A new method for measuring daytime sleepiness: the Epworth Sleepiness Scale. Sleep 1991;14:540–5.

33. Ayap I, Norman RG, Krieger AC, et al. Non-invasive detection of respiratory effort-related arousals (RERAs) by a nasal cannula/pressure transducer system. Sleep 2000;23:763–71.

Index

Note: Page numbers of article titles are in **boldface** type.

Sleep Med Clin 7 (2012) 571–576
http://dx.doi.org/10.1016/S1556-407X(12)00090-2
1556-407X/12/$ – see front matter © 2012 Elsevier Inc. All rights reserved.